T·H·E

BIRTH BOOK

By the same authors

300 Questions New Parents Ask
The Fussy Baby
Nighttime Parenting
Creative Parenting
Becoming a Father
The Baby Book

T·H·E

BIRTH BOOK

Everything You Need to Know
to Have a Safe and Satisfying Birth

WILLIAM SEARS, M.D.
AND MARTHA SEARS, R.N.

LITTLE, BROWN AND COMPANY

Boston ◆ *New York* ◆ *Toronto* ◆ *London*

First Edition

This book is intended to help the reader become a wiser consumer of medical care. Since every parent's obstetrical situation is unique, the information in this book should not replace regular visits to a health care professional. Always consult your doctor for your obstetrical care and decisions.

Library of Congress Cataloging-in-Publication Data

Sears, William, M.D.
    The birth book : everything you need to know to have a safe and satisfying birth / William Sears and Martha Sears. — 1st ed.
        p.   cm.
    Includes bibliographical references and index.
    ISBN 0-316-77908-3 (hc)
    ISBN 0-316-77907-5 (pb)
    1. Childbirth.   I. Sears, Martha.   II. Title.
RG651.S43   1994
618.4 — dc20   93-5748

10 9 8 7 6 5 4 3 2 1

MAR

Drawings by Deborah Maze
Designed by Jeanne Abboud

Published simultaneously in Canada by Little, Brown & Company (Canada) Limited

PRINTED IN THE UNITED STATES OF AMERICA

To our births

James
Robert
Peter
Hayden
Erin
Matthew
Stephen
Lauren

and our grandbirths

Andrew
and
Lea

Contents

A Word from Dr. Bill and Martha

YOU'RE GOING TO HAVE A BABY! Soon you are sharing the news with friends and family. Now, along with growing your baby, come the many choices you need to make about birthing your baby. *The Birth Book* will help you make informed choices. While you can't totally orchestrate the perfect birth — birth is full of surprises — you can create the conditions that increase your chances of having the birth you want. Determining the birth you want and finding out how to get it is what this book is all about. This is a system-fixing, not a system-bashing, book. As a doctor and nurse we are in the medical system and proud to be. At this writing, our oldest two sons are in medical school, and a third is considering it. The problems we expose and the solutions we propose are included because we value our profession and feel obligated to do our part to improve it. The medical way of birth, while necessary or desirable for some mothers, is neither necessary nor satisfying for others. We want parents to take responsibility for their birth decisions, and we give you the tools to do so. In addition to empowering you with wisdom to get the birth you want, we equip you to enter your labor knowing your body, reading its signals, and trusting your responses. Therein lie the keys to a positive birth experience.

We wish you the best in your baby's birth.

William and Martha Sears
San Clemente, California
January 1994

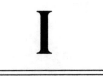

PREPARING FOR BIRTH

Besides being a time for growing a baby, pregnancy is a time when you grow as a person, healing memories or fears about birth, working out a birthing philosophy, assembling the right team, and selecting the right birth place for you. In no time in history have women enjoyed more birthing options. In this section we will help you sift through available resources and work out your own approach to birth. While few women get all their birth wishes, in general, the better you prepare, the more satisfying your birth.

Let's get started!

Our Birth Experiences —
What We Have Learned

EW MOMENTS IN LIFE are as memorable as your baby's birth. Over the past thirty years we have delivered seven babies of our own, assisted at the birth of our eighth child, our daughter by adoption, and been involved with more than a thousand births in a professional capacity, Bill as a pediatrician and occasionally Martha as a labor-support person. We come away from births with a variety of feelings. Many are happy: "What a wonderful birth! If only they could all go that way." Other times, we feel that parents have a less than satisfying birth experience and that it could have gone better: "If only they had known this.... If only they had tried that...." We have found that many couples see birth as an ordeal to be survived. They don't realize that birth can be satisfying and even enjoyable. We want to tell you everything we've learned about how to make the most of your labor and birth. We've found that when birth is experienced as a positive, enriching event, life with baby gets off to a better start. And often this better start makes a crucial difference in the life of the new family. Birth matters.

OUR EIGHT BIRTHS: MARTHA'S STORY

Jim was born in 1967 at Boston Lying-In Hospital. We felt safe and secure delivering our baby in the teaching hospital of Harvard Medical School. At that time fathers were not allowed in either the labor or the delivery room and the standard method of birth included spinal anesthesia, episiotomy, and forceps delivery. Early during my pregnancy I had attempted to discuss unmedicated birth with my doctor, but he dismissed me with a patronizing pat on the shoulder, saying, "Why would you want to suffer if you don't have to?" Since I was young and naive and not in the practice of arguing with doctors, I said no more. This exchange set the tone for a birth that on the surface turned out fine, but underneath I felt angry, frustrated, and betrayed because of what was imposed on me against my will. I had wanted an unmedicated birth, but I had no intention of "suffering" through it.

Labor began with my water breaking at 3:00 A.M. It progressed quickly, and by the time we were ready to leave for the hospital around 4:00 A.M., my contractions were coming close together and were quite strong. I concentrated so hard on my breathing that I hardly realized that my husband was there. In the admitting room, after I was shaved and examined, we were told that my cervix was completely dilated, unusual for a first labor. For this reason I was not given an enema (standard practice at the time), but was whisked off to the labor ward where Bill and I had to say good-bye. At this point, I felt overwhelmed. But fortunately, I also recognized that I was beginning to feel the urge to push. Pushing helped — I began to recognize an urgent force within me that demanded a response. But there was absolutely no need for what happened next. Just as I was really getting into pushing, I was instructed to roll over onto a table to receive a spinal anesthesia. Almost immediately my body felt like a sack of potatoes from the waist down, and then my legs were placed in the stirrups again. A nurse announced that she could see a patch of black hair, and that made me determined to help birth my baby. I tried to push with each contraction, but the only way I could tell my uterus was contracting was to feel my abdomen with my hand; the spinal anesthesia had blocked out all feeling. In order to insert the forceps to grasp the baby, the doctor cut my perineum. Within minutes it was all over. I held my breath as I saw our baby boy held up feet first in the hands of the doctor. He was born at 5:13 A.M., just slightly more than two hours after my labor had started. As wonderful as that moment was, there was a very helpless, hollow feeling, a sense of not having participated. Because of my spinal, I felt like my very nature (as a birth-giving woman) had been denied. I was a passive bystander, a powerless observer at the birth of my own child.

When I realized that the top half of my body could move, I propped myself up on my elbows and looked over at the tiny pile of flesh emitting a few small sounds across the room. The nurse placed him in a bassinet and wheeled him around to "let him get a look at his mother." I gazed into my son's face and saw a huge nose, a pointed head, and a large mouth opened wide screaming. All too quickly he was taken away to be washed and wrapped, and only after that was I able to hold him for a few minutes before he was taken away again. The doctor dialed the waiting room and handed me the receiver so that I could tell Bill the good news. How strange that I should be telling my husband that we had a baby boy — and over the phone! How wrong! Instead of holding my baby and my husband, I was left holding a phone. Bill and I met as I was being wheeled off to the recovery room. Just then a bassinet appeared and Bill was "allowed" to sneak a peek at our baby. I then spent several hours alone in the recovery room, numb from the waist down, trying to make sense of what had happened. In my mind I knew I had given birth, but I didn't know it in my body. I also felt strangely disconnected from my baby. I lost out on that heightened time for bonding when my baby had just been born. When my hormones were highest I was incapacitated and separated. Not only did I not experience the sensation of giving birth, but I also lacked its immediate reward. The next time I saw Jim was through the nursery window after I had been moved into a room on the postpartum floor. To me, this experience epitomizes the cold, mechanical, inhumane attitude toward birth that was prevalent in the sixties. I was determined that things would be very different for our next baby.

Two years later Bob was born at the Bethesda Naval Hospital with the help of a doctor who had no problem with my desire for an unanesthetized birth. This hospital allowed fathers in the labor room, but not in the delivery room. Labor began at 6:45 A.M. with a series of contractions that steadily progressed to being five minutes apart and lasting forty-five to sixty seconds. But by 8:00 A.M. this pattern was gone. I decided to lie down and concentrate on my labor before Bill left for work. The contractions intensified, so we quickly dressed, packed, and headed for the hospital. By 9:00 A.M. I was settled in my labor bed and found to be only 3 centimeters dilated. Already this was different from the first labor. After an enema, the contractions began coming every two minutes, lasting at least seventy seconds. Bill and I used the next half hour to concentrate on relaxation and on coping with each contraction. It was so good to have him there. By 10:00 A.M. I was beginning to feel a new pressure, so I asked to be checked again and was found to be 8 centimeters dilated. Soon it was time to go to delivery, and while I panted and blew to avoid pushing, my legs were put up into the stirrups, and an I.V. (standard procedure) was started in my arm. The contractions were enormous and had a sharper edge than I had experienced with Jim. And I made sounds that paralleled those sensations. Just before the doctor broke my water, he checked with me to see if I still wanted to go all the way without a spinal. I said I did, thinking to myself, "The worst is over now. Just let me push and I'll be fine."

The doctor had determined that the baby's position was posterior, with the back of his head facing toward my tailbone (which explained the intense sensations), so I was given a local anesthetic to enable the doctor to use forceps. After the first push the doctor cut my perineum. After two more pushes he inserted the forceps and used them to rotate the baby's head from the posterior to the anterior position, the preferred way for a baby to come down the birth canal. However, he did not need to use the forceps to get the baby out — one more push and I felt an incredible surge as my baby's head moved through my vagina and was born. What relief! With the next push the shoulders were free, and then I could see two little legs and an arm flailing around. The moment of giving birth was so much more real to me than my first birth. Even though the sensations of this posterior labor were so incredibly overpowering, I remember thinking to myself how much better it was to possess the full knowledge of having given birth, of having felt everything, so that I could use that information in the processing of all that was happening to me in becoming this baby's mother. Even considering the fact that I could not touch Bob right away due to the wrist restraints (another unnecessary standard procedure) that were in place, I felt so much more connected with this baby than I had initially with Jim.

The sensations I had with Bob's birth were so intense and overwhelming that for several days afterward I kept saying, "Never again." Years later, as I trained to be a childbirth educator, I came to realize just what I had accomplished in this unanesthetized birth. This baby had been in a posterior position, giving me a terrible backache, yet the time that had elapsed during this labor was remarkably short considering the position of the baby's head. In his eagerness to give me a spinal anesthetic to help me be comfortable, this doctor could have "helped" me miss the most intense experience of my life, that of giving birth for the first time with complete awareness and sensation. I would not trade that experience for a million dollars. I know now I hurt more than I needed to — there are a number of commonsense substitutes for spinal anesthesia and forceps rotation that would have helped me be more comfortable. True, the use of forceps may have shortened the pushing stage, but I eventually learned the wisdom of having my body upright and mobile and taking more time to let the natural course of birth unfold.

I was astounded by the unbelievable difference between my two labor and my two birth experiences. I planned someday to become a childbirth educator, and six years later, there I was — studying to become that childbirth educator while Bill and I took a childbirth class in preparation for our third baby. We were in Toronto, Canada, this time, and the climate in the world of birth had changed. Couples were becoming better informed, and doctors were more willing to listen to their "patients." Women were no longer willing to accept the role of patient — after all, pregnancy is not a disease. Of our three hospital births, this one would come closest to the ideal. Bill was allowed to be with me throughout labor and birth, and we were by now aware of the importance of immediate breastfeeding and rooming-in, that is, having the baby stay with us in our room. This labor began at midnight when my membranes ruptured and some long, hard contractions followed, coming close together. We got to the hospital by 12:45 A.M., and much of the time in the labor room was spent having my pubic area shaved and being interviewed — irritating and distracting procedures because I wanted only to attend to my contractions. I was just beginning to get relaxed and confi-

dent in the handling of my contractions when, to my amazement, I felt the pushing urge. My cervix had still not been checked, so that was done quickly, and I was found to be 5 centimeters dilated and "going fast." The next several contractions were huge, and the pushing urge got stronger and stronger, so we were rushed to delivery. I was so busy blowing to avoid pushing that I didn't even think of looking around for Bill until I was being moved over onto the delivery table.

The moving about from home to hospital, labor room to delivery room, and wheelchair to bed to delivery table, plus dealing with disturbing routines, were the hardest parts of this labor. How much nicer it would have been to be in a comfortable nest and not to be harried and hassled. Once my legs were up in stirrups and I was given the go-ahead to push, I found great relief. Just at that point, a doctor appeared next to me offering me some gas to breathe that would "take away 70 percent of the pain." I was simply too busy to pay attention to him. Thank goodness Bill told him that I did not need any help. We wanted to avoid an episiotomy, but at the last minute the doctor decided to do one. Then one more push and I felt the baby's head being born. I was told to stop pushing then and Bill was holding my hand, all excited by the sight of his baby's head. Remember, he had not witnessed our first two births. He urged me to sit up a bit so that I could see it, too. I had a minute or two of rest then, and together we drank in the sight of our baby still half enclosed in my body. The high at that moment will never be forgotten, although we only began to realize the strength and beauty of it afterward. At the time we could only look on in awe. My next push, at 1:25 A.M., was the most creative, actively productive effort I had ever made. One shoulder, the other shoulder, then the baby's blue and white body was being held face up, with the evidence of him for all to see. "Hello, Peter," I said, and he was placed on my abdomen wrapped in a green towel, his little red face turned toward my face. Bill and I relaxed together and marveled at our new son. At that moment we learned firsthand that being present at his baby's birth is very important to a father's feelings of attachment.

Just before the doctor left, I asked him how soon I would be able to feed Peter. To my pleasant surprise, he told the nurse to let me feed the baby right away. I could have danced for joy. This would be the first time I was to be allowed to feed my baby right after birth. Once I was cleaned up, the nurse brought Peter to me, and we had our first meeting as a breastfeeding pair. Later that night as I lay awake thinking of the birth, it seemed so strange that he was not with me. The knowledge that I had actually held him and fed him helped me firmly grasp the fact of new motherhood. The closeness we had established in that first feeding was very important to me. Being separated from Peter like this for the rest of the night was unnecessary. He wasn't brought to me for feeding and rooming-in until 9:00 A.M. This was precious time lost between us when I wasn't able to sleep a wink anyway.

Our fourth baby, daughter Hayden, was born at our home in Hilton Head, South Carolina. The obstetrical department in the local hospital had not yet opened, and the nearest obstetrical unit was an hour away. With my history of short labors, we didn't want to run this race. We deliberated for months over our situation. We were excited about the "daring" prospect of a home birth, but it was unknown for us personally, so it took a while for us to feel comfortable about

it. My obstetrician's solution to our dilemma had been to induce my labor artificially, but we felt this procedure had far greater risks (prematurity, painful labor, possible surgical birth) than a well-planned home birth. So, we enlisted the help of a family practitioner who had attended many home births in the past. As it turned out, this labor lasted only sixty minutes from start to finish. Our instincts had been right!

When my water broke and labor began at 5:00 A.M., I experienced great comfort in knowing that I could lie back and relax and safely await the progression of my labor. True to form, my labor progressed quickly and the doctor arrived fifteen minutes before our baby was born at 6:00 A.M. She was gently and quietly born, beautifully pink all over immediately. One small cry and she was placed on my abdomen and covered with a blanket. I soothed her quiet cries, and she was at peace. As soon as I could, I turned onto my side and she had her first feeding. She took my breast immediately and sucked hard and well. She stayed like this a long time, through the champagne toast and greetings from friends. Her first two hours of life were very special. There were no hospital routines to comply with. She stayed right with me, right in my arms, eyes wide open, busy looking us over. There was no separation to interrupt the beautiful flow of bonding going on between Bill, Hayden, and me, and the other children as they came in to join us. To have a baby born to you in your own bed, in your own familiar home, with loving people around you, with no stirrups, no drapes, no episiotomy, no hassles, is an experience I wish every woman could have. I distinctly remember feeling at peace with the fact that I didn't have to run around getting dressed, checking my suitcase, packing the children off to someone else's care, focusing my energy on getting away from my nest to the hospital. Instead I could slowly and comfortably, and at my own pace, feather my nest and climb into it and climb out again when I felt that I needed to move around. I was in total harmony with my own body.

Bill notes: The time had come for us to practice what we preached and take responsibility for our birthing decisions. Birth carries a risk no matter how carefully you prepare to have your baby. You have to look for the least risky decision. We considered all of our options: preterm induction in the hospital one hour away, trying to race to the hospital after the first contraction, or staying home. At this point I was a charter member of the medical establishment and could easily have been voted the husband least likely to approve of home birthing. I thought home births were for poor people and hippies. Of course, "what if?" fear set in. After all, my training and exposure had defined birth as a medical complication waiting to happen. I filled our bedroom with all the necessary emergency equipment, prearranged emergency transport, and prepared for a long list of possible emergencies. As soon as Hayden took her first breath, I breathed easier, too. Our home birth made the front page of our local newspaper, much to the chagrin of my medical colleagues, who feared we might start some sort of counter-culture movement.

It was at this birth that I reached a turning point in my own attitude and feelings about birth. Fear of childbirth had never been a problem for me. I have always had a quiet confidence in my body's ability to give birth. But with our hospital births, fear had

been present, stemming from the doctors and the nurses and from the hospital setting itself. In this home birth there was none of that fear surrounding me. Bill managed to keep his fear to himself. I felt at peace and inwardly quiet during this birth, and these feelings were reflected in our baby. We had finally experienced birth at its best, and now there was no turning back.

Our next three babies were born in California, all at home, all attended by the same wonderful midwife. Our fifth baby, Erin, came after a five-hour labor. Even though it was longer than my other labors, this one was less hectic and less intense. I found that I enjoyed this slower labor since I had time to reflect upon the process of labor and birth as I was going through it. I enjoyed this special time moving around in the comfort of our home, helping the children get breakfast, deciding what I wanted to wear, and actually relaxing through contractions. I was learning firsthand how different a contraction felt when I relaxed my abdominal muscles instead of bracing them to "get through it." I actually had the time to try out all the relaxation techniques I had been teaching, and saw for myself that labor did not have to be painful. This was the first birth at which we were privileged to have all of our children in attendance, and we captured the whole beautiful family event on videotape. We have since used this video in teaching numerous couples the joys of birth in a natural setting with the benefits of total relaxation and loving support.

Baby number six, Matthew, was born after a relaxed morning of thinking I was only in prelabor. A reporter from a local newspaper had been at our home with a photographer, doing a story on our family. By the time I realized I was in labor (you'd think I would have known after five babies), I had just enough time to summon Bill back home and get the waterproof sheets down on the bed before the baby started to come. In fact, our midwife did not make it in time for this birth, though she attended by phone, and Bill had the privilege of catching this baby. It is interesting that Bill has always felt a special bond with Matthew, in part, he feels, as a result of this first touching. I learned how much easier for me birth is in the side-lying position than in the semisitting position reclining against pillows, which I had adopted for Erin's and Hayden's births. Being completely off my back made a big difference.

Stephen came after a labor of about five hours, the first four hours of which were so mild I was barely convinced that I was really in labor. Things changed dramatically in the last hour, and in this birth we learned the benefits of using water to achieve enough relaxation to deal with unexpected pain. (See "Water for Birth," page 152.) Our midwife was on hand once again, and she helped Bill deal with the compound presentation (hand alongside the baby's head) so that he could catch this baby, too. In Stephen's birth we learned the importance of absolutely no unnecessary interruption in the mother-baby bonding. If we had been in a hospital, the discovery that Stephen has Down syndrome could have caused everybody to focus more on his "problem" than on the normal needs of this new little person.

Our eighth baby, Lauren, who came into our family by adoption, was born in a hospital. The same wonderful midwife who had attended three of our home births acted as a professional labor assistant for our baby's birth mother. Though I wasn't giving birth to Lauren, by acting as a labor-support person, I did give her biological mother the benefit of my birth experiences. As it turned out, this was the third baby of ours that Bill was privileged to catch, as the obstetrician did not make it in time for the birth. Being back in a hospital setting with this baby's birth, we saw with fresh awareness how much still needs to be improved in the typical hospital birth. For instance, the nurse in charge was very reluctant to allow our baby's mother the freedom to choose her own comfortable positions during her labor, and certainly would not allow her to use any alternative position for giving birth. After all, it would not be "convenient for the doctor," the nurse insisted. But this informed birth mother persisted, "Who's having the baby — me or the doctor?"

Fortunately, she was a very determined young woman in her attitude toward giving birth, and she did not have any internal fears to disturb her; but she did have to cope

---

Imagining Your Baby's Birth

Here is an exercise that will increase your likelihood of having a satisfying birth experience. If this is your first baby and it's early in your pregnancy, you may not have worked out your birth philosophy. It helps to imagine your baby's birth. Better, write the story of your baby's birth, underlining the parts that are most important to you. As you read this book, make a list of the things you must do to have those birth-day wishes happen. Update this list periodically as your B-day nears. The story and the list will help you formulate a birth plan that will help you get the birth you want (see "Composing Your Birth Plan," page 231).

with the effects of the fearful mind-sets of others. We were reminded during Lauren's birth how important it is when going into a hospital setting for birth to have a supportive, well-trained caregiver who understands your desires and who will work with you to have the kind of birth you want. Ideally this will have been communicated to the hospital staff ahead of time with a complete birth plan. (See "Composing Your Birth Plan," page 231.)

TEN TIPS FOR A SAFE AND SATISFYING BIRTH

Based on our experience with birth, here are ten ways you can increase your chances of having a safe and satisfying birth. In the following chapters we discuss each one of these in detail.

1. Trust your body. For the majority of mothers, birth is a normal physiologic process and the system works well, as long as you don't interfere with it. By understanding how your body labors to give birth, and how you can work *with* it instead of against it, you lower your chances of having to suffer or be drugged to give birth. Trust that your body is built to give birth.

One of our goals in this book is to take the fear out of birth. It is normal to be somewhat apprehensive about labor, especially if this is your first baby or if you have had a previous unsatisfying birth experience. But prolonged and unresolved fear will interfere with how your body functions during birth. Be aware as well that the medicalization of birth sets you up to distrust your body and fear birth. You choose a doctor for fear that something will go wrong; you choose a hospital for fear of an emergency;

you succumb to a battery of prenatal tests and spend much of your pregnancy fearing that something will go wrong. This fear interferes with the biological system, and really is unfounded. For 90 percent of women who prepare for birth, birth goes right. Around 10 percent of women need varying amounts of medical help to deliver healthy babies, but even for these women, having confidence in themselves will enhance their births. (See "Fear — Labor's Foe," in chapter 8.)

2. Use pregnancy as a time to prepare. It's a good thing that pregnancy takes so long; it gives you time to get ready for the momentous event — both physically and emotionally. Preparing for birth does not mean simply filing in and out of a six-week childbirth class clutching your pillows and a pile of handouts. It does not mean cramming yourself full of facts and breathing techniques. We believe that preparing for birth means being "studied up," as Martha says in her childbirth class: learning about all of the childbirth options available to you, selecting what best fits your birth-experience goal and your individual obstetrical situation, coming to birth equipped with a philosophy and a plan for the birth you want, and having the wisdom to be flexible to adjust if, due to circumstances beyond your control, your birth does not go according to plan. The process of exploring birth choices can be therapeutic. It compels you to examine yourself, your strengths, your weaknesses, and your fears, and to look at memories from your past that may affect your birth. See chapter 3, "Choices in Childbirth."

3. Take responsibility for your birth choices. If you don't, someone else will take over and make your choices for you. If you simply say, "Doctor, tell me what to do," and check into whatever system of birth your attendant promotes or your insurance plan allows, you set yourself up for a less than satisfying birth. If you need tests, technology, or a surgical birth, you are most likely to have no regrets if you actively participate in these decisions. Why do we place such a strong emphasis on birth responsibility? Because over the years we have learned that how a woman gives birth is related, for better or for worse, to her overall self-worth. Giving birth is the most powerful act you will ever perform, and it should leave you feeling good about yourself. We will show you how to come to your birth empowered to make the choices that will give you the birth you want.

4. Formulate your own birth philosophy. Early in our birthing experience, we were more caught up with the end *product* of birth — delivering a baby — than the *process* — the whole experience. As you will see in chapter 14, "Birth Stories," giving birth is the fullest expression of a woman's sexuality, the memories of which last a lifetime. How a woman approaches birth is intimately connected to how she approaches life. What kind of birth experience is right for you? What, besides a healthy baby, do you expect from your baby's birth? Early in your first pregnancy you may not know the options available to you, so you may not yet know what you want. Realizing this, we will take you through the pros and cons of the most common birth choices.

Being around birth has taught us that the term *positive birth experience* means different things to different women. A woman who chooses to make full use of modern epidural anesthesia may feel satisfied with her birth experience: "Because it didn't hurt

so much, I have mostly pleasant memories." Another woman's dream birth experience may be a drug-free labor and a drug-free baby: "It hurt some, but I did it!" Both of these women achieved the birth they wanted. Both deserve bragging rights.

5. Choose your birth attendants and birth place wisely. Birth attendants should do just that — attend the birth. Most women need continuous support during labor. But different attendants attend birth differently, and some are more likely to try to control the natural processes. Some women feel more comfortable with the medical model of birth, others prefer the midwifery model with its motto of "watchful waiting," and some do best with a combination of these approaches. Unlike other medical situations (such as having your appendix removed), with birth we want you to have more than a doctor-patient relationship. This is a partnership and we will equip mothers to be participating partners more than passive patients.

There is no one right place to birth a baby — only the right place to birth *your* baby. The best place for you may be at home, at a birth center, or in a hospital. Explore these options. And be prepared to change birth places if your circumstances or your goals change during your pregnancy. We will help you explore all of these options to help you choose the right attendant and the right place for your baby's birth. See chapter 3, "Choices in Childbirth."

6. Explore the best positions for your birth. There is no one right position for laboring and giving birth; there is only the one that works best for you. Many women's minds are stuck in the scene of mother lying on her back with her feet up in stirrups while the doctor waits, hands extended quarterback-style, to catch the baby. This is a scene from birthing's past, and one that new insights show is neither healthy for baby nor comfortable for mother. We will walk, kneel, and squat you through various labor and birth positions so that you will be able to find the ones that work for you and your baby. See chapter 11, "Best Birthing Positions."

7. Use technology wisely. We would like to take the focus off the riskiness of birth. For the majority of women, birth is not a medical matter; it is a natural, biological event. If used wisely, technology can detect problems and provide solutions should nature fail. If abused, technology can actually become the problem. In birth, nature causes fewer complications than humans do. Whether you need or desire a high-tech birth depends on your birthing philosophy and your individual obstetrical needs. If you learn about the benefits and risks of tests and technology, you can be part of the decisions about using these modern tools wisely. In labor, like life, things sometimes don't go as desired. And because of circumstances beyond your control, you may need a high-tech birth. This "high-risk" label (often overused and unnecessary) does not mean you must become a passive patient. Instead, you must play an even more responsible role in your birthing decisions. Even high-risk births can be satisfying. See chapter 5 for information on using tests and technology wisely.

8. Learn some of the many self-care techniques to ease the discomforts of labor. Women do not have to suffer or be drugged to give birth. So many overdrugged or unnecessarily agonizing births could have been better if only a mother had known this. . . . *If only* she had been free to change positions. . . . *If only* she had realized what pain relief was available. We will get all of these *if only*s off our chest in chapters 8, 9, and 10 of this book.

It is neither safe nor healthy for a woman to be disconnected from her sensations during labor. Pain has a purpose. It compels a woman to do something to relieve it, and in making helpful adjustments in her body she often makes adjustments that help her baby's well-being.

Pain can be your own internal monitor. By appreciating that pain has a purpose, you can make these sensations work for you to accelerate the progress of labor. Unmanageable pain, for example, is not normal during labor. Instead, it is your body's signal that you need to make a change. Teaching you how to read your body's signals and what changes to make is one of this book's goals. We will explore all the safest and most researched methods of pain relief for childbirth to help you create the pain-management system that works best for you and your baby.

If you leave pain relief up to your doctor, you are likely to be disappointed. *A pain-free birth without risks is a promise your doctor can't deliver.* There is no pain-relieving drug that has ever been proven to be totally safe for mother and baby. But by understanding the benefits and risks of medication during childbirth, and by understanding when and how to use medical pain relief wisely, and by doing your part to lessen the need for drugs, you increase your chances of having a satisfying birth and a drug-free baby. The easing of the discomforts of labor and birth works best when it occurs within a partnership between you and your birth attendant. You use your own natural labor-easing coping mechanisms, and your birth attendant offers medical and/or midwifery help should it be needed or desired.

9. Learn ways to help your labor progress. "Failure to progress" is frequently cited as the reason for a cesarean birth — but the problem is usually avoidable. Different labors progress at different rates. Some take hours, some piddle along for days. It is your reaction to your individual labor that counts. Fear and tension stall labor. Confidence and knowledge of what's happening and how to work with your body help labor progress. Like your cardiovascular, gastroin-testinal, and endocrine systems, your birthing system is affected, for better or for worse, by how your mind and body work together. Birth is a mind-body experience, an intense physical process whose outcome is closely tied to emotions and mental attitude. There is a harmony to birth — an interconnection between mind and body and birthing systems. Throughout Part 2 of this book we will point out safe and effective ways to use both your mind and your body to keep your labor on track.

10. You can prevent a cesarean section — most of the time. With the cesarean-section rate in the United States averaging 25 percent women are beginning to question the American way of birth. In approximately 5 percent of births, a cesarean section may be necessary, occasionally even lifesaving, but women have the power to prevent the remainder of surgical births, which are unnecessary. In chapter 6, "Cesarean Births," we will show you how to minimize your likelihood of having a cesarean. And if you do need a surgical birth, we will show you how to make it a birth first, an operation second.

Every birth is different. Why is it that some women agonize through lengthy labors, while others breeze through birth? Many factors determine the length and intensity of labor: your previous birth experience, your usual perception of pain, your physical and mental preparation for birth, the position and size of the baby, your choice of birth attendants, and the support you receive during labor. We have come to appreciate that there is no one way to birth babies. But there is a best way for each mother to birth her own baby. Finding that way is a chal-

---

There Is a Rhythm to Every Labor

Our family hobby is sailing. As in birth, in sailing there are conditions you can change and those that are beyond your direction. The wind and waves we cannot control, but we can trim our sails to ride with these conditions. When trimmed right, the boat functions beautifully, is speedier, and less rocky (in sailor jargon, the craft is "in the groove"), but when not trimmed properly, the boat is out of harmony with the forces of nature. The ride is slower, uncomfortable. Also like in birth, a rough ride and slower progress is a signal that we need to trim the sails, shift the weight, change sails, and so forth. Then we're in the groove again.

lenge, and this book will help you meet that challenge. Our desire is not to judge ways of giving birth, but rather to inform you about them. It is up to you to choose what you believe is best for you and your baby.

Even with the best of knowledge and preparation, you will seldom be able to orchestrate the perfect labor. Far from being predictable, each birth is a wondrous creation, full of surprises. Therein lies the mystery and the beauty of birth. Even after our twenty-seven years of birth experience, we are still in awe of this event.

2

Birth — Then and Now

TO APPRECIATE WHERE birthing practices are going, it helps to know where they have been. Many changes have occurred in birthing, some of them for the good, some not. Gone is the fear of death for baby and mother in childbirth. Today's mothers nearly always come through childbirth alive, as do most of their babies. Proponents of the new obstetrics boast that at no time in history has a laboring mother been more safely cared for. Opponents counter that with approximately 25 percent of mothers ending up with cesareans, the American way of birth is not as good as it should be. And many parents feel that today's high-tech approach to birth deprives them of a sense of control and interferes with the human experience of birth. Here's how modern birthing practices evolved and what parents can do to make them better.

BIRTH BEFORE 1900: HOME, SWEET HOME

In earlier centuries birth was a social event held in the home. Female friends and family came to help and it was usually a women-only affair. In fact, a sixteenth-century male physician was burned at the stake for posing as a female midwife. Experienced mothers helped ease the discomfort and steady the progress of the laboring novice, and after birth these friends continued to lavish their attention on the new mother during her "confinement." Mother gave birth in the presence of familiar caregivers and in the comfort of her own home.

The midwife mind-set. Until the 1900s, nearly all births were attended by midwives. These women were noted for their gentle touch, and their skills came, not from universities or books, but through learning from other midwives, from hands-on experience, and from a personal knowledge and understanding of birth as the healthy event it usually is. Her tools were her hands, and her focus was on the whole person going through labor, not just on the birth canal. The mother usually gave birth in a vertical position, and the midwife accommodated. And the physicians of the time stayed clear of birth; it was women's business and it was surrounded with ideas the doctors deemed "magic" or "superstitious."

But birth was not all that simple in those

days. Women dreaded birth because of the possibility of death. The church advised women to repent and make themselves right with God during pregnancy in case they didn't survive childbirth. Church teaching predominated even in matters as personal as birth. Women were conditioned to believe that birthpain was an unavoidable consequence of original sin. Women were unfairly and incorrectly tagged with the "curse of Eve" found in Gen. 3:16: "I will greatly increase your *pains* in childbirth; with *pain* you will give birth to children."* Physicians at this time also believed the concept taught by the church that pain in childbirth was inevitable. (Fortunately, in the 1930s British obstetrician Grantly Dick-Read would challenge this dismal view of birth by proclaiming: "Childbirth does not have to be painful.")

Ripe for change. As the age of science and reason came to hold sway, birth became a subject of inquiry. This led to a desire to understand the natural process of birth, and, more significant, to control it. It also brought doctors into the picture.

In the early 1800s the all-male medical schools in Europe attracted American men who wanted to become doctors. Courses in childbirth were only a minor part of medical training. Midwives still controlled normal childbirth. Doctors, scared off by the rituals surrounding birth, felt that anything magical

was beneath their professional dignity. Midwives called the doctors only when complications arose. Cesarean sections, done by physicians, were performed only to save the life of the baby after the mother had died or was going to die.

Men at birth. Unlike Europe, America was more receptive to doctors being present at birth. A turf battle (one that continues today) developed between female midwives and male doctors. Doctors returning from European medical schools with book knowledge of birth needed employment. Their first marketing strategy was to convince women that educated men could improve upon the natural process of birth and possibly prevent it from going wrong. It became fashionable to be delivered by a doctor, and women paid handsome fees for this status. Eventually, middle- and upper-class women flocked to doctors for assistance in childbirth, leaving the poor and uneducated to be attended by midwives. Childbirth became the doctor's entry into caring for the whole family. Attending women in labor became a way to build a medical practice and gain social acceptance as a respected professional. According to the physician's logic of the times: birth is a medical matter; doctors are medically trained; therefore, women need doctors at birth.

Tools of the trade. With the advent of males in a formerly female sphere, childbirth inevitably became mechanized. To many, the female delivery system was little more than a mechanical pump, so they developed tools to make it work better. Enter the forceps. Introduced in the 1700s, and initially used only to extract stillborn babies, this cold, metal tool became man's entry into the previously female-dominated

---

* *Note that the words of Adam in Gen. 3:17 read, "Through* toil *you will eat of the earth all the days of your life." The original Hebrew word for "toil" (*etsev*), spoken to Adam, is the same one that is used speaking to Eve. Male translators injected their own bias by incorrectly translating the word* etsev *to read "pain" for Eve but "toil" for Adam. Biblical scholars now believe the word should be translated "hard work" in both verses for both sexes.*

arena. Pulling the baby through the birth canal with forceps became standard operating procedure for "modern" deliveries. Men were trained to use them at what would be the modern equivalent of trade schools; they entered the market as "male-midwives." Forceps were considered to be tools unbecoming to the "unskilled" female midwife. These iron hands gave men — and eventually doctors — an edge in the competition for market share. And forceps brought other substantial changes to how babies were born. With a forceps delivery, a woman had to lie on her back so that the male-midwife or doctor could use his instruments. An episiotomy, surgical enlargement of the opening of the vagina, was needed in order to make room for the forceps.

The rise of obstetrics and the fall of midwifery. In Europe male obstetrics and female midwifery began to coexist as a shared enterprise. The schools for birth trained both. Midwives attended uncomplicated births (home and hospital) and the obstetricians assisted births requiring their special training. And in some countries, namely Holland, this model is still working today, with the best statistics in the world for safety of mother and baby. But in America this commonsense approach to birth-attending roles never materialized.

The final blow to the art of midwifery came in the form of licensure. By the beginning of the twentieth century, licensure became synonymous with competence, and the midwife had to prove her skills to a state licensing board, which was controlled by the increasingly influential medical profession. Ideally, licensing should have upgraded and popularized midwifery, but it didn't. By this time, midwives had lost their autonomy and their clout as a profession, and they

were practicing under the supervision of physicians. Even the "professor of midwifery" at Harvard Medical School was male. Society tended to downgrade the art of midwifery and value university credentials more than traditional experience. Midwives empowered women to give birth, trusting in nature and taking the time to let birth happen, in a way that couldn't be scientifically measured. The physician, on the other hand, was trained as a scientist, didn't trust nature, and tried to make things happen.

Whose fault? How could women let this happen? you may wonder. Birth practices don't just happen; they evolve over time and are influenced by many social circumstances. To understand why it happened, you must look at the prevailing beliefs of the era. This was a time when women feared death and suffering in childbirth. Any new methods that appeared to offer better odds of survival at childbirth and a shortened, less agonizing labor were eagerly embraced by women. Their quest for a safer and painless birth mattered more than the sex of the birth attendant. So strong was this desire that women even overcame their Victorian modesty and were able to expose themselves to male doctors. Fear of death or the agony of prolonged labors made women open to any promise of a better birth.

The new science of obstetrics did offer the services demanded by the public. But women wanted what doctors couldn't deliver — a painless birth without risks. Chloroform and ether, sometimes fatal to mother and baby, were certainly not without risk. Women and their doctors made the best decisions they could considering social customs and what they knew about birth at the time. Doctors believed they were offering women what they wanted. True, doctors may have been opportunists, but women gave them the opportunities. The missing ingredient here was that women should have been educated rather than medicated. Unfortunately, the knowledge they needed was not yet available. Somewhere between folk wisdom and science lay a body of knowledge not yet formulated.

It is fashionable for birth books to engage in historical system-bashing. But the authors of these books overlook an important fact of history. To expect women and doctors of the past to have done other than what they did is to expect eighteenth- and nineteenth-century people to have made decisions with modern minds. Nineteenth-century women were different from us. The first woman in town to have a doctor at her birth was taking responsibility for a choice different from her friends' choice. By her standards hers was a better birth. How could she know that today's women may judge it differently? One mother recently told us, "My grandmother's first two children were born at home, her third in the hospital. She has never understood why I chose to birth my kids at home. When they could finally afford it, she went to the hospital. The home/hospital thing means something entirely different to her than to me." If we could fast-forward the birth history tape, can you imagine a woman of the 1900s seeing the wired-up woman of the nineties giving birth? She wouldn't think we were too smart, either.

For better or worse. The changes in birthing practices during the eighteenth and nineteenth centuries were a mixed blessing. On the positive side, the new science of obstetrics removed many of the superstitions surrounding birth. Making birth a mechanical science demystified the process. A scientific knowledge of normal birth pro-

cesses led to a deeper understanding of why complications occur and how to fix them. On the other hand, the decline of the midwife and the rise of the scientific obstetrician dehumanized birth into an exercise of time management, and allowed men and machines to take over and "manage" what nature had been doing pretty well on its own.

BIRTHING PRACTICES 1900–1950: BIRTH THE AMERICAN WAY

By the year 1900, women believed that doctors could give them safer and speedier births than midwives could. Women had little understanding of how their bodies worked to give birth and, more important, they had lost confidence in their bodies. They surrendered even more power over their bodies with the next birth-changing event: taking birth out of the home and putting it into the hospital.

Your place or mine? The mother's home was the last remnant of birth that was under her domain, and by the early twentieth century, the time-honored tradition of giving birth at home was going the way of the midwife. Prior to the 1900s fewer than 5 percent of babies were born in hospitals. This number increased to 75 percent by 1936 and to 99 percent by 1970. The hospital was geared toward routines, efficiency, and profit. Note that in 1890 (as in 1990) there was no proof that births attended by doctors were any safer than home births attended by skilled midwives. Mothers and doctors just *perceived* them to be safer, a perception that continues to this day. In fact, according to childbirth historians, birth at home under the midwives had been much safer. When birthing went from home to hospital, the maternal death rate from "childbed fever" (overwhelming infection) went up. Crowded wards and the lack of hand-washing by doctors caused this tragedy since the microbial basis of disease was not yet accepted nor had antibiotics been discovered.

By the early 1900s, the family doctor practicing midwifery was becoming more competent. He had the tools and pain-relieving medicines (chloroform-and-ether anesthesia was established) in his bag. He believed that nature was competent but slow, and that he could either improve upon nature or at least speed its progress. To spend all those hours acquiring medical skills and then not use them was beyond his patience. "Don't just stand there — do something!" became the mind-set for assisting at birth. The midwife, on the other hand, trusted in the wisdom of nature and had the patience to wait. For better or for worse, the entry of men into the childbirth arena and the transferring of birth from home to the hospital were the most significant turning points in the history of birth — and ones that still affect birthing practices today.

Birth fashions. It became fashionable to have babies in a hospital, a turnabout from earlier decades, when hospitals had served the poor and rehabilitated the unfortunate. Historically, the middle and upper classes have set the standard of medicine, so by 1940, a hospital birth became the standard. Women no longer were willing to be confined at home. Maternity fashions flourished, allowing the pregnant woman to go out proudly in public. Giving birth in the hospital was part of this trend away from the

home. This was the new obstetrics and "new" was perceived as better.

The following excerpt from a 1926 magazine story illustrates the thinking of the times:

"But is the hospital necessary at all?" demanded a young woman of her obstetrician friend. "Why not bring the baby at home?"

"What would you do if your automobile broke down on a country road?" the doctor countered with another question.

"Try and fix it," said the modern chauffeuse.

"And if you couldn't?"

"Have it hauled to the nearest garage."

"Exactly. Where the trained mechanics and their necessary tools are," agreed the doctor. "It's the same with the hospital. I can do my best work — and the best we must have in medicine all the time — not in some cramped little apartment or private home, but where I have the proper facilities and trained helpers. If anything goes wrong I have all known aids to meet your emergency."

Who could argue with that?

Painless birth. Pain relief during birth was a more urgent issue to women than the place of birth or its attendant. Since hospitals and doctors controlled the anesthetics, they got the birth business. Shortly before the turn of the century, doctors in Germany had developed a method of painless childbirth called *twilight sleep,* which used a triple-whammy of drugs. The woman got a shot of morphine at the beginning of labor to dull the pain, followed by the amnesiac scopolamine, which caused her to escape from her body and forget her birth trauma, topped off with a whiff of chloroform or ether to put her out during the baby's final passage through the birth canal. With the advent of twilight sleep, the mother was demoted from the person in control to semi-conscious patient.

Martha notes: At the start of my nurse's training in the early sixties, women finally began to get suspicious. I remember my instructors describing women under "twilight" behaving like deranged animals and having to be tied to their beds. On their backs, they were in agony, but they could do nothing to help themselves; when they woke up, they couldn't even remember it. I'm sure that the nurses caring for these women didn't know it could be any different, and that the telling of these horror stories were responsible for at least my generation of girls' having an exaggerated terror of childbirth, which lasted for decades after "twilight" was gone.

American doctors initially rejected these anesthetics as unreliable and unsafe. But women pushed for their use. Influential women even traveled to Germany for a painless birth and returned to extol the virtues of twilight sleep and popularize its use. Male doctors, cautious about these new drugs, were accused of being unsympathetic to women; being liberated from the pain of childbirth was part of the whole women's rights movement of the time. Hospitals picked up on consumers' demands and turned twilight sleep into their reason for being in the birth business. Twilight sleep became the hospital's selling point during the 1920s, as "family-centered birth" would become in the 1980s, and it became the standard in maternity care. But rather than dealing with the root causes of pain (fear and tension), hospitals played on the fear of pain and offered drugs as a way to cover it up.

Birth the hospital way. While women made gains in their quest for a painless, sanitized birth, they gave up their ability to take an active part in childbirth. Anesthesia brought profound changes in birthing practices that had prevailed since the beginning of womankind. The shift from a vertical to a horizontal position for birthing — a change that still infects the hospital birthing scene today — was an absolute necessity because the woman was now so heavily drugged that she could no longer walk during labor or help push her baby out. Because of the anesthetic she had little control over her body and needed arm restraints and leg stirrups. To this new and unhelpful birth posture were added the humiliating (and unnecessary!) practices of enemas and pubic shaving. The mother was made into the perfect surgical patient, clean and asleep.

Meanwhile, since the woman was in no position to give birth, someone had to take the baby from her body. This meant the use of forceps, an episiotomy, and sometimes drugs to augment labor. The unkind cut of the episiotomy was marketed as necessary for a faster second stage of labor and to prevent a ragged tear.

Following the birth, the patient was wheeled into a recovery room to awaken from the anesthetic after the "operation." Hours later she awoke in her hospital room to find out if she had a boy or a girl. Meanwhile, babies were also recovering from a birth script they never would have written. After birth, the baby was placed in a metal box and wheeled to the nursery to join other anonymous babies in metal boxes, and left to bond with a box. The drugged baby and his mother were then periodically reunited on a rigid four-hour feeding schedule, but they spent most of their time apart so that mother could rest and baby could be cared for by the "experts" in the nursery. Mother gave up not only her role in giving birth, but initially also her part in giving care to her baby, thinking this was for her own good — and her baby's.

There was one bright spot in these birth changes. Mothers were relying on doctors to give them a safer birth, and this put pressure on the doctors to deliver. Doctors became better trained and hospitals began to provide better care. The male doctors who specialized in birth acquired a more fitting title. "Male midwife" was confusing, and perhaps perceived by the medical profession as demeaning. A doctor specializing in delivering babies was now called an obstetrician, which, ironically, comes from the Latin *ob* and *stare* — "to stand by." Rather than stand by the mother in case they were needed, some stood in the way of the natural birth process.

Managing birth — managing babies. By now women had lost confidence in their ability to give birth and had turned over their responsibility to childbirth specialists. This loss of trust in their birthing abilities carried over to their mothering abilities. If specialists should manage their births, specialists should manage their babies. Mothers began asking their doctors questions like, "What do I do when my baby cries?" and "How do I feed my baby?" They wanted answers based on scientific principles, measurable and controllable. Hence, the advent of rigid schedules and regimented parenting, practices that were supposed to prevent spoiling children. The most absurd flip-flop was the switch from breastfeeding to bottle-feeding. Many believed the milk that scien-

Birth as an Illness

In the early 1900s birth came to be viewed as a pathological process requiring medical help. Influential obstetrical textbooks taught that a healthy birth occurred naturally (i.e., without doctors and their intervening tools) in only a minority of mothers and that most births needed to have the natural process improved upon. Early obstetrical schools taught that all women should have the benefit of an episiotomy and forceps delivery. It took the next sixty years to reverse this view and accept the reality that specialized obstetrical intervention is needed in only a minority of births. The pathological view of birth and the obstetrician's duty to rescue women from the "dangers of nature" were epitomized by a prominent obstetrician of the 1920s, Dr. Joseph DeLee: "I have often wondered whether nature did not deliberately intend women to be used up in the process of reproduction, in a manner analogous to that of the salmon, which dies after spawning."

tists formulated in a can was better and easier to deliver than what mothers made in their bodies. Doctors would decide whether a mother was "fit" to breastfeed her baby by taking a sample of her milk, swirling it around in a bottle, holding it up against a light, and seeing how thick it was. The change from breast to bottle seemed to please both pupils and teachers. The mother was liberated from her responsibility to feed her baby herself. Bottle-feeding suited doctors since, unlike breastfeeding, formula was something they could prescribe, control, and change. They could *do something.* Prescribing artificial baby milk became another way for mothers to need doctors. Like the new obstetrics, bottle-feeding became the standard for the educated and affluent. A great-grandmother shared with us her "managed-babies" story: "My doctor did the 'How thick is your breast milk?' test on me with each of my four children. Two times he said I was 'fit to nurse.' The other two he told me I would hurt my babies with my inferior milk. I was in wonderful health with each of my children. I can't believe I didn't even think to question his pronouncement."

Mothers allowed themselves to succumb to these marketing practices, and by 1960 breastfeeding rates had declined to a pitiful 20 percent. Even women who did breastfeed yielded to pressure to wean early. Changes in birthing and feeding practices led to other changes in how babies and children were parented. Babies were put on schedules. They no longer slept with their mothers. As with birth, mothers came to rely more and more on child-rearing experts who wrote books, and less on their own judgment and knowledge of their child. Women trusted their traditional wisdom and intuition about birthing and raising children less than the preachings of whatever baby-care guru reigned at the time.

For their own good? In hindsight it's apparent that the whole birthing and mothering scene was a mess, but it was truly no one's fault. Mothers believed all this intervention was for their own and their babies' good, and doctors believed they were saving women from the agony and mortality of childbirth. And things *had* improved: mothers could assume that when they entered the maternity ward, they would leave alive and with a healthy baby. The fear of death or disability, which scared laboring women, was a memory of generations past. (This was, however, more the result of the discovery of the microbial basis of infection and the use of antibiotics than a change in birth place or attendant.) Yet by the 1950s women began questioning whether this medicalization of birth was really for their own good. For the next several decades they would look at the birth scene and ask, "What's wrong with this picture?"

BIRTHING PRACTICES 1950– 1990: WOMEN ON TOP

A turning point in birthing history occurred in the 1960s when mothers finally began taking responsibility for their birth choices. The time had come, some mothers thought, to have a better birth. They sensed that something important had been taken from them, and they were determined to get it back. Over the next four decades, they struggled to do so. But birth had become so medicalized that it was difficult for these women to push their birth needs through the obstetric establishment.

Another obstacle to birth reform was the lack of birthing alternatives. Midwives were all but extinct. By 1970 obstetrics had become such a respected science that a healthy baby and a healthy mother were virtually expected every time. Most women felt powerless to challenge the medical-technological establishment, and, quite honestly, were not quite sure they wanted to. Less-resigned women were passionate, nearly militant, about change. While not wanting birth to revert to the Dark Ages, they felt modern obstetrics, under the guise of progress, had thrown out the baby with the bath water.

Birth schools. In the sixties, women began teaching each other about birth. Prepared childbirth classes empowered women to manage their own births and demonstrated that it was healthier for mother and baby to do so. As women began taking more responsibility for their birthing decisions, they began to humanize what went on in the delivery room. Mothers also began demanding that fathers be allowed a role at birth. Before 1970, the very person who helped make the baby was banished from the birth. Consumer demand brought men into the delivery room, to witness the birth of their babies and to support their wives. "Choices" and "alternatives" were the buzzwords of the sixties; witness the motto of the International Childbirth Education Association (ICEA): "Freedom of choice through knowledge of alternatives."

Pain relievers. The central issue in childbirth was still pain, but now women began learning that it was within their power to influence their perception of pain, using methods popularized from Grantly Dick-Read's *Childbirth Without Fear;* Dr. Robert Bradley's *Husband-Coached Childbirth;* and the writings of French obstetrician Fernand Lamaze. Even as early as the 1930s Dr. Dick-Read had challenged the traditional teachings that pain in childbirth was inevitable. Dick-Read's approach to dealing with pain in labor was to use the combination of relaxation and education. He taught that with proper education and support, normal childbirth was not designed to be painful. Twenty

years later, childbirth educators, realizing he was right, began to teach this to more women.

Two schools of thought in childbirth education emerged. One approach was to teach a mother, by diversion and distraction, how to escape from her body and her pain. But dissatisfaction with escape methods and a new emphasis on getting in touch with one's inner self led to another approach of labor management: rather than trying to flee from labor pain, women were taught to understand the physical processes of birth, to listen to their inner signals, and to work with them. This method was considered more in tune with a woman's sexuality. Birth was a "psychosexual experience" women really didn't want to miss. While techniques differed, the new childbirth revolved around the central issue that a woman could manage pain in labor or at least tell others how she wanted it managed. Most important, she could take charge of her own birthing. In fact, it was her responsibility to do so.

Au naturel. The back-to-nature philosophy of the early 1970s, along with the willingness to challenge authority that came out of the late sixties, affected child-birthing. People had become more skeptical about scientific progress and all establishments, including the medical one. Natural childbirth was assumed to be better, and a sign of accomplishment for mother. While in the early part of the century it was fashionable to be asleep during childbirth, in the sixties and seventies it became desirable to be awake. Birth sensations, like sex, were to be experienced, not diluted by depressing medications or undermined by hospital routines. While women embraced natural childbirth as a desirable goal, the birthing establishment viewed it as a trendy but impossible dream.

The great masquerade. As the postwar baby boom ended and birth rates fell, hospitals, fearing they would be caught with their delivery rooms empty, listened to the real consultants — those who were having the babies. Motivated more by consumer pressure than by a real desire for change, hospitals began to advertise alternatives. Their first offering was the alternative birthing center, or ABC, a room that created a homelike environment, a place to give birth that was like a home away from home. Commendable, but not enough. Behind the flowered curtains of the ABC room the medical mind-set prevailed. Still ingrained into obstetricians and obstetrical nurses was the belief that birth was a potential medical crisis ready to happen, not a natural process that required understanding and support. In fact, the 1970s brought even more technology to childbirth.

Back home. A few women realized that the obstetrician-hospital medical attitude was unchangeable and dropped out entirely, choosing to have their babies at home or in freestanding (that is, "free of hospital control") birthing centers. Those who dared venture from the safe and sanitary hospital were considered "irresponsible" by many people, but these women countered that the very reason they sought an alternative was that they were being responsible.

High-tech births. In the seventies, the electronic fetal monitor (EFM) entered the birth scene, a device that would affect birthing practices for years to come. Proponents touted EFM as a lifesaving device that could detect when the baby was in distress during labor and alert the obstetrician to intervene before damage or death occurred. Opponents countered that EFM would cause more problems than it solved. Never mind that babies had, for millennia, managed to leave their wombs without electronic surveillance. Both sides were right. Electronic fetal monitoring has saved the brains and lives of some babies, but it has also caused many unnecessary surgical births and perpetuated the belief that every birth is just one monitor bleep away from a life-or-death crisis. Nevertheless, EFM's popularity became firmly established long before its usefulness or safety had been proven.

Surgical births. Between 1970 and 1990 the cesarean rate jumped from 5 percent to 25–30 percent. Think about it. Can the birthing organs in 30 percent of women have gone wrong in just twenty years? Could the problem be not in the delivery system of the mother but in the delivery system of the new obstetrics? The increase in cesareans has many causes, among them the use of EFM and the malpractice crisis in obstetrics.

Legal births. The fear of liability that looms over delivery rooms has had a great effect on what goes on during a birth in the late twentieth century. When a less-than-perfect baby arrives, even through no one's fault, someone has to pay. Over the past twenty years physicians' premiums for malpractice insurance have tripled, as has the number of surgical births. There is money to be made in misfortune. A legal cloud hangs over the birthing room, a cloud that influences decision making. Doing what's best for mother and baby used to be the basis for an obstetrician's decisions. Now the main objective seems to be staying out of legal trouble. "Did you do everything to prevent the baby's injury?" the court asks the accused doctor. "Everything" means employing every test and intervention that, regardless of whether they are in the best interest of mother and baby, will clear the doctor in a lawsuit. We believe that until obstetricians receive some relief from the fear of being sued and a better way is found to compensate birth injuries (such as a Birth Injury Fund, a sort of Workmen's Compensation for babies), mothers will not get the births they want.

Painless births. Even through the 1980s the central issue remained pain relief. Although childbirth classes prepared women to use their bodies to lessen pain, or at least to handle it, many women opted for birthing practices that offered the greatest promise of pain relief, which by now included the popular epidural anesthesia. Specialists in obstetrical analgesia had so perfected their techniques that they could turn their pain-relieving medicine on and off at various stages of labor allowing mothers both some sensation and some movement. The "you can have it all" philosophy of the eighties had made its way into the birthing room.

THE 1990S AND BEYOND: WHAT'S AHEAD

We believe that the nineties will be a decade when women realize their choices in birth — what's best, what's available, and what's the most comfortable. The "you can have it all" philosophy will give way to the realization that actually you can't. Women must make informed choices and realize every option has its price.

Women helping women. One trend that we are certain will become important in the 1990s is a recognition that women need women at birth. We have already seen the beginning of a new profession — the professional labor assistant. This woman, usually a midwife, childbirth educator, or obstetrical nurse, is specially trained to support the laboring mother knowledgeably during birth. From experienced veteran to novice, a flow of energies empowers the mother to move in harmony with her body, to recognize and act on her own body signals so that labor can progress more comfortably and efficiently. The labor assistant also acts as a liaison between the laboring couple and the medical and nursing staff, helping the mother participate in birthing decisions should interventions be considered. As we discuss in chapter 3, this labor-support person does not displace the father.

Money and birth. Every decade has its driving force and for the nineties it is money — or, more specifically, the lack of it. The growing cost of medical care and the demand for universal health care in America mean that choices must be made. While some women are covered by traditional insurance plans with high premiums that allow them to choose their obstetricians, many have lost the freedom to choose and have to settle for whatever doctors happen to be signed up with their plan. The public isn't aware of what is happening behind doors on the insurance scene. Since companies may soon be required to insure their employees, the American free-enterprise system is opening the door for a whole parade of insurance brokers, all claiming more for less. Employee health care is being auctioned off to the company that promises to deliver the lowest health costs, resulting in a lack of choice of physicians that employees feel powerless to change and employers can't afford to change. The good news is that people are insured; the bad news is what they get for their buck.

Obstetrics is just one of the many specialties affected. The justified pride a doctor feels at being selected by a patient because he or she has a reputation for delivering competent and caring medicine no longer applies. Now the rationale for the choice is simply "You're on my plan." But since many plans drastically cut the doctor's fees, the obstetrician must see twice as many women or spend half as much time with them. The paradox is that women are finally demanding more time with their birth attendants but, due to economic forces, at a time when they are unwilling or unable to pay for it.

On the bright side, economic forces have a way of compelling people to take inventory of what's important, affordable, needed, and wanted, and then figure out how they can get it. People are beginning to question whether all this high-priced help and technology is necessary in order to have a safe and satisfying birth. We predict that most women (or "the plan") will choose the following model as the most satisfying and economic birth: a midwife as the primary birth attendant with an obstetrician as consultant. In the last five years of the twentieth century, as America comes to terms with its priorities, we will see a long overdue sorting-out of what really is the best birth buy.

A change in birthing philosophy. Expect a shift in attitude from one that regards birth as a disease to one that respects its nor-

malcy. The emphasis and resources will focus on the 90 percent of mothers who can and should deliver their babies with the minimum of intervention, making possible improvements in obstetrical care for the 10 percent who need specialists.

A change in birthing positions. Baby catchers, prepare to change your style! The sitting doctor and the back-lying patient is a scene from birthing's past. Active labors and vertical births are in.

More midwives are coming! There will be more emphasis on midwife-obstetrician teams. The midwife will give routine prenatal care and attend normal births, freeing the obstetrician to do that for which he or she is trained — caring personally for those mothers who have birth complications. The benefit to the consumer will be an upgrading of care as obstetricians, professional labor assistants, and midwives work together to give each mother the safest and most satisfying birth.

Back home? Home birth could become an option for more women depending on two factors: the ability of midwives to organize and maintain a high standard of training, licensure, and self-regulation — and be *perceived* as doing so; and the willingness of obstetricians and hospitals to provide medical backup. Some women will always prefer to give birth at home. Licensing, instead of outlawing, the attendants and providing medical support will make home birth even safer. Midwives attending home births could then practice within the law and the medical system.

Natural or managed birth? There will be many women who feel the hospital setting robs them of their femininity and power. They will choose to give birth at home, at a birth center or will be assertive enough to get the hospital birth they want in order to have the full "experience" of birth. There still, however, will be women who prefer managed births. These are women who are delighted with the present American way of birth and who want some of the "experience" of birth, but prefer the packaged delivery of scheduled induction, Pitocin augmentation, electronic fetal monitoring, and epidural analgesia. Both styles of birth will be available according to what women need or demand.

More labor-friendly technology. In essence, the technology will be used only when necessary and in such a way that it doesn't interfere with natural processes. Also expect surgical births to be cut in half over the next ten years, if, and only if, there is legal reform, technological reform, and the wise use of midwives as primary birth attendants.

WHAT YOU CAN DO

Women need to take more responsibility for their birthing decisions. At no time in history has obstetrics been more ripe for change. Health-care excesses are on the hit list of every political reformer, mothers are better informed than ever before, and obstetrics as it is now practiced is becoming less satisfying. Be a wise consumer. Exercise your options. Based on your personal needs and wants, choose the birthing attendants and place best for you and your baby. If these options are not available in your community, lobby for them. *Doctors and insurance companies should not determine birthing practices — women must.* It's up to the baby bearers of the next generation to determine how they want to have their babies. Parents, the best birthing years are yet to come. We envision the nineties to be the golden decade of obstetrics — and a great time to birth a baby.

Choices in Childbirth

W OMEN IN THE NINETIES have more birth choices than ever before. But choice has its price. Making the right choice implies that a woman has done her homework to understand all the alternatives available to her, and, having explored all these alternatives, chooses what's best for her. To do otherwise is to lose this advantage. Take pain relief in childbirth, for example. Because epidural anesthesia is such a popular choice, many women elect to go directly to a high-tech birth rather than take the time and energy to explore more natural but less risky methods of pain relief. Making the right choice is best summed up in the motto of the International Childbirth Education Association: "Freedom of choice through knowledge of alternatives." We wish to guide you first through the best of the modern alternatives. Then, having explored them all, you will be empowered to make wise birth choices. Taking responsibility for your birth decisions increases your chances of having a satisfying birth.

One day we were chatting with a group of obstetricians and nurses about how much women differ in their birth preparation. The general consensus of these birth attendants was that the more informed women are, the easier they birth. Even well-read, well-fed, and well-toned mothers may have birth complications, but they tend to have fewer problems and are better prepared to cope with unforeseen circumstances by remaining part of the decision-making process should the birthing situation become less than ideal. Your baby is born only once — make the experience special.

WORKING OUT A BIRTHING PHILOSOPHY

Before you set out to interview birth attendants and choose a birth place, spend some time interviewing *yourself.* It helps to know what you want before you talk to others. What kind of birth do you want? What do you expect from your health-care providers? What are your feelings and beliefs about childbirth? In essence, have you worked out your own birth philosophy? If this is your first baby and your first major encounter with the health-care system, you may not yet know the answers to all these questions.

Appreciate that your birth experience, whether wondrous or unpleasant, will be remembered for the rest of your life. It only makes sense to put time and effort into the choices that increase your chances of making birth a fulfilling experience. But you may be so scared about giving birth that you haven't yet developed a birthing philosophy. These feelings are normal. Birth (and its anticipation) can be an intimidating experience, especially for first-timers. In this chapter we will discuss some considerations to help you work out a birthing philosophy that works best for you.

Women in charge. Some expectant mothers are up on the new obstetrics. They subscribe to lots of magazines that cover health issues. They have read all about birth. They know their options and they know what they want. They believe that the only reason for having an obstetrician is in case something unexpected (and perhaps beyond their control) happens. Yet they don't honestly believe anything like this can happen to them because they have absolutely everything under control. All will go as planned because they have done everything "right."

Doctors in charge. At the opposite extreme is the newly pregnant woman who is totally new to the birth scene. She is overawed by the medical establishment and has read no books on birth (except perhaps a pamphlet picked up at the doctor's office), but she has exposed herself to the parade of veterans only too eager to share their own horror stories about birth. She imagines herself most comfortable with a delivery system where "we do it all for you." She envisions her pregnancy and delivery progressing with little input from her under the benevolent control of an experienced authority figure who is a bit gray at the temples. She assumes that decisions made for her must be better than any decisions she would make for herself.

Both of these mothers are likely to have a less-than-satisfying birth experience. On the one hand, being entirely closed to the suggestions of your birth attendant may deprive you of the valuable experience that a professional has to share with you. On the other hand, taking no responsibility for your birthing decisions devalues the power of womanhood and the specialness of birth.

It is most rewarding to plan your birth in partnership with your birth attendant — allowing your birth philosophy to evolve during your journey through pregnancy. Books, classes, and conversations with other mothers will help you discover your needs and feel comfortable conveying them to your birth attendant, who, in turn, will respect your wishes. Together you formulate a birth plan that is best for you and your baby. In this way you avoid the "my way versus doctor's way" conflict that can arise at crucial moments during your pregnancy and delivery.

A first-time mother who empowered herself with all the tools to increase her chances of a satisfying birth experience told us about her partnership with her birth attendant: "I wanted to be in complete control of my faculties, no drugs or intervention unless there was distress. I wanted the security of a doctor's knowledge. I wanted to know from the nurses and doctors what was going on at all times and why. I didn't want to be left out of the decisions but at the same time I didn't want the sole responsibility for making them." This mother took the best from herself and the best from her birth attendants and had a satisfying birth experience.

CHOOSING YOUR BIRTH TEAM

Choosing Dr. Right

When beginning your search for a doctor, the best source of referrals is other women. Talk to friends, childbirth educators, obstetric nurses — anyone who has recently given birth or who has lots of contact with expectant and new mothers. It's best to get referrals from mothers who share your own birth philosophy. Narrow the list down to two or three prospects and then make plans to interview these physicians. When making the appointment, let the receptionist know it's for an interview only. Ask the receptionist about fees, office hours, and insurance coverage over the phone. Make a list of what's important for you to ask the doctor. A prepared list ensures that you cover all your questions and also respects the doctor's time. The very fact that you are interviewing a doctor conveys to him or her that you care enough to seek the best for yourself and your baby. If possible, both expectant parents should attend this interview. Let your prospective doctor know your referral source. His or her best advertisement is satisfied parents. Sources such as "the yellow pages" or "You're on our insurance plan" do not make good first impressions.

Beginning Your Interview

Introduce yourself to the front-office personnel and, more important, the back-office nurses. Many times throughout your pregnancy you will have questions for them and need their support. After introductions, a good opener is to ask the doctor about his or her birth philosophy. You want to discover what your doctor's attitude about birth is. Best (for most parents) is a partner-

A Sample Prenatal Interview List

While quizzing your prospective doctor, be sure you know where he or she stands on these important topics:

- labor management (chap. 12*)
- pain management (chap. 8)
- natural childbirth (chap. 3)
- walking during labor (chap. 12)
- improvising various labor and birthing positions (chap. 11)
- electronic fetal monitoring: continuous, intermittent, telemetry, none (chap. 5)
- labor-support persons: professional assistant, baby's father (chap. 3)
- routine intravenous fluids (chap. 12)
- episiotomy: how often performed, alternatives (chap. 5)
- forceps and vacuum extractors (chap. 10)
- birth plans (chap. 13)
- criteria for cesarean birth (chap. 6)
- vaginal birth after cesarean (chap. 7)
- use of water during labor (chap. 9)
- epidural anesthesia (chap. 10)
- childbirth classes (chap. 3)
- pregnancy health: exercise, nutrition, weight gain, etc. (chap. 4)
- hospital affiliations (chap. 3)
- routine prenatal screening tests (chap. 5)
- call schedule (group or solo practice; birth philosophy of the covering doctors) (chap. 3)
- vacation schedule (in case it's during your due date) (chap. 3)
- fees, insurance plans (usually handled by office staff) (chap. 3)

* Because early in pregnancy many expectant couples have not yet worked out all of their birth needs, a discussion of these topics of concern is found in the chapter listed after each topic.

ship attitude: "Birth is most commonly a healthy and uncomplicated process, and I will do my best to help it progress that way. You do what you do best to grow and birth your baby, and I'll do what I do best to safeguard the health of both you and your baby. That's our partnership."

After you have determined how this doctor approaches birth, next find out how he or she manages a birth. It is unfair and unwise to ask questions that are too specific, such as, "How will you manage my pain?" since at this point neither you nor your doctor knows what your situation will be on the big day. More helpful are general questions: "How do most mothers in your practice cope with pain in labor?" "In what position do most mothers in your practice give birth?" "What do you do and what do you suggest women do if labor is not progressing?" Look for a balance of natural methods of pain control and medical management. Basically you want to find out if the doctor is flexible. Is his or her birth mind-set stuck in the horizontal position, or is the doctor knowledgeable about the value of walking around during labor and birthing upright? Also, ask about the doctor's cesarean rate, and what percentage of women in the practice receive epidurals, episiotomies, and electronic fetal monitoring. The answers to these questions will reveal something of the philosophy the doctor brings to birth.

Avoid Negative Openers

In this initial interview, and later on during your prenatal visits, don't come armed with a nonnegotiable list of "I don't want"s. Ease into these preferences. Otherwise you will come across as a graduate fresh out of the school of those birth books and childbirth classes that paint, to the detriment of all, the doctor as an adversary — which he or she is not. As you wish your doctor to be open to your individual wants and needs, don't close your mind to other viewpoints that may be worth considering. The person with whom you are speaking is a highly trained medical professional with justified pride in his or her profession and extreme interest in the medical safety of your birth. Express your desires and the reasons behind them, and then be willing to listen to the doctor's answer. For example: "Doctor, I don't want to be confined to bed during labor because of continuous fetal monitoring. I would like to be able to move around and work with my body. Would you help me make this possible?" Expect an answer something like, "I respect your desires and am willing to use monitoring only if necessary, but I would reserve the right to intervene medically should the need arise. I would explain interventions that may become necessary, and you would have a voice in these decisions." In other words, the doctor will ask the same respect and flexibility of you that you are asking of him or her. You want to establish a relationship of mutual trust.

Other Questions to Ask

Find out how the doctor's call schedule works. Some doctors have a single practice and attend all of their own births unless they are sick or out of town. Other doctors share calls on a rotation basis, so you may get one of three or four doctors as your birth attendant. Ask if all of the doctors share the same philosophy of birth. Beware of the obstetrician who talks like a midwife but thinks like a doctor. Obstetricians know what today's savvy mothers are reading and thinking and may woo you with all the right answers. Best to ask for names and check with the doctor's clients. Does this doctor practice what he or she preaches?

Is your doctor a team player? If you wish to have a professional labor assistant or a midwife involved in your birth, how will your prospective doctor accept and work with this attendant to help you get the birth you want?

After the Interview

Choose a physician with a philosophy similar to yours. Choosing a doctor is a bit like choosing a marriage partner. If you go into this relationship believing, "We think quite differently, but I'm drawn to his personality. I'm sure he'll change for me," you are making a mistake. Chances are that this doctor will click into his or her own birthing mind-set at the first irregularity on the fetal monitor, at a vulnerable time when you are unable or unwilling to negotiate. If you feel you have to change your obstetrician's mind, change doctors.

Using a Midwife

It took us three births to realize that, with all due respect to the medical profession, the majority of laboring women, especially first-time moms, need more than an obstetrician has to offer. With our last five babies we had the ideal: a midwife and an obstetrician working as a team. We took the roles of each literally: obstetrician means "one who stands by" and midwife means "with woman." One is not better or more qualified than the other. They are different professionals with different philosophies and different roles.

A profile of an obstetrician. A physician goes through four years of premedical training and four years of medical school to learn the science of the body. After graduation he or she decides to specialize in obstetrics and gynecology, requiring at least four more years of training. Much of that time — especially in gynecology — is spent as a surgeon. The obstetrical training concentrates on complicated pregnancies and deliveries. The doctor develops a surgical mind-set, and birth becomes a procedure in which the surgeon is the star of the show. The physician is geared to pathology, the abnormal, the complicated. Patients with problems pose the intellectual and technical challenges he or she was trained to handle. Much obstetrical training takes place in a charity hospital where the majority of the patients receive no childbirth education and may play no part in determining the course of their care.

When the surgeon leaves the inner-city medical center for the world of everyday obstetrics, he or she experiences a role reversal. Here, mothers are the center of attention. They deliver; the doctor attends. And most births are exasperatingly simple. They involve a lot of waiting around for events completely out of the doctor's control. Only when something goes wrong is the doctor on his or her familiar turf again. He or she is again in control, feeling competent, comfortable, and valuable — intervening in the birthing room or moving to the operating room.

No childbirth movement, birth book, or mother armed with birth plans will completely erase this surgical mind-set — nor should it. We need competent physicians who specialize in complicated births. But 90 percent of births have no complication and should not need the doctor's surgical skills.

A profile of a midwife. The midwife comes from a different background from the

Who's Who in Birth Attendants

Obstetricians/Gynecologists have an M.D. or a D.O. (Doctor of Osteopathy) degree and have completed at least three years of specialty training in obstetrics and gynecology. If the M.D.s have passed an exam given by their professional society, they may display the credentials F.A.C.O.G. (Fellow of the American College of Obstetrics and Gynecology).

Family physicians care for the medical needs of the whole family. Their family-practice training includes obstetrics, though they don't have the specialized training of an OB/Gyn physician. They refer mothers with anticipated complications to obstetricians.

Certified nurse-midwives (C.N.M.) have a degree in nursing, experience as a labor and delivery nurse, and at least one year of additional hands-on training in midwifery. To become certified and practice midwifery they must pass an exam given by the American College of Nurse Midwives and be licensed by the state in which they practice. Midwives care for the mother throughout the course of normal pregnancy and delivery and may also provide basic gynecological care. They must have backup for birth from a physician on-call. C.N.M.s practice in hospitals, birthing centers, and attend home births in states where they are licensed to do so.

Perinatologists are obstetricians/gynecologists who have extra training in caring for mothers with complicated pregnancies (called high-risk) or anticipated problems at birth. These specialists practice at major medical centers. They may care for the mother during her entire pregnancy and attend the birth, or may function as a consultant to a mother's regular obstetrician.

Neonatologists are pediatricians who specialize in the care of premature and sick newborns. They practice in a newborn intensive care unit and attend high-risk births if the obstetrician anticipates a complication.

Licensed midwives (also known as lay- or direct-entry midwives) have midwifery training but without the prerequisite of a degree in nursing. They must have completed some type of midwifery training (state requirements vary) and passed the exam given by their state licensing department, if available. At this writing only a few states license these midwives.

Unlicensed midwives have varying degrees of training. Most have learned their skills by apprenticing with another midwife. Some are highly skilled, but others are not. Some have physician backup, but others may not. In many states these midwives attend home births illegally, or at least not sanctioned by law. Because so many states refuse to license direct-entry midwives and make it nearly impossible for them to practice, many practice without state recognition. Their own professional organizations are trying very hard to gain official licensing policies across the country.

Professional Labor Assistants (also called labor-support persons) are midwives, childbirth educators, obstetrical nurses, or other qualified persons who are trained to support the laboring mother during childbirth. A PLA makes no _doula_ medical decisions but attends to the mother, easing her discomfort and helping her work with her body toward progress in labor. She may also make follow-up home visits, assisting the mother with the transition into parenting, caring for the baby's siblings, breastfeeding, and infant care issues, and helping the mother care for herself.

obstetrician's. She is trained to assist mothers with normal, uncomplicated pregnancies and labors, but she also knows how to recognize a potential problem that needs obstetrical consultation. To her, birth is a natural process. She patiently blends into the birth scene, sometimes just sitting back and listening, and at other times giving hands-on support that eases the discomfort and accelerates the progress of labor, all the while safeguarding the health of the mother and baby by close, continual observation.

The midwife's philosophy is different from the obstetrician's — not better, not less, just different. An obstetrician manages labor; the midwife supports labor. The obstetrician makes things happen; the midwife lets things happen. The doctor trusts technology and is wary of nature. The midwife trusts nature and is cautious about technology. The obstetrician fears a birth may go wrong. The midwife expects the birth will go right.

The midwife is a catalyst for the mother's body chemistry, helping the laboring woman use her energy wisely. She communicates peace and relaxation. There is no need to fear or be in a hurry. Believing that fear is the most contagious disease to infect a laboring woman, she banishes all thoughts and personnel that may bring this unwelcome intruder into the birth scene.

Getting the best of both. Our wish for you is to have the science of obstetrics and the art of midwifery working together in your birth. We predict that obstetricians wishing to stay in the baby business will soon include midwives as members of their practice. If there are any complications during your pregnancy, labor, or in the final stages of birth, you are in excellent hands with an obstetrician, but you will get to those final stages most comfortably and expeditiously with a midwife. Our hope is that mothers not regard an obstetrician or midwife attendant as an either/or decision. There are ways to obtain the best of both specialties.

One option is to be under the care of a certified midwife and an obstetrician throughout pregnancy, labor, and delivery, with the midwife as the primary birth attendant and the physician as backup to be called upon only in the event of complications. If you have any current or anticipated complications, consider using a physician as your primary caregiver, but also employ a midwife to comanage your labor. A third alternative would be to have a physician as your primary birth attendant and hire a professional labor assistant to support you during labor.

You may ask, "Won't the obstetrical nurses give me the support I need?" Depending on how many other women they have to care for, you may or may not receive all the hands-on attention you need. They also have administrative and technical duties that demand their time. The amount of labor assistance and the level of experience you will get from your nurse is hard to predict. Some are mothers themselves and have had experience working as or with midwives. Others may have limited midwifery experience. And, of course, most mothers labor through one or two changes of nursing shifts.

With an obstetrician-only–attended birth, many mothers do not get the personal attention they pay for, such as in this birth scenario: You enter the hospital in labor and are evaluated by the obstetrical nurse. Meanwhile, the doctor is back in his or her office juggling the schedule hoping to be there in time for your birth yet relying on the nurses to keep posted on your progress. The machine monitors your progress in the hospital, the doctor monitors your progress by phone, and a valuable pair of hands is missing. The midwife or labor-support professional will supply this missing ingredient.

Questions to Ask a Midwife

- What is her training and experience? Where did she train, how long has she been a midwife, and how many births has she attended?
- Does she have obstetrical backup? With whom? Call the doctor to confirm.
- If the backup physician must assume your care due to complications, what will her continued role be in your labor and birth?
- Is she a licensed lay midwife or a certified nurse-midwife? (Not all states license lay midwives. See "Resources for Alternative Childbirths," page 45, to find out which states do.)
- Does she practice with other midwives? What is her coverage if she is occupied with another mother in labor or on vacation? Does she carry an electronic pager?
- What is her plan of action should it be necessary to transfer you or your baby to a hospital or to an obstetrician's care? Under what conditions would she consider such a transfer? Does she have an arrangement with the hospital that allows her to comanage your labor in the hospital?
- Does she perform episiotomies? If so, what are her criteria for so doing? In case of tears, is she trained in suturing the perineum?
- Is she certified in neonatal resuscitation? What resuscitation equipment does she have?
- Can she provide references of mothers she has recently attended?
- What are her fees and will insurance cover her services?

For more information on choosing and using a midwife see "Who's Who in Birth Attendants," page 33, and information on choosing a midwife-attended home birth, pages 43–50.

Choosing a Labor-Support Person

When women began to shun drugs in favor of being awake and aware during childbirth, they woke up to the fact that an important person was missing from the birth team. This missing woman is the labor-support person.

Who is she? The labor-support person *must* be a woman *and* a mother. Since she is a relative newcomer to the childbirth team (or, more accurately, a rediscovered tradition), the terms describing her are unfamiliar. *Labor-support person* is a general term that refers to any knowledgeable and nurturing woman who cares for the laboring mother's needs before, during, and after her birth. A *doula,* from the Greek for woman's servant, has no special medical training, but provides companionship, and ministers to the needs of the laboring and postpartum mother. She can be a good friend or a person hired for her services. Doula services (primarily to provide postpartum help) are springing up throughout the land. The professional labor assistant (PLA) (also called a monitrice) is a labor-support person who provides the companionship and comfort of a doula but also has special obstetric training. She is a midwife, obstetrical nurse, or laywoman with training in midwifery. For most mothers, a PLA is your best birth buy.

What does she do? A PLA is not just a nice woman to have around to rub your back and fetch you juice. She does a lot more. She is an anchor offering emotional support to the laboring mother as well as praise, pep talks, encouragement, and empowerment. She helps keep your birth wishes in perspective if complications set in and difficult compromises and decisions need to be made. She affirms and works through joyous accomplishments and disappointments in the post-partum period. This special person is also a teacher, instructing the mother in labor-saving techniques, answering questions, explaining labor events as they occur, and preparing the couple for what is ahead. The anticipatory guidance she provides can alleviate most of the fear of the unknown. The PLA is also a diplomat, the mother's advocate, acting as a liaison between parents and the medical staff, conveying the couple's wishes and seeing that they are honored whenever possible. She makes no medical decisions but helps interpret the suggestions of the medical attendants to the parents. She assists the parents in asking the right questions so that they are informed enough to take an active part in the decisions. She also helps ensure that interventions are avoided or at least decided on mutually. She has a sensitive presence, knowing when actively to assist the mother and when to retreat quietly into the shadows and leave the laboring couple alone so that the mother does not feel watched or judged. Best of all she is a comforter, touching and tuning in to the mother during contractions, helping her relax, and assisting her in using her natural resources to ease her discomfort and steady the progress of labor. And when the mother's strength seems gone, her own strength is offered to the woman, encouraging her beyond her perceived limits to meet her goal of birthing her baby.

Not only does the labor-support person make for easier labors, but woman-supported births are better for mothers and babies medically. Studies have shown that mothers who were supported during their labors had shorter labors (up to 50 percent in some studies) and were less likely to need cesareans (8 percent in the supported group versus 18 percent in nonsupported), and fewer needed forceps deliveries or epidural analgesia. Supported women also needed fewer episiotomies and experienced fewer perineal tears. The mothers in the supported group made an easier transition into motherhood, tended to breastfeed longer, and their babies experienced fewer newborn problems requiring special care.

An obstetrical nurse and professional labor assistant for many mothers in our practice has compiled the following statistics of her experiences over the past three years: Of the forty women she attended, 7.8 percent had a cesarean (the local rate is 30 percent); 12 percent had an epidural (in most hospitals at least 60 percent of mothers have an epidural); fifteen of the mothers were planning VBACs (vaginal birth after a cesarean); thirteen (86 percent) had a VBAC; only one needed forceps delivery; and all babies and mothers had healthy outcomes. The average age of these mothers was thirty-three years.

As with other birth attendants, interview prospective PLAs before choosing one. Meet with your chosen PLA a few months before the birth. She will help you work out a birthing plan that best fits your situation and increases your chances of getting the birth you want. As you get to know how she operates and she gets to know what you need, you'll form a trusting relationship with each other. Some PLAs will come to your home when labor begins, and assist you as long as you are comfortable staying there. Most women go to the hospital much too early, before active labor has actually begun. The result may be either a frustrating trip back home or premature admission to the hospital, which opens the door for a long list of procedures that might not have been necessary if the mother had labored for a while longer at home. The labor assistant monitors your labor at home and helps you decide when to leave for the hospital, neither leaving home too soon nor remaining home too long.

Questions About Professional Labor Assistants

Where do I find one of these gems, and what do they cost?

Because this is a relatively new field, you may not find PLAs in the yellow pages (and that might not be the best referral source anyway). Get referrals from your childbirth class, obstetrician, cesarean awareness group, or hospital. Network with mothers in parenting organizations such as La Leche League International. (See "Resources for Labor Assistants," page 37.) The best source is other women who have used a PLA at their birth. If mothers demand these specialists, the supply will soon follow.

Expect to pay between $250 and $500 for the services of a PLA; she is worth every penny. If you push hard enough, insurance companies will often cover this fee, but you may have to build a case for yourself and show them that studies have shown the

---

Resources for Labor Assistants

National Association of Childbirth Assistants (NACA)
205 Copco Lane
San Jose, CA 95123
(408) 225-9167

Doulas of North America (DONA)
Pennypress Inc.
1100 23rd Avenue
Seattle, WA 98112
Fax for DONA: (206) 325-0472
Phone for Pennypress: (206) 325-1419

Childbirth and Family Education
415 Boxauxhall
Katy, TX 77450-2203
(713) 497-8894

---

presence of a PLA at birth lowers the total costs, mainly by lessening the chances of a cesarean. We have had several VBAC mothers whose insurance companies promised to cover the cost of the PLA if the PLA helped them avoid a repeat cesarean. Deals like this are both good medicine and good business. Even if you do have to pay her yourself, you can't put a price tag on the benefits you incur by keeping your birth as natural as possible. Many of these benefits are lifelong for you and your baby. Be aware that even "routine" but possibly unnecessary interventions quickly add up (e.g., I.V. = $110; internal fetal monitoring = $125; epidural anesthesia = $850–$1500). So even if she helps you decrease some simple interventions you may easily make up for her fee.

Won't my husband feel displaced by this extra person in the birthing room?

The PLA does not replace the father at birth. Instead she takes the pressure off him to "coach," freeing him up to do what a man does best — love his mate. In fact, a PLA should empower both the mother and father to perform their roles. Nor does the PLA take the place of the obstetrician or staff nurse, but rather she fills in the gaps in the health-care team to provide consistent, continual care. This allows the obstetrician to be used more efficiently and frees him or her to make the best medical decisions. Even if you have a nurse assigned only to you, she can't be there constantly, and during delivery she will be helping the doctor.

A mother notes: Because my husband was freed from the primary role of guiding me through labor, he and I were able to labor lovingly together. I didn't rely on him to somehow save me from the pain of labor, so there was no tension between us from expectations. He said he was glad to be part of the experience rather than carrying the burden of the experience.

I've chosen a midwife and home birth. Do I also need a professional labor assistant?

Usually not. In most cases your midwife will function as your PLA. Mothers need a PLA mainly if they choose a hospital-obstetrician style of birth, because, in reality, obstetricians attend births, not labors.

Martha notes: Even with my seventh labor I benefited from the labor support of my midwife because she knew what to do when I experienced intensely painful contractions requiring complete physical relaxation. Her presence kept my mind relaxed so I could better help my body relax and birth comfortably.

I am categorized as high-risk because of high blood pressure, and my doctor is worried about toxemia. Would using a PLA help in my situation?

Definitely! PLAs are especially valuable in high-risk pregnancies (such as pre-eclampsia), where you need every person and tool at your disposal to lessen your risk. This is especially true if you have high blood pressure since monitoring and intravenous medications may restrict your freedom to move during labor. It takes a lot of knowledge and creativity to encourage you through a complicated labor safely. The PLA can provide this resource. Being at high risk makes you especially vulnerable to the fear–tension–pain cycle, because you are more likely to expect something to go wrong. The PLA can help you labor in ways that ease the stress you and your baby feel during labor. In our experience, continuous labor support is especially valuable in mothers seeking a VBAC, a situation that many medical staff still view as high-risk.

CHOOSING A BIRTH PLACE

When putting together your birth team it is important to consider not only the attendants but also the place. Your feelings about the place are important, as are the attitudes of the people who work there.

Choosing a Hospital Birth

In recent years hospital obstetrical units have become more labor-friendly. Hospitals competing to stay in the baby business have yielded to consumer pressure and have developed LDR rooms, meaning the mother labors, delivers, recovers, and spends her postpartum hospital stay all in the same room. Gone are the days when mother was treated like a surgical patient, laboring in one room, being wheeled into an operating room–like area for delivery, and recovering in a room separated from her baby after the birth. Admittedly, there are surgical-type delivery rooms still around, but I suspect these will soon be completely phased out.

The problem. Two requirements top the list for choosing a birth place: an *atmosphere* conducive to giving birth, and an *attitude* that birth is a normal healthy process most of the time. Interior designers have labored hard to create a home-away-from-home atmosphere in LDR rooms. But wood and wallpaper alone do not make a room conducive to giving birth. People make the difference, and all too often attendants in the LDR facilities have inherited the surgical mind-set. Behind the *House Beautiful* decor sits all the shiny medical and surgical equipment just waiting to be pulled out and used, sometimes routinely, as soon as the second stage of labor begins. Some of these "family birth centers" are really high-tech hospitals in high-touch disguise. When choosing a hospital don't be oversold by the appearance of the room. It is the skills and the attitude of your doctor and birth attendants that are most important to the well-being of you and your baby.

The solution. Just as parents lobbied to get the right birthing facilities into hospitals, they must use parent power to get the right attendants into these rooms — midwives. Imagine what would happen if today three

million expectant women in the United States called the hospital of their choice and asked, "Do you have midwives on your obstetrical staff to care for me during labor?" New midwifery schools would open immediately and hospitals would compete intensely for their graduates. The modern model of birth — an LDR birth place with midwives and obstetricians as birth attendants — is a realistic goal. And here is where good medicine is good business. Obstetrical costs would decrease because surgical deliveries would decrease and many currently routine but costly interventions would be avoided. For hospital administrators and the medical staff to change from the old surgical-type delivery facility to the LDR concept was a business decision, not a birth decision. By asking for midwives in addition to obstetricians, women, as they have in so many other fields, can influence the way birth business is done.

How to Check Out a Hospital

Here are some considerations for evaluating a maternity department in a hospital.

PERSONS

- What are the qualifications of the nursing staff? Have they had any midwifery training?
- How specifically will the nurse attend to your labor and delivery? Will there be one nurse assigned to care for you? Will her care be continuous or intermittent, and how much hands-on labor support will you get? Will one nurse be assigned to help care for mother and baby postpartum (called couplet nursing), or will there be separate obstetrical and nursery nurses? Above all, are the birthing philosophies of the nurses in accord with yours?

- Does the hospital provide a lactation consultant if needed or desired?
- Do they welcome your bringing in your own labor-support person, and will they work with her?
- Does the hospital provide a nurse to visit your home after discharge?

PLACES

- Does the hospital have an LDR room or suite? What are the criteria for using it?
- What is the level of emergency obstetrical care? Is 24-hour anesthesia coverage available, in hospital or on-call? Are there facilities for elective or emergency cesarean deliveries?
- What is the level of newborn nursery care? Level I means there is only care for healthy newborns and for non-serious illnesses; Level II means facilities and staff care for moderate illnesses and conditions, such as infections and prematurity, and specially trained nurses and neonatologists are available; Level III means there is a nursery with a full-service intensive care unit, and seldom is there any reason to transfer babies to another hospital.
- Where is the night entrance and what is the easiest route to the labor area?
- What degree of privacy will you have during labor?
- What facilities are available (such as an extra bed or couch) for your partner and/or labor-support person?

POLICIES

- What are the policies regarding visitors (baby's siblings and others)? Also, can baby's siblings be present at the birth? Is there an age restriction?

- What are the routine policies on the use of fetal monitoring (electronic or nurse-at-bedside using a fetal stethoscope), enemas, stirrups, I.V.?
- How much freedom will you have to move during each stage of labor? What positions will you be allowed for birth?
- Is the nursing staff open to your birth plan?
- Do they permit snacks and drinks during labor?
- Are there any restrictions on taking photos and videos?
- How do you preregister?
- What are the options and routines of newborn care, bonding after delivery, routine newborn procedures, rooming-in, supplemental feedings?
- Does the hospital provide labor-easing aids, such as labor tubs, VCR, videos, and relaxation tapes?
- What classes are provided on childbirth preparation, breastfeeding, infant care, and postpartum adjustments?
- What are the usual costs and extras? Does the hospital participate in your insurance plan? What percentage of your bill will be covered?

Choosing a Birth Center

Another birth-place option is the alternative birth center. These facilities provide a low-tech, high-touch environment for laboring women at low risk for obstetrical complications, and parents are encouraged to participate in the management decisions. For some parents who have reservations about a hospital birth, yet do not wish to give birth at home, a birth center is a safe compromise. There are two types of these facilities.

Children at Birth

Our older children have been present at the birth of our last four babies. In our experience children aged three and older can handle the theatrics of labor and respect the dignity of birth. If you choose to have your children present — *and if they want to be there* — here's what to consider:

- If your hospital or birthing center does not allow children at birth, request it. Hospitals advertise family-centered birth, and children are certainly part of a family.

- Assign a caregiver to the children. You don't want to be distracted by children's antics. If a child seems disturbed by your birthing noises and contortions, the caregiver will explain what's happening and/or temporarily escort the worried child out of the birthing room.

- Prepare the children for what to expect in terms they can understand: "Mommy's face will get red and she will make loud and funny noises (demonstrate), but it's okay; she's just working hard to push the baby out."

- Video-capture this unforgettable family scene. Expressions on the children's faces and their spontaneous dialogues are priceless. During one of our family births our four-year-old dressed up like a nurse and the seven-year-old like a doctor (with a football helmet on). Their sensitivity in caring for their mother's needs by bringing her juice, wiping her brow, and speaking softly would make any professional birth attendant proud.

- Read the valuable resource *Children at Birth* by Margie and Jay Hathaway, Academy Publications, Box 5224, Sherman Oaks, CA 91413. (Also available in video)

We have noticed a special sibling bonding that occurs when older children witness a birth. Sharing the birth experience is the best way to start them off as siblings without rivalry.

Free-standing birth centers. These centers are located outside the hospital environment, "free" of hospital rules and attitudes. Most are staffed by certified nurse-midwives with obstetrician backup; a few are operated by obstetricians or by family physicians with certified nurse-midwives as assistants. Opponents charge that free-standing birth centers expose a laboring woman to added risk, since the full range of emergency care that can be given only in a hospital is not immediately accessible. Proponents counter by claiming that the freedom to manage the birthing process in a low-tech, personalized way makes it far less likely that the mother will need emergency care. Besides, to become licensed, a birth center must have easy access to a hospital that offers high-level obstetric and neonatal care; specifically, there must be a "decision to incision" time of no more than thirty minutes, in case an emergency surgical birth is needed.

Do we think free-standing birth centers are safe? Yes! In 1983 the National Association of Childbearing Centers (NACC) was formed to establish national standards for free-standing birth centers, specifically regarding staff credentials, the physical environment, the overall educational services provided to the parents, and criteria for

Hot Beds!

In 1992, the University of California, Irvine, opened a free-standing birth center in Anaheim, primarily to serve the overflow of indigent obstetrical patients. To their surprise, women of means flocked to this center to deliver their babies. The demand for this high-touch birthing service exceeded the supply, prompting the local newspaper to dub this birth center "Hot Beds!" This facility boasts such labor-friendly statistics as a 5 percent cesarean section and a 6 percent episiotomy rate. Mothers have continuous labor support, freedom of movement, electronic fetal monitoring only when necessary, and use of a labor tub as desired. Certified nurse-midwives run the center along with obstetrical consultation and a close (but not too close) affiliation with the university hospital's department of obstetrics. Each midwife is on the faculty of the university. Medical students and family-practice residents from UCI rotate through the Birthing Center, opening their eyes and their minds to the many ways to deliver a healthy baby. Clients are carefully selected before delivering in this center. There is 24-hour emergency hospital transport. If a mother is transported to the university hospital, a midwife may accompany the mother and comanage her labor with the obstetrician in the hospital. We hope this facility serves as a model for midwives and obstetricians working together and points the direction for future maternity care in this country.

licensure and regulation. In 1989 the *New England Journal of Medicine* reported a study of nearly twelve thousand women admitted for labor and delivery to eighty-four free-standing birth centers in the United States. The study concluded that birth centers offer a safe and acceptable alternative to hospital births for low-risk women. The cesarean-section rate for the women in the study was 4.4 percent, far below the national average. There were no maternal deaths, and the neonatal death rate was well below average. The best odds for a safe birth in a birth center were among women who had a "proven pelvis" — that is, those who had previously delivered babies vaginally. In this study, 25 percent of the women who were having their first baby were transferred to a hospital, whereas only 7 percent of women who had had a previous birth needed transfer. (Because free-standing birth centers are under scrutiny by the medical profession, some centers may be overcautious in transferring mothers to a hospital. As birth centers, obstetricians, and hospitals learn to work cooperatively, this high transfer rate should be reduced. In our local birth center, the transfer rate for first-time mothers is 10 percent.) Economically, birth center costs average around 50 percent less than hospital costs. Some insurance companies are catching on to the economic advantage of birth centers, offering 100 percent coverage with no deductible if you deliver with a certified nurse-midwife in a birthing center.

In-hospital birth centers. These facilities, with a birth-center philosophy and a staff made up primarily of nurse-midwives, are located near or adjacent to hospital obstetrical units, in case emergency transfer is necessary. Opponents of in-hospital centers argue that the medical mind-set prevails, resulting in a higher transfer rate than in free-standing centers. Proponents believe that in-hospital facilities offer mother and baby the best of both worlds — the low-tech birth center atmosphere with easy access to emergency care.

How to Check Out a Birth Center

Here are some considerations for evaluating a birth center.

- Do you have any obstetrical risk factors that might jeopardize the safety of either you or your baby if you choose an out-of-hospital birth? (VBAC is usually not a risk factor.)
- Is the birth center licensed and a member of NACC? (See "Resources for Alternative Childbirths," page 45.)
- Are the midwives licensed? Is there adequate obstetrical backup in case unanticipated complications occur during labor or delivery?

- How accessible is the nearest hospital, and what would be the routine if a transfer were to become necessary?
- What percentage of mothers delivering in the center need transfer to the hospital? What are the criteria for their transfer? As an added precaution, ask for the names of mothers who have recently labored at the center and talk to these women. (You might want to talk to some who needed to be transferred.)
- Does the backup doctor at the birth center continue your care if you are transferred to the hospital? Will the midwife who has attended you during labor at the birth center accompany you and stay with you at the hospital?

The main advantage of a birth center is not the physical facility itself but rather its attitude toward birth as a normal process, along with the woman-to-woman support from midwives that is lacking in most hospitals.

Choosing a Home Birth

In 1900 fewer than 5 percent of births took place in hospitals. This increased to 75 percent by 1936, and by 1970 approximately 99 percent of mothers delivered in hospitals. But is this progress? Illustrating the differing perceptions of home birthing are these two mothers discussing their birth choices: "You are brave to have a home birth," said a concerned mother. "You are brave to have a hospital birth," replied the other.

Advantages of Giving Birth at Home

Here are some of the advantages of having your baby in your own home.

- You are free to move with the flow of your body during labor, a plus toward helping labor progress. You have the privacy of your own nest, and can retreat into quiet corners. And you are familiar and comfortable with the birth setting.
- You eliminate the internal fear factor that comes from just being in a hospital, and avoid the anxiety projected by staff and generated by policies and routines.
- You can invite those you wish. No strangers are there.
- You participate in the decisions. There is no intervention without your approval and you follow your own script.
- Your labor is not interrupted by trivial hospital routine nor dampened by depressing medications. You can tune in to your instincts and move in the direction your body tells you.
- Your birth attendant is usually a midwife, providing a woman-to-woman connection that is vital in easing the discomfort and smoothing the progress of labor.
- You can emote without worry that you are embarrassing the personnel or disturbing the patient in the next room. (If you live in an apartment, prepare your next-door neighbors for the normal sounds of labor.)
- There is less concern about timing. No one is in a hurry, and there are no other "patients" demanding the attention of your birth attendants.
- There is little intervention since the technology is not right at hand. The midwife or physician attending you at home, however, will have equipment to monitor the health of both you and your baby, and emergency resuscitation equipment if the need arises.
- There are no foreign germs. Risk of infection is lower with home birth. (The hospital, on the other hand, is home to a whole host of foreign germs. Some hospitals even have women sharing rooms and bathrooms postpartum.)
- The cost is usually less than with hospital births.
- Mother-infant and family bonding is better. Naturally, baby rooms in with mother.

Disadvantages of Home-Birthing

If you're considering a home birth, you should be aware of the following factors.

- At present, the health-care delivery system in most areas of the United States is not set up for home-birthing. There is no organized transport system, and obstetrical backup is frequently lacking.
- Because of the current attitude among medical professionals toward midwives ("either choose me or choose a midwife"), sometimes there is no collaboration between midwife and obstetrician to enable mother to get the best of both professions. If there is no prenatal care from the obstetrician, it can be difficult for the midwife to consult an obstetrician when questions or problems arise. Also, because the availability of licensed midwives doing home births is limited, some mothers choose unlicensed midwives where there is no governing body or peer review to assure proper standards of care and competency. This can increase the risk of home-birthing.
- If obstetrician backup is lacking and a crisis develops, the mother must be rushed to the nearest emergency room to be attended by an anonymous physician. Take the time to choose qualified attendants with proper backup, for the safety of both you and your baby and to avoid such a scenario.

- Unforeseen complications may occur. No matter how thoroughly a mother is screened, unanticipated complications may arise requiring lifesaving assistance that can be done only in a hospital or a birthing center set up for emergencies. Examples of such crises are meconium aspiration (inhaling of thick intestinal secretions into baby's lungs) or a prolapsed cord (the umbilical cord comes down before the head, pinching off the baby's oxygen supply in the birth canal).

- Adequate emergency care may not be available during a transfer from the home to the hospital.
- The cost to the parents, in some instances, may actually be greater in a home birth, since many insurance plans do not cover midwife fees or the cost of home birth. Check with your insurer.

Is a Home Birth Safe?

Home-birthing organizations shout, "Yes"; the obstetrician-hospital-complex system

---

Resources for Alternative Childbirths

NAPSAC (National Association of Parents and Professionals for Safe Alternatives in Childbirth)
Box 646
Marble Hill, MO 63764
(314) 238-2010

National Association of Childbearing Centers
3123 Gottschall Road
Perkiomenville, PA 18074
(215) 234-8068

American College of Home Obstetrics
P.O. Box 508
Oak Park, IL 60303
(708) 388-1461

Association for Childbirth at Home International
P.O. Box 430
Glendale, CA 91209
(213) 667-0839

California Association of Midwives (CAM)
P.O. Box 417854
Sacramento, CA 95814
(800) 829-5791
(Request their publication *Midwife Means "With Woman,"* an informative 56-page booklet about choosing and using a midwife.)

American College of Nurse-Midwives (ACNM)
1522 K Street N.W., Suite 1120
Washington, DC 20005
(202) 347-5445

Informed Homebirth and Parenting
P.O. Box 3675
Ann Arbor, MI 48106
(313) 662-6857

MANA (Midwives' Alliance of North America)
600 Fifth Street
Monett, MO 65708

says, "No." And both sides have statistics to support their view. The people in white coats boast that the chances of a mother dying in childbirth was much higher in 1935 than in 1980, and that this is the result of technology available only in the hospital. Home-birth supporters argue that there is no reason to believe that there is a cause-and-effect relationship between birth in the hospital and lower mortality rates. Today's women have better access to prenatal care and more is known about safe birthing. Antibiotics are available to treat infection, and most aspects of health are better now than they used to be. Hospitals actually have higher mortality rates than home births, in part because mothers with the highest risk of life-threatening medical problems deliver in hospitals. Statistics that show poor outcomes in home births are equally misleading since these studies lump all out-of-hospital births together, whether they're planned, properly attended home births or involve foolhardy couples with no prenatal care doing it on their own.

Our interpretation of the current home-birth statistics, especially those from Europe, leads us to conclude that if the mother has been properly selected (that is, she is low-risk) and the home birth expertly attended, there is no increased risk (or perhaps even less) either to mother or baby when delivering at home. The home-birth experience in the Netherlands, a country where around 35 percent of all births occur at home, and where the national cesarean rate is 6 percent, could serve as a model for the United States. The birth attendants are licensed midwives, obstetricians, or general practitioners. Midwives deliver babies in the hospital as well as at home. There is a protocol that determines when birth attendants need to refer a woman with obstetrical problems to the hospital, a prearranged transport system, and good medical communication between home and hospital. Laboring mothers in these countries can have the best of all worlds: an obstetrician, a midwife, the choice of a home birth, and a willing hospital should a complication arise. Our conclusion after surveying reputable studies (an exercise we needed to do to make our birthing choices) was that it is not the place of birth that determines the health of the mother and baby, it is the overall system of care.

Are You a Candidate for Home Birth?

In considering a home birth four important persons enter into your decision: you, your baby, baby's father, and your birth attendant.

- Why do you want to have your baby at home? Is it because you are afraid of hospitals, afraid of needles, afraid of surgery? It is better to have a home birth because you truly believe you belong at home rather than because you don't like hospitals.
- What is your obstetrical history? Is this your first baby? Although first-time mothers can and do deliver safely at home, the odds of avoiding transfer are best if you have a "proven pelvis" — a previous vaginal delivery. A history of obstetrical problems (e.g., uterine abnormalities) may make home birth an unwise choice, but every birth is different, and this pregnancy and delivery may not have the same complications as the last one. It is certainly possible to have a VBAC at home.
- Even if you qualify physically for a home

birth, is your mind equally low-risk? Fears about birth or about something going wrong can keep you from progressing in labor.

- Do you feel prepared enough to handle the challenge of labor? (Labor itself is the final test of this.) If you feel pressured by your mate to give birth at home, this is not good. If he is the reluctant one, you may yet be able to convince him. But you need to be in agreement.
- What is your history of handling pain and stress? You do not have the option of pain medications at home, because they increase the risk of problems, particularly for the baby. When medications are not available, you won't even think about them, unless in your heart you don't want to be at home; if that's the case, you'll think about them plenty. The relaxation, creativity, and the freedom to move and use water at home really does make up for the loss of a medication option.
- Are you convinced a home birth is for you? If you are afraid of home birth, you shouldn't try one. If you have doubts, you probably belong in a hospital or birth center. This must be *your* decision (not pressure from peers), based on strong inner conviction that home-birthing is best for you. If you can put aside the fear factor and trust your body and your birth attendant, then a home birth may be for you. A decision-making technique that has proven helpful for us is to make a "pretend decision." Make a decision about your place of birth and your attendant. Live with this decision for a while. If a month or two later you still feel you made the right decision and your obstetrical situation remains low-risk, stick with your original choice.

Is Your Home Near a Hospital?

Even if you are set on having a home birth, you should realize that sometimes transfer to a hospital is required. Make sure you live close enough to deal with an emergency.

- Is your home close to a hospital that has an obstetrical unit? Ideally, it should be no more than ten or fifteen minutes away.
- Are transport ambulances available in case you need to be rushed from home to a hospital?

Is There a Qualified Home-Birth Attendant in Your Community?

To find one, talk to childbirth educators or contact The National Association of Parents and Professionals for Safe Alternatives in Childbirth (NAPSAC); American College of Home Obstetrics (ACHO); and Midwives' Alliance of North America (MANA). (See "Resources for Alternative Childbirths," page 45, for addresses of these resources.) Check out the credentials of physicians and midwives attending home births. See "Questions to Ask a Midwife," page 35, before interviewing prospective birth attendants.

Lessen Surprises.

Your labor, delivery, and the appearance of your baby will bring plenty of surprises to the birth day. You don't want to set yourself up for any more. Avoid this birth scene: You decide to have a home birth but are so fearful or distrusting of the medical-hospital complex that you fail to make arrangements for medical backup. But to your surprise and through no one's fault a complication arises, and suddenly you and your baby need the unfriendly system you have rejected. Unannounced, you rush to the hospital emer-

Birth Problems

Birth is risky, just as life is. No matter how well planned, unanticipated problems can arise, though this is less likely to happen when mother is well educated about the birth process and has taken good care of herself during pregnancy.

What Could Go Wrong

- *Placenta previa.* The placenta is located partially or completely over the cervix and is prone to sudden and life-threatening hemorrhage before or during labor. Chances of this happening: 0.2 percent* of primips under age 25; 1 percent of multips over age 35.

- *Abruptio placentae.* The placenta partially or completely detaches from the uterus before or during labor. This can result in life-threatening hemorrhage. Chances of this happening in varying degrees: 1 percent.

- *Shoulder dystocia.* The shoulder gets wedged during passage through the birth canal. Most common in babies over 9 pounds. Chances of this happening with varying degrees of difficulty: 0.15–1.7 percent.

- *Prolapsed cord.* The umbilical cord gets squeezed between baby's head and the pelvic bones, decreasing oxygen supply to baby. Chances of this happening: 0.5 percent.

- *Fetal distress.* The fetal monitor detects that baby's heart rate becomes persistently abnormal, often due to compression of umbilical cord or inadequate functioning of the placenta.

- *Meconium aspiration.* Baby passes meconium before birth and then inhales this thick, sticky stuff into his windpipe, blocking the passage of air.

What You Can Do to be Prepared

- Notify your birth attendant immediately if you have bleeding. A prenatal ultrasound can confirm the site of the placenta.

- Choose a birth place within 15 minutes of a hospital. Notify your birth attendant if you experience sudden, severe uterine pain and tenderness with or without bleeding.

- The more prepared and relaxed you are during birth, the less the chances of this happening. Good nutrition, avoiding excessive weight gain, and consistent exercise during pregnancy lessen the chance of having a very large baby.

- Don't allow artificial rupture of your membranes if baby's head is not fully engaged (see explanation page 200). If delivering at home or at a birth center, be sure your birth attendant knows how to handle this emergency and that transport facilities are available.

- Change positions. Get off your back onto your left side, then into the all-fours position. Avoid exhaustion and dehydration.

- Fetal distress and consequent meconium aspiration occur less frequently during prepared, progressing, and relaxed labors. If having an out-of-hospital birth, be sure your birth attendant is experienced and skilled in sucking out meconium immediately when baby's head emerges. Passage of thick meconium during labor warrants transfer to a hospital.

*These percentages are gleaned from current obstetrical textbooks. Many are old statistics, before modern screening tests such as ultrasound were used.

Birth Problems (cont.)

- *Failure to progress.* Your cervix does not open and/or your baby does not descend.

- *Cephalopelvic disproportion* (CPD). Baby's body is too large to fit through mother's pelvis. True CPD is rare — this problem is usually due to mismanagement of labor causing failure to progress.

- *Premature rupture of membranes.* The longer the time between the rupture of membranes and delivery of the baby, the greater the chances that an infection may occur within the uterus or the baby. The worry and the risk of such an infection begins 24 hours after rupture of the membranes. Many obstetricians advise an induced labor if the membranes ruptured more than 24 hours ago.
  Chances of this happening: 5 percent.

- *Baby's breathing is slow to start.* For a variety of reasons, some babies are born blue, limp, and not breathing on their own. Resuscitation is necessary.

- Walk during labor. Assume vertical positions. Stay off your back. Rest and relax between contractions. Drink and snack. Avoid epidural anesthesia early in labor (see additional tips, page 204).

- Try vertical laboring. Squatting widens the pelvis (see page 187). Different positions may help a persistently posterior baby to rotate and descend.

- Be sure to notify your doctor when your water breaks or begins leaking. Note color, consistency, and odor. If considering an out-of-hospital birth, be sure your birth attendant is knowledgeable about monitoring for signs of infection in mother or baby, such as maternal fever, fetal distress, or infection signs in the amniotic fluid. Keep vaginal exams to a minimum since they can introduce infection.

- A well-managed labor (by mother and birth attendant) with no drugs or timely dosing (see page 170) if drugs are used lowers the risk of this happening. Be sure your birth attendant is certified in neonatal CPR and has the equipment and skills to resuscitate a newborn.

gency room, where you are quickly labeled "one of those irresponsible home-birth fanatics." You are assigned an anonymous obstetrician (whoever is on emergency call), and the hospital staff is less than welcoming and sometimes even punitive. Because you are a stranger to the doctor, there is nothing known about your past obstetrical history, and you are at a higher risk for a surgical birth because the doctor and the hospital do not want to take any more risks. You get the medical care you need, but are unlikely to get any sympathy or support during what is perhaps a very

distressing, even frightening, time. A bit of preplanning can avoid this scene.

If you are planning a midwife-attended home birth, be sure to meet the backup physician ahead of time. Your midwife may have a regular backup physician, or you may have to find someone on your own. Depending on a doctor's sympathy for home-birthing and the legal standards of the community, he or she may not be willing to back up a home birth. Schedule a couple of prenatal visits with the backup doctor, one in the first trimester of your pregnancy and the other a few weeks before your due date. Tell this physician why you have decided to have a home birth, but emphasize that you are responsible and are not taking any foolish risks. You are coming to the doctor for two reasons. First, you don't want any surprises. Is there any detectable medical reason why you shouldn't deliver at home? If warranted, the doctor may advise an ultrasound (see the advantages of ultrasound, page 82) to confirm the position of the baby or placenta (even experienced hands cannot always detect these situations). Ultrasound removes the guesswork. Second, you're asking the doctor to become your birth attendant should an unanticipated problem arise necessitating transfer from home to hospital, which happens in around 10 percent of out-of-hospital births.

CHOOSING A CHILDBIRTH CLASS

A childbirth class should do three things: It should help you learn the kind of birth you want; it should equip you with the means to have the birth you want; and it should also prepare you for other possible labor and birth situations, since births seldom go exactly according to plan. Childbirth classes have something to offer everyone, both first-time parents and veterans. You can learn things from the instructor and from other people in the class that you won't learn by reading a book. Taking a childbirth class increases your chances of delivering naturally. But you shouldn't feel that you have failed if you discover that natural childbirth is not for you or if medical complications require a departure from your original birth plan.

Making Your Selection

As you search for a birth philosophy you are likely to encounter two schools of thought. Both have something to offer the pregnant shopper. The "politically correct" school presents all the options available in childbirth without making value judgments about what is best. These classes tend to be offered through a hospital, and their philosophies tend to be in accord with the prevailing medical policies on birth at that institution. Teachers of these classes are more oriented toward preparing parents for hospital routines than toward reforming the system.

In the other school are the birth-reform groups. They tend to be independent of hospitals, and their birthing philosophies may conflict with the usual medical routines. The teachers are intent not only on preparing parents to have a satisfying birth experience but also on empowering them to improve the system.

Wise birth consumers would do well to extract the best of both schools. Learning only from books and classes that teach the medical way of birth may deprive you of many tools you need to get the birth you want. Too much of the antiestablishment school may confuse you and undermine the trust between you and your doctor.

There are many different kinds of childbirth classes; they are not all alike. Here's how to begin your search:

What's available. Find out what classes are available in your community. Quiz friends and your obstetrician or midwife. Check with national childbirth organizations. If you belong to a health maintenance organization or choose a birth center, childbirth classes may be offered as part of the total package.

What Is Natural Childbirth?

Having a "natural" birth means different things to different women. One mother told us for her a natural childbirth was going to the hospital without her makeup on. With the increasing prevalence of cesarean births, mothers now regard any vaginal delivery as natural. For this reason, birth-savvy mothers who value totally unmedicated and intervention-free births have a new term for it — *pure birth.*

With so many birth options, has the term "natural" lost its meaning? Dr. Grantly Dick-Read, author of *Childbirth Without Fear,* regarded natural childbirth as a physiological childbirth in which no physical, chemical, or psychological interventions disturb the normal process of birth. Yet even Dr. Dick-Read acknowledged that natural childbirth was not synonymous with either painless or nonmedicated birth.

When the natural childbirth method (not really new, but a rediscovery of what birth was meant to be) became popular, many obstetricians and some childbirth educators accepted it as a trendy but impossible dream. Some approached it like dentistry — why would people want to feel pain if they didn't have to? While some childbirth organizations, in particular ASPO/Lamaze, have changed their promotion from natural to "prepared" childbirth (meaning anything goes as long as a mother has a positive birth experience), Bradley instructors cling to the root meaning of natural — a drug-free birth.

It's not what's in a name, but what's in a birth that counts. The important issues are the well-being of the baby and mother and the birth experience they have. Just because the ideal of a drug-free birth is not achievable or desired by all women, we shouldn't lose sight of what an ideal birth can be. We prefer the term *responsible childbirth.* Despite its unappealing ring, this is a goal all women can attain if they want to. Responsible childbirth means you have explored available options, formulated a philosophy and plan of birth, assembled your best team and place, and prepared your mind and body with the necessary information and techniques to enter birth. With this powerful package, you can call your birth anything you wish — and brag accordingly.

In-hospital vs. out-of-hospital classes. Ideally, schools should prepare students for the real world in a variety of circumstances. In-hospital classes prepare you for the birthing policies of that hospital. On the other hand, out-of-hospital classes have the advantage of describing a variety of birth choices so that you can prepare for the birth you want — but one that the hospital may not be willing to deliver. Ideally, birth place, birth attendant, and childbirth educator should all share the same birth philosophy, but where this is not the case, a good childbirth class should help you understand your doctor better and enable you to work with him or her and the hospital staff to achieve a birth that is safe and satisfying. Look for an instructor who emphasizes flexibility and good communication between parents and professionals.

An "early bird" class. While most classes begin around the sixth month and run six to twelve weeks, try to attend a class in the first few months of your pregnancy. This helps you through the stage where you're selecting birth environments and birth attendants and prepares you for the rapid emotional and physical changes of pregnancy. Attending this early class also helps you discern if this style of class and the philosophy of the childbirth educator will be right for you when it's time to take the regular class.

The smaller the better. To ensure individualized attention and a lot of hands-on instruction, a class size of six couples is ideal and eight couples is the maximum. If possible, choose a class at a time and location convenient for both you and your birth partner (someone else of your choosing if baby's father will not be involved). It is important that you both attend *all* the sessions. Give it priority in your schedules.

The experience of the instructor. Has she experienced birth herself? Is she up-to-date on all the options in childbirth? It's best if she is involved as a labor-support person herself. Is she using her teaching to work out her own biases and experiences, or is her first concern her students? Get references from friends and acquaintances.

The class content. Avoid classes taught by instructors who have had negative childbirth experiences and who are down on the medical profession. These classes leave you confused, undermine your confidence in your doctor, and spend much of the time teaching you what you don't want rather than preparing you for all the things that may happen. Choose a class that teaches you how to relax and tune in to your body, rather than to use external gimmicks to teach you to escape from your body. These are unrealistic and easily forgotten during the heightened excitement of labor.

Teaching methods. Adults, like children, learn better when the material is presented in an interesting way. Expect a lot of visual aids: slides, movies or videos, and large charts; some discussion time; some lectures; and lots of hands-on practice sessions, especially of relaxation skills. A lending library of additional reading is helpful because there is much to learn that can't be taught in actual class time. Make your reading choices carefully — follow a recommended list or get suggestions from trusted sources — so that your reading will be constructive and not confusing.

Show and tell. A few weeks after birth, graduates return with their little "diplomas" to share their birthing experiences and discuss problems adjusting to and caring for a new baby. Sometimes during this class, family planning is discussed and postnatal exercises are taught. The friends you make in this class may become a valuable support group as life with baby goes on. Enjoy your weekly night out with your expectant friends. You owe it to yourselves and your baby. It's good preparation and it's fun.

Confessions of a Childbirth Educator

There is frustration among the ranks of childbirth teachers. For what kind of birth are they supposed to be preparing mothers?

Some hospital-based birth educators, constrained by their own hospital's birthing policies, prepare parents more to be compliant patients than to be informed consumers. If these teachers arm their pupils to question the rigid hospital birthing practices, they may be out of a job. Independent childbirth educators, on the other hand, sometimes are more geared toward home birth and may not prepare parents to cope with the medical way of birth. As a result, the mother's list of "I don't want"s and her obstetrician's list of "you must have"s are in conflict. At each prenatal visit, friction develops and sparks fly.

Childbirth educators are also confronted with a variety of mothers who have different goals. Some mothers are intent on having a birth free of drugs and interventions, and want the full experience of birth. Other women don't want to experience labor and delivery to such an intensity and want to know all their options for both self-help *and* medical pain relief. And even the best childbirth educators have their personal biases. When Martha began teaching childbirth classes, most women were strapped to delivery tables. "The very thought of this back-birthing scene brought out the lioness in me," Martha confided, as she emphasized the importance of freedom of movement to her class.

Childbirth educators want to prepare, not scare. For this reason they may tend to minimize the intensity of labor sensations. Telling it like it is ("It can hurt like ...") may scare some women into calling in the anesthesiologist before labor even begins. It's politically incorrect to even mention the *P*-word during class. Rather than "pain," educators are apt to say "contractions." But some women prefer no surprises and feel that they would have been better off being

Resources for Childbirth Education

Each of the following organizations has books and other printed resources valuable to expectant parents.

The American Society for Psychoprophylaxis in Obstetrics (ASPO)
1840 Wilson Boulevard
Suite 204
Arlington, VA 22201
(800) 368-4404

American Academy of Husband-Coached Childbirth (AAHCC-Bradley)
Box 5224
Sherman Oaks, CA 91413-5224
(800) 423-2397; (800) 42-BIRTH in Calif.

International Childbirth Education Association (ICEA)
P.O. Box 20048
Minneapolis, MN 55420
(612) 854-8660

Apple Tree Family Ministries (AFTM)
P.O. Box 2083
Artesia, CA 90702-2083
(310) 925-0149

NAPSAC (National Association of Parents and Professionals for Safe Alternatives in Childbirth)
Box 646
Marble Hill, MO 63764
(314) 238-2010
(Request their consumer guide to childbirth education organizations.)

told how overwhelming the birth feelings could be. Perhaps a statement like "In a small percentage of women it hurts incredibly . . ." would keep women from being caught off guard. Appreciate these problems for what they are. Childbirth classes are starter courses. Read birth books, interview veteran mothers, and take responsibility for educating yourself beyond the class material.

Who's Who in Childbirth Education

Pregnant parents shopping for childbirth education will find a variety of approaches to meet their needs. There is something for everybody. Basically there are two approaches to birth preparation and all the current childbirth classes adopt one or the other, or a combination of both. The main difference is the approach to pain relief. Classes in the Lamaze tradition emphasize distraction techniques to escape from pain and gain control over labor. Opposing schools (e.g., Bradley and others) teach the woman how to accept and experience the birth process, to work with her body to prevent and manage pain, and how to release muscle tension and surrender to the working of her body rather than escape from it. To give credit where due, Lamaze, Bradley, and all spin-off methods from these schools owe much of their material to the teachings of Dr. Grantly Dick-Read.

Not all childbirth classes are created equal. Some are wimpy in their approach to women's rights in birth; others take a stand. The type of childbirth class you select depends on the birth you want and the type of person you are. Because couples have a variety of birth wishes and needs, there must be a variety of childbirth methods to

meet these needs. In conducting your search, try to make a wise match. If you are not certain about what you want, do your homework before classes begin. Talk to graduates of each school and read their manuals (see "Resources for Childbirth Education," page 53). Here are the most popular methods from which to choose.

ASPO/Lamaze. This method has its roots in Russia, where obstetricians used conditioned responses to ease labor pain. At the first sign of a contraction, women are conditioned to relax instead of tense and to divert their attention away from any discomfort. In the early fifties French obstetrician Fernand Lamaze brought the Russian conditioned response exercises to Western Europe, added breathing exercises, and provided labor support from a labor-support person, or *monitrice.* The package became known as "Painless Childbirth." When the Lamaze method came to America, it became known also as *psychoprophylaxis,* implying the preparation of the mind for labor. In the 1960s, the American Society for Psychoprophylaxis in Obstetrics (ASPO) was formed to accredit childbirth educators. The organization is now known as ASPO/Lamaze, and its teachers are known as ASPO-certified childbirth educators or ACCEs. Central to Lamaze is a particular approach to pain relief. Besides preparing the woman for how her body works during labor and telling her what she can do to lessen pain, Lamaze emphasizes reducing a woman's *perception* of pain. A pupil is taught how to trick her brain in order to take control of her contractions. Through breathing techniques and focusing on real or imagined diversions, the mother disassociates her attention from her contracting uterus to convince her mind that her body doesn't really hurt.

Critics of the Lamaze method charge that the system of "mind over labor" often doesn't work. At the height of her contraction, a Lamaze grad is likely to forget her rigidly rehearsed breathing and welcome a medically managed birth. She may be overwhelmed by the contraction if the breathing technique isn't adequate to divert her attention. Many have said that the contrived breathing patterns actually created tension instead of helping them relax. To be fair, most of today's Lamaze instructors, fortunately, have relaxed their reliance on the rehearsed rapid pant that a woman is supposed to turn on by reflex. Instead they teach "paced breathing," based on a woman's own individual respiratory preference.

Lamaze opponents are also skeptical of encouraging a woman to escape from her body during contractions or to try to control her labor. They believe that it is better for a woman to get her mind *into* her labor rather than *away* from it, and that yielding to her body's forces is more helpful than trying to control them. They believe that nature has an important message: it is more effective for a woman to listen and work with her body signals than to manipulate them. Lamaze detractors believe that birth, like sex, is not an experience you should control, that it's better for a woman to get involved with her labor than to distance herself from it. Critics feel that the Lamaze method prevents a woman from achieving her fullest birth experience because many Lamaze mothers readily accept medication, and, even without drugs, they are trying to distance themselves from their bodies. But some women may not want a "full" birth experience — they just want a baby.

A final criticism of ASPO/Lamaze is that the organization takes a timid approach to shaking up the obstetrical-hospital estab-lishment. The classes, especially the hospital-based ones, prepare mothers to be compliant patients rather than discerning consumers. But this weakness may be its strength. Because they are politically correct on childbirth issues, they attract more pupils and offend fewer doctors. Hospitals will sponsor them and obstetricians will recommend them. ASPO/Lamaze focuses more on preparing women to deliver within the current delivery system than on arming their pupils to go out and change the birth world.

The Bradley Method®. Developed in the 1940s by Denver obstetrician Robert Bradley, this approach teaches women to be involved in their labors rather than to escape from them. Dr. Bradley believed a woman should "give birth" to her baby rather than be delivered, quite a turnaround for an obstetrician. Unlike childbirth classes that suggest that all options are equal and no matter what happens, birth is a wonderful experience, Bradley takes a stand. The method gives couples the goal of a nonmedicated, natural childbirth and the tools to get it. Bradley classes convince parents that they can reach that goal and teaches the reasoning behind the value of such a goal. It is these convictions that carry them through difficult labors. In a twelve-week course the Bradley Method® teaches women that they can trust their bodies and the natural processes of labor, that natural is the healthiest and safest for mother and baby. While "natural" has different meanings to different people, Bradley instructors mean by "natural childbirth" no medication and no unnecessary interventions. Therefore, they may gloss over the options of medical pain relief. More than 90 percent of Bradley graduates go on to have unmedicated births, though this may be credited more to the clientele who are motivated to take responsibility for their birth decisions than to the method itself. The rest may well represent the small percentage in any population who will need medical help.

Bradley grads are not expected to tough it out with stoic determination, but rather they come to birth armed with an impressive amount of information and with their body's own tools to ensure contractions are manageable. Because of their motivation and preparation, Bradley moms are passionate about achieving natural childbirth, yet there is no stigma attached if medication or intervention is needed. Bradley pupils are taught the risks of "managed births," so that the woman is not robbed of her chosen birth experience and has the satisfaction of a drug-free birth and drug-free baby as her reward. The Bradley philosophy is not simply antidrug — its main purpose is to inform mothers that, in most cases, the risk of a medicated childbirth is greater than the benefits.

Bradley breathing is more natural, more relaxed, and more physiological than the patterned breathing of Lamaze. The Bradley belief is that the body knows how to breathe and how to birth; a woman need only learn the signals and how to respond to them. Rather than try to control their reactions to labor, Bradley laborers are encouraged to release and yield to their instincts. Like Lamaze, Bradley brings fathers into the birth scene as "labor coaches," a role not all men are comfortable playing. In fact, the organization is called the American Academy of Husband-Coached Childbirth (AAHCC). (See "Resources for Childbirth Education," page 53.)

A Bradley couple is likely to enter the birth place as wise consumers wishing to participate in the birthing decisions, and well equipped to do so. If these are your desires and natural childbirth is your goal, Bradley is the class for you. But Bradley's strength is also its weakness. Because of their depth of preparation and commitment, Bradley couples are not always looked on kindly by the medical establishment. Unfortunately, many doctors do not enjoy being questioned by their "patients"; they seem threatened by what appears to be a lack of trust — and their own lack of time. Because Bradley teachers take a stand for natural childbirth instead of "equal options," they can be perceived as troublemakers. So, parents, protect your childbirth educator. Be sure your doctor realizes your requests are truly *your* birth wishes. Never say, "But my childbirth educator said...."

Critics claim that Bradley-teaching prepares couples better for an out-of-hospital birth than for one in the hospital. We disagree. If a mother truly wants a natural childbirth and wants to deliver in the hospital, Bradley classes give her the best odds of achieving the birth she wants. However, we do believe that some Bradley teachers need to keep their personal biases private and support the mother-doctor trust rather than undermine it. If you find that your previously secure relationship with your doctor is being sabotaged, either you have the wrong instructor or you have the wrong doctor.

The International Childbirth Education Association. ICEA is an umbrella organization that promotes many childbirth methods and in some ways incorporates the best of all of them. The ICEA trains and certifies teachers, holds national conventions, and maintains a mail-order bookstore. The

Don't Fire the Coach

In the 1960s men were snatched off the Little League fields and promoted to "labor coaches," a role neither befitting some men nor helpful to some women. They were given stopwatches for timing contractions, clipboards for taking notes, and maybe even a T-shirt with "coach" across the chest. While many men admirably perform this role and thrive as coach, others do not want to be put in charge, as the role of coach implies, and some women don't want their husbands "telling me what to do" during labor.

Birth reformers came up with the job title "coach" as a way to get fathers into the delivery room, thinking that most men would identify with the word because they understood sports. Like sports, birth is challenging and there are rules and time-tested strategies. Unlike sports, however, few men understand birth and no man has ever labored out a baby. My first experience as a birth coach came nearly twenty years ago. At the height of the game of labor I totally forgot what I had learned at practice and did what I naturally do best — love my wife. Once I dropped the role of coach and took on the role of lover, the whole process became easier for me.

It's the nature of many men to want to rush in and "fix" a prolonged and painful labor rather than to let it "flow" patiently and naturally. The normal sights and sounds of labor can trigger the man's desire to rescue his mate from pain. A caring mate is likely to panic or feel "something's wrong." "It is difficult to see someone you love hurting," volunteered a laboring mother. She embraced her husband for emotional support yet relied more on her professional labor assistant for woman-to-woman empathy and for helpful suggestions. Some men function better as teammates rather than coaches during birth. They make best use of their abilities as a player, one who knows his position and comes through during tough times. "My husband was very supportive, but he can't think and feel like a woman," confided a veteran mother. "The nurses and my labor-support person knew what I wanted before I had to ask." Most husbands — and obstetricians — have trouble with their own *P*-word at birth — patience. Some men, in their rush to help, actually interfere with the harmony of labor, breaking a woman's concentration during birth. Also, birth partners take note: Employing a labor assistant does not mean you can watch television while the women do all the labor. You have an important role at birth. (See page 38 for clarification of the roles of father and PLA; also see "Coach of the Year" birth story, page 255).

If your mate doesn't want to coach, find another job for him in the organization. Sometimes the birth partner can be a cheerleader and pump up the mother with "you can do it" encouragement. A birth partner can also be a masseur, giving a loving touch, a rock to hold the mother steady, a pillar to lean against, and a servant to deliver juice and snacks. Most of all, partners are there as lovers.

strength of the ICEA is its list of board members, which reads like a Who's Who of childbirth education. ICEA's well-researched "position statement" pamphlets on every aspect of childbirth are, in our opinion, the best in the business. ICEA is a credible source of information for consumers and childbirth educators seeking to upgrade their skills. If you have an obstetrical question on anything from VBAC to herpes, you will find this organization a valuable resource. Their motto, "Freedom of choice through knowledge of alternatives," truly fits the desires of parents today. To find an ICEA-certified childbirth instructor in your area, contact the organization's headquarters. (See "Resources for Childbirth Education," page 53.)

All of the above. Many freelance childbirth educators have selected the best of Lamaze, Bradley, ICEA, and other methods to formulate their own childbirth-preparation package. But "independents" do not have the supervision or the resources of the major childbirth organizations. For example, any teacher can claim to be a Lamaze instructor but not be certified by any organization. The term *Lamaze* is not a registered service mark but rather a generic name. ASPO teachers do need to be certified to teach Lamaze. Back in the days when our living room was filled with couples practicing for the big event, our classes were a compilation of these "big three," together with our own birth experiences and philosophies.

Getting Your Body Ready for Birth

BESIDES PREPARING YOUR mind for birth it's necessary to prepare your body. Just as you would prepare for an athletic event, you should tone your body for birth. Exercise will also help you cope with the discomforts of pregnancy. The muscles you use most during birth are the ones that need most attention. Here are some useful conditioning tips to prepare your body for birth.

ASSUMING THE RIGHT PREGNANCY POSTURE

As the baby grows, your center of gravity changes. The extra weight in front can cause a swayback posture that puts uncomfortable strain on your lower back. Try these head-to-toe tips for posture that is kind to your back.

Keep your head up. Naturally you will affectionately peer down at the bulge. But habitually looking down throws off your posture. Keep your chin level. Imagine your birth partner holding each side of your head and lifting you toward the ceiling. When your head is held correctly, your shoulders and back will fall into place.

Drop your shoulders. Relax your shoulders to a natural position. Avoid throwing your shoulder blades back, since it strains the lower back muscles.

Avoid tensing and swaying your lower back. As the weight of your baby grows in the front, your back muscles contract to counterbalance the forward shift in gravity. The constant muscle tension may cause backache. While a slight curve of your lower back is normal, avoid exaggerating the curve into a swayback posture. If you had chronic back pain before pregnancy it may be worse now. Chiropractic attention may be necessary.

Tilt your pelvis forward. Pull in your abdominal muscles, tuck in your buttock muscles, and tilt your pelvis forward. This posture counteracts the arching tendency of your lower back.

Relax your knees. Bend them slightly; avoid locking your knees.

Keep your feet shoulder-width apart. Support your weight equally, and avoid leaning back on your heels. Also, avoid high, spiked heels. Most women find medium-height wide heels more comfortable and stable during the latter months of pregnancy.

GOOD BODY MECHANICS

Pregnancy hormones naturally loosen ligaments and joints, which makes it possible for your pelvis to be more flexible during birth. This loosening is responsible for the waddle walk of later pregnancy. Try the fol- lowing suggestions to avoid strain or injury during normal daily activities.

Stand smart. To lessen ankle swelling and promote good circulation, avoid standing for long periods, especially in the same position. To maintain good circulation, periodically exercise by flexing your calf muscles. Change positions frequently. Rest one foot on a support such as a low stool or shelf; switch to the other foot occasionally.

Lift lightly. Your back is not designed to be a crane, especially when you're pregnant. Don't lift heavy objects. For light lifting, use your arm, leg, and thigh muscles, not your

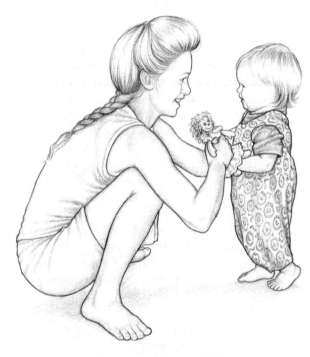

Squat to address a child

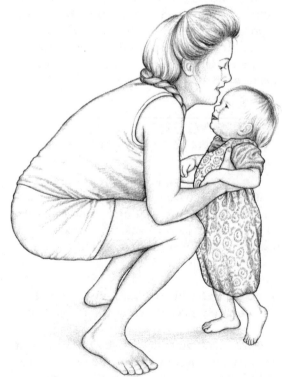

Lift with arms and legs, not with your back

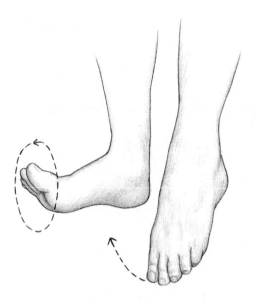

Foot exercises

back. Squat (don't bend) close to the object. Keep your head up and your back straight; lift by pushing up with your legs and flexing your arms. Avoid the natural urge to bend over to pick up a toddler. Instead, squat down to the child's eye level or sit on the floor and cuddle.

Sit sensibly. To maintain good circulation, avoid sitting for more than a half hour at a time. Straight-back chairs with a small pillow behind your lower back are kinder to your spine than soft, deep chairs. Use a footstool. Shift positions frequently and avoid crossing your legs. Whenever possible, sit cross-legged on the floor (see "Tailor Sitting," page 63). Periodically exercise your calf muscles by pointing your feet forward and then flexing them back. Draw circles with your large toe and then with your heel. When going from a sitting to a standing position, avoid lunging forward and doing the work with your back. Slide toward the edge of the chair, plant your feet on the floor, and use your leg muscles to lift yourself off. Don't forget to reach out for assistance from someone willing to offer a pregnant woman a hand. While riding in a car, elevate your legs and exercise your calf muscles frequently.

Sleep on your side. During the last four to five months of your pregnancy, side-lying is the most comfortable position for mother and healthiest for baby. To feather your nest in the third trimester, you will likely need at

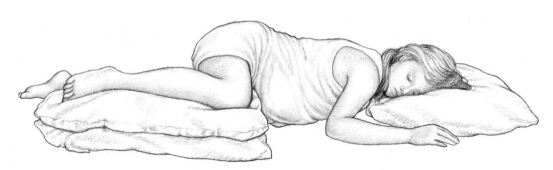

Feathering your nest

least four pillows, two under your head, one supporting your top leg, and perhaps another behind your lower back. If you feel off-balance lying on your side, shift slightly onto your stomach by moving your top leg forward so it is completely off your lower leg, and let your abdomen snuggle into the mattress, as shown in the figure on page 61. See page 66 for why not to sleep on your back.

Rise properly. Don't sit up suddenly when the alarm clock rings; you'll strain your lower back and abdominal muscles. Instead, roll over on your side, but don't yet swing your feet over the side of the bed. (This motion twists the lower back ligaments.) Now, using your arms, first push yourself up to a sitting position, and then gently swing your legs over the side.

BEST BIRTH EXERCISES

During pregnancy two general types of exercises are considered. *Conditioning exercises* help the muscles and other tissues directly involved in birth. *Aerobic exercises* are ones that use up oxygen and condition the heart muscle.

Conditioning Exercises — Exercising for Birth

Conditioning exercises are helpful to the mother and not harmful to the baby. Here are the most useful postures:

Pelvic Floor Exercises (Kegel Exercises)

Increasing the tone and elasticity of your pelvic floor muscles during pregnancy will help them work better for you during birth and return to their original condition postpartum. These muscles attach to the pelvic bones and act like a hammock to cradle and support your pelvic organs. During pregnancy these muscles stretch and sag due to the effect of pregnancy hormones and the increased weight of your uterus. During birth the muscles that encircle the birth canal stretch to their maximum. To become aware of these muscles, try stopping and starting the flow of urine, or contract and release these muscles while inserting your finger into your vagina or while having intercourse. The sensations during intercourse come from the nerve endings from the muscles beneath the vaginal wall. The degree of response from these nerve endings is directly related to the tone of your pelvic floor muscles. Veterans of the Kegel exercises (named for the doctor who invented them) confide that not only do they experience less leaking of urine (a common nuisance during pregnancy and postpartum), but also sexual enjoyment is enhanced for them and their partners.

Practice Kegel exercises in all positions: lying down, standing, squatting, or tailor sitting. Tense your vaginal muscles (the same ones used for control of urination and during intercourse) and hold for around five seconds. Contract and release these muscles at least two hundred times a day (four sets of fifty), or as often as you think about it. Pick a cue time to help you remember: while talking on the phone, waiting in line, stopping at traffic lights, and so forth. To keep your motivation high, try a variety of movements. Our favorite is the *elevator ride:* Your vaginal muscles are arranged like a stack of rings that can be tightened. Think of each ring as a different floor you would pass on an elevator. Start on the first floor

Lining Up

Chiropractic care during pregnancy can not only improve musculoskeletal alignment and relieve areas of muscle tension, but it can also influence the quality of your birth experience. Studies show that women who suffered from low back pain during previous labors and then received chiropractic care in subsequent pregnancies reported significantly reduced low back pain in their subsequent labors.

Practitioners of SOT (sacro occipital technique) have especially effective techniques for pregnant women. Martha had the benefit of this attention weekly in the last trimester of our sixth pregnancy. This technique recognizes that the "wobbly" pregnant pelvis, especially the sacroiliac joint, needs to be stabilized. By the use of foam wedges (blocks) the pelvis is balanced using low-force adjustment (the women's own body weight does the work rather than direct manipulation by the practitioner). If you can't locate a practitioner of SOT, consult a chiropractor who has a lot of experience working with pregnant women.

The uterus works best in a framework of ligaments and bones that are balanced and aligned. This allows the baby to travel more easily through the birth passage, avoiding long, difficult back labors and "failure to progress," and reducing the incidence of cesarean section. Many women are advised incorrectly that they must put up with the low back pain, nausea, and headaches of pregnancy. Through chiropractic care, however, women can experience relief from these so-called "normal" discomforts, and enjoy a healthier pregnancy and birth.

---

and gradually have your elevator lift to the second floor, then third, and so on, all the way to the sixth floor. Hold it there as long as you can, then gradually lower the elevator through each floor back to first. That is the toning part of the exercise. Now, drop down to the basement. That is the letting go part of the exercise, which will help you sense how to keep tension away from these birthing muscles. You want to be "in the basement" when your baby comes down so you don't resist the birth. Being "in the basement" feels lovely and loose, similar to the total release you have when you are ready for penetration in intercourse, and especially similar to how your vagina feels once you've completed lovemaking — slightly bulgy and full. You always end the elevator exercise with your muscles returned to the first floor, with that slight amount of tone you maintain unconsciously.

Variations. Contract the area around your vagina and urethra then release. Start contracting from anus forward to pubic bone, release from pubic bone to anus. Make your tempo wavelike to build elasticity. Contract the pelvic floor muscles gradually, count to ten, hold, then gradually release to a count of ten.

Tailor Sitting

Sit cross-legged while reading, eating, or watching television. This posture loosens

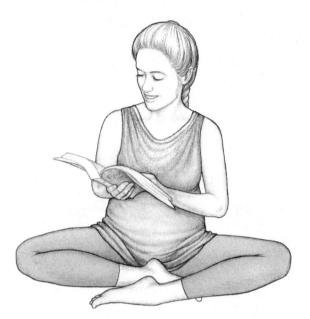

*Tailor sitting: Sit on floor throughout pregnancy
instead of on a chair*

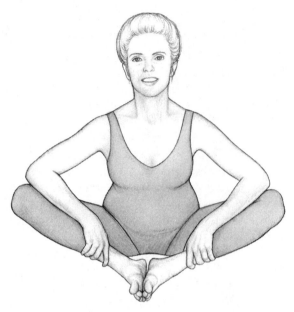

Variation of tailor sitting

perineal tissues and stretches inner thigh
muscles, strengthening them for birth. It
also brings your uterus forward, taking pressure off your back. Sit tailor-style for at least
ten minutes several times a day, and gradually increase the duration.

Variations. Sit upright leaning against a wall
or couch and bring the soles of your feet
together. Bring your knees increasingly
wider apart as you contract and release your
pelvic floor muscles. Gently push down on
one knee and thigh and then the other. You
will notice that each week you are able to
stretch your thighs more comfortably and
wider apart. Also try making shoulder circles: While sitting tailor-style, rest your
hands on your knees and shrug both shoulders toward your ears and release. As you
lift both shoulders, inhale and circle them

toward your back and down, and while
exhaling, move them toward the front. This
exercise can condition and relax neck and
upper back muscles that may be strained
during labor.

Squatting

This posture stretches ligaments to widen
the pelvic outlet, prepares thigh and leg
muscles for this valuable birth posture, and
conditions you to squat instead of bend over
to pick up objects. Squat at least one minute
ten times a day, and build up squatting for
longer periods so this position will be very
natural for you in labor. You can "squat
around" instead of sit around. (See squatting
tips, page 187.) Toddlers and young children squat a lot as they go about their
"work," but in our culture, this posture has
disappeared from the routine of adults. You

will have to relearn this skill and overcome a feeling of awkwardness or even slight embarrassment in assuming this "primitive" posture. Could it be that women who squatted around the cooking fire and at the stream had a much easier time giving birth because squatting was so natural for them? If you have a toddler, spend as much time as possible squatting with him or her.

All-Fours Exercises

The *pelvic tilt* prepares pelvic tissues, strengthens abdominal muscles, and promotes spine alignment to lessen backache. Get on your hands and knees with your hands directly below your shoulders and your knees below your hips. Keep your lower back flat. Relax. Don't arch or sag your back. Take a deep breath, then, while slowly exhaling, drop your head, keep your back straight, tuck in your buttocks, and draw in your abdomen (imagine a puppy tucking in her tail). Hold this posture for a count of three, then exhale and relax. Do your tilts in sets of fifty three or four times a day, or whenever you have a backache. During this exercise you can also tighten your pelvic floor muscles. In this position you can increase the mobility of your pelvic structures by doing the *pelvic rock* — rolling your hips hula hoop–style. These movements will also be useful in labor if you have backache and/or if baby has a posterior presentation.

Variations. Stretching the pelvic floor muscles can be helped by what we call the *leap frog* position. Get on all fours and spread your knees as wide as you comfortably can and rest forward on your hands. Contract and relax your pelvic floor muscles at least ten times. Or try pelvic rocking and tighten-

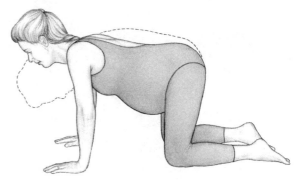

All-fours exercise

ing exercises, leaning forward on your elbows. Finally, spend some time getting used to the knee-chest position (see figure on page 191) — one you may later need to ease the pain of back labor. (To lessen the

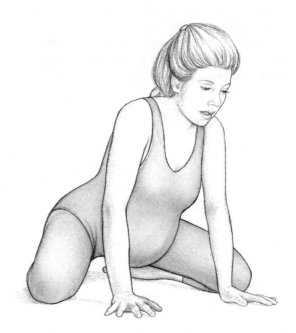

Leap-frog exercise

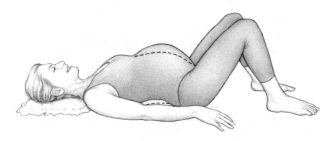

Pelvic tilt

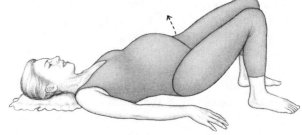

Pelvic rock

feeling of blood rushing to your head, lower your head into the knee-chest position very slowly and raise it again if you have an uncomfortable feeling. As you get used to this exercise these unusual sensations will lessen.)

Back-Lying Exercises

Avoid exercising while lying on your back after the fourth month of pregnancy. Because the weighty uterus presses on the spine and major blood vessels in the latter half of pregnancy, lying on your back may be uncomfortable for you and unsafe for baby. In the first four months, try these exercises

to condition your back and pelvic muscles. Do the *pelvic tilt:* lie on your back with your knees bent and feet flat. Place a thin pillow under your head. Slowly breathe in deeply, let your abdomen rise, then, while exhaling, pull your abdomen in tightly and press the small of your back flat against the

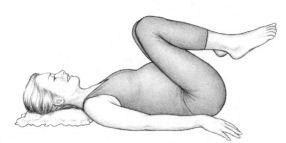

Buttocks curl

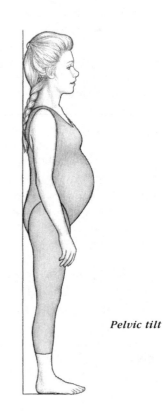

Pelvic tilt

floor. Then do the *pelvic rock:* keeping most of your upper back pressed against the floor, raise your hips and buttocks slightly and gently rock them in a circular or hula hoop motion. Do the *buttocks curl:* slowly and without jerking, draw your knees up over your abdomen and tighten your belly as you press your lower back against the floor as you did in the pelvic tilt exercises. Hold for a count of three, then slowly return your feet to the floor.

Standing Exercises

Try the *standing pelvic tilt.* Stand with your back against the wall and your heels about four inches from the wall. Press the small of your back against the wall by pulling in your abdominal muscles and tucking in your buttocks muscles. Keep your chin level and raise your chest so that your upper back is flat against the wall. Hold for a count of five. Repeat three to ten times. Now walk away and try to maintain this posture during the day.

Aerobic Exercises — Exercising for Two

Aerobic exercises include everyday exercises such as walking and swimming. Are these exercises helpful to the pregnant mother and safe for the baby? The answer is yes — in moderation (in excess, no).

Best Pregnancy Exercises

- swimming
- stationary cycling
- brisk walking
- low-impact aerobics

Benefits to mother. Aerobic exercises increase the performance of your cardiovascular system, making it more efficient. Aerobic exercise causes your heart to work faster to deliver more oxygen to working muscles. After repeated exercise, your heart rate gets used to delivering extra oxygen without working so fast and hard. The resting heart rate of a long-distance runner, for example, is lower than that of a sedentary person. Besides making your circulatory system work better, exercise makes a pregnant woman feel better. It lessens leg swelling and helps prevent varicose veins, improves overall muscle tone, helps you maintain and regain your desired figure, enhances sleep, and gives your whole self a physical and emotional boost that helps you handle the stress of labor and delivery as well as life with a new baby.

Effect on the baby. To adapt to the increased demands for blood and oxygen during pregnancy, your blood volume increases 40 percent, the amount of blood pumped by your heart (called cardiac output) increases 30–40 percent, and your heart rate increases. So, your cardiovascular system is already exercising simply because you are pregnant. If you put on an oversized jogging suit and join the pack of morning runners here's what happens. When you exercise, your body automatically redistributes the blood from internal organs to the exercising muscles. This means there may be less blood flowing to the uterus. That's the main concern with exercise during pregnancy. When your heart rate increases, so does your baby's, and perhaps the same physiological changes that occur in you may also occur in baby. The increased fetal heart rate that has been measured while a mother exercises suggests that her fetus senses when mother is exercising and he or she reacts with his or her own compensatory cardiovascular mechanisms.

Whether or not this is good or bad for baby is not known. Some research studies suggest babies of strenuously exercising mothers have lower birth weights; other studies show no difference. One interesting study showed that mothers who exercised regularly showed a greater cardiac reserve. This means that their hearts were so used to the increased demands of exercise that they operated more efficiently and, consequently, needed to shunt less blood from internal organs, including the uterus, during exercise. In essence, a fit mother could enjoy strenuous exercise without compromising the nourishment to her baby. Because the results of studies on babies of exercising mothers are conflicting and not always helpful, we are left to rely on common sense. Based on these considerations, here is a commonsense guide to exercising during pregnancy.

First, consult your doctor. Do you have any medical problems such as heart disease, high blood pressure, or diabetes that may compromise your baby if you exercise too much? In partnership with your doctor, work out an exercise routine that is best for you and your baby based on your obstetrical and medical history and your current level of fitness. Most obstetricians discourage jogging during pregnancy because they believe this exercise may add harmful stress on the uterine ligaments that are already being stretched by pregnancy.

How fit are you now? If you were fit before pregnancy you will be able to tolerate more strenuous exercise during preg-

nancy without compromising yourself or your baby. (Your cardiac reserve is better; see explanation above.) If you are a person who hasn't been exercising, but now that you're pregnant feels obligated to join the crowd in sweat suits, you will need to build up your fitness program *gradually* and *slowly.*

Know when to say when. As a common-sense physiological guide, if the exercise is too strenuous for you, it's too strenuous for baby as well. Try the *pulse test.* Place your fingers on the artery just under your jaw and take your pulse for ten seconds, then multiply by six. If your pulse reaches 140 beats per minute while you are exercising, slow down. Listen to your body's stop signs: pounding pulse, shortness of breath, dizziness, headaches. The athletes' axiom "no pain, no gain" doesn't apply to a pregnant woman, and trainers are rethinking this advice even for athletes. If any part of your body hurts, stop exercising it. Or try the *talk test.* If you are too winded to carry on a conversation during exercise slow down until the words flow easily.

Keep the exercise short and frequent. Small, frequent doses of exercise are easiest on your body, and on the little one inside you. Try ten- to fifteen-minute bouts twice daily, three times a week and gradually build up to your level of fun and fitness (with a heart rate less than 140 and no shortness of breath during the exercise). Regular exercise is more body- and baby-friendly than sporadic bursts.

Keep the weight off your feet. Studies have shown that upright weight-bearing exercises (e.g., jogging, running) are more likely to bother baby's heart rate than horizontal non–weight-bearing activities (e.g., swimming). Less bouncy exercises (e.g., swimming, cycling) are easier on your body (and baby's) than bouncy ones. If you are an avid runner, consider walking briskly instead, especially in the last few months of pregnancy.

Keep cool. Studies suggest a mother's fetus could be harmed by prolonged elevated body temperatures of 102° F or higher. If you are getting hot during your exercise, slow down to cool down. This is why the self-cooling exercise of swimming is best while pregnant. Exercise during the cool times of the day, especially in hot, humid weather. For the same reason, pregnant women should avoid saunas and hot tubs. If you like warm baths, keep the water around body temperature (99° F). The harmful effects of overheating are highest in the first three months of pregnancy.

Slow as you grow. In the final months of pregnancy your body has less cardiac reserve, meaning there is little cardiovascular energy left over for exercise. Runners, start walking; cyclers, start swimming.

Warm up and cool down. Spend a few minutes stretching and easing into the exercise before going full throttle. Gradually wind down the exercise until your breathing and heart rate return to normal. Abruptly stopping strenuous exercise may cause your blood to pool in the exercised muscles.

Give baby a postexercise rest. After exercising lie for ten minutes on your left side. Major blood vessels (aorta and inferior vena cava) run along the right side of your spine and may be compressed by the weight of your uterus while you're lying on your back. Lying on your left side takes all the pressure off the vena cava and promotes circulation to your placenta and uterus.

Replace fuel and replenish your fluids. Don't exercise with an empty stomach or when you feel hungry. Quick-energy carbohydrate foods (e.g., honey, fruit) are nonfilling preexercise foods that provide fuel. After exercising, eat to satisfy hunger and drink at least two eight-ounce glasses of water or juice.

Dress for the occasion. Wear pants with a comfortable elastic waistband, and wear supportive shoes. Wear a supportive bra or even two if your breasts are heavy. The fashion for exercise during pregnancy is cool and comfortable. As during labor, comfort comes before glamour.

EATING RIGHT — FOR TWO

During pregnancy you are growing a human being. The better you eat, the better your baby grows. Women who wisely nourish themselves during pregnancy are more likely to give birth to healthy babies. Babies of well-fed mothers tend to be less premature, grow at an appropriate pace, have fewer congenital defects, and show better brain growth. Mothers who eat right during pregnancy are less likely to experience gestational diabetes, toxemia, anemia, leg cramps, heartburn, obesity, and complicated labors. And if you eat wisely, you will have less weight to shed postpartum.

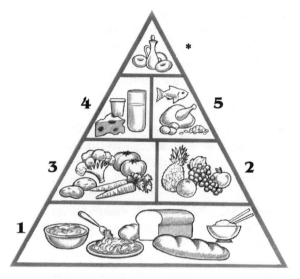

1. bread, cereal, rice, and pasta
   (5 servings)
2. fruit
   (2–4 servings)
3. vegetables
   (3–5 servings)
4. milk, yogurt, and cheese
   (2–3 servings)
5. meat, poultry, fish, dry beans, eggs, and nuts
   (2–3 servings)
* fats, oils, and sweets
   (use sparingly)

Five basic food groups

Eleven Suggestions for Eating Right While Pregnant

1. Make every calorie count. To nourish yourself and your passenger, you will need to eat approximately three hundred more calories than you normally do each day, somewhat less during the first trimester, more during the last. That's not much extra food (e.g., two glasses of skim milk, an egg, and four ounces of pasta). But not all calories are created equal. Push away empty calories, foods that provide little nutritional value, such as sweets. Reach for nutrient-dense foods, those that pack a lot of nourish-

---

Daily Food Needs During Pregnancy

Bread, cereal, rice, and pasta. 5 servings (one serving = 1 slice of bread, ½ cup of rice, pasta, or cooked cereal, ½ cup of potatoes or beans, or ¾ cup of dry cereal). Use whole grains whenever possible.

Vegetables. 3 servings (one serving = 1 cup of raw or ½ cup of cooked). Use fresh whenever possible; organic is best.

Fruits. 2 servings (one serving = ½ cup of fruit or 1 cup of juice). Use fresh whenever possible; organic is best.

Dairy products. 4 servings (one serving = 1 cup of milk, ½ cup of cottage cheese, yogurt, or ice cream, or 1 ounce of cheese). If allergic to dairy, see alternative sources of calcium, page 73.

Meat, poultry, fish, dried beans, eggs, and nuts. 3–4 servings (one serving = 3 ounces of meat, fish, or poultry, 2 large eggs, 2 tablespoons of peanut butter, or 1 cup of cooked legumes).

---

ment into each calorie. Try these ten good nutrient-dense foods: avocado, brown rice, plain low-fat yogurt, eggs, fish (be sure the fish don't come from waters high in mercury), kidney beans, vegetables, tofu, turkey, and whole-grain pasta.

Limit fats to 30–35 percent of the calories in your diet (e.g., 80–90 grams of fat); 50–55 percent of the calories should come from carbohydrates, and 10–15 percent from proteins. The healthiest fats are found in avo-cado, fish, nut butter, and olive oil. However, some animal and dairy fat is also needed. A sweet tooth is common during pregnancy, but you should limit your intake of sweets. Some sugars are healthier than others. The best sugars are complex carbohydrates, better known by grandmother's term "starches." These include: whole-grain pasta, legumes, potatoes, whole grains and cereals, and seeds. These supersugars provide slow, steady energy and give you a feeling of full-ness longer, without the high and low feel-ings of fast-acting sugars such as sucrose.

2. Choose fresh foods. Pregnancy makes you more selective about what you put in your shopping cart. Try spending more time in the fresh produce aisle than in the canned goods section. Stick to freshly prepared foods rather than those that are processed. If you can't buy organic foods, peel fruits and vegetables to eliminate pesticides.

3. Eating for two doesn't mean eating double. While it's unhealthy to undereat during pregnancy, it's also unhealthy to overeat. An occasional binge goes with the emotional territory, but if you habitually indulge during pregnancy, you're likely to pay for your excesses during and after deliv-ery. Find some foods that are nutritious as well as emotionally comforting. Overeating (eating junk food for example) is likely to result in an oversized baby who may need intervention at birth.

4. How your weight adds up. Weight gain during pregnancy depends a lot on your body type. Ectomorph (tall and lean) moth-ers tend to gain less, endomorphs (short and pear-shaped) tend to gain the most, and mesomorphs (average build) are somewhere in between. A healthy woman who was at her ideal weight before pregnancy will nor-mally gain twenty-five to thirty-five pounds. A woman who was previously underweight could gain more, an overweight woman would be wise to stay within the twenty-five to thirty-five range. A healthy pattern is to gain around four pounds during the first twelve weeks, and roughly a pound a week thereafter. You may have one monthly weight check that seems to "go tilt," adding eight or nine pounds even though you are eating wisely. This will probably not become a pattern — many women have it happen once in their pregnancy. Nearly half of your pregnancy weight gain (the baby, the pla-centa, and the amniotic fluid) will be shed at birth. If you are feeling well, baby is grow-ing well, and you have no excess swelling, you are probably eating just right and gain-ing the right amount of weight for you. Even if the amount exceeds the above guidelines, if you are eating nutritious foods only, the weight gain should not be a problem. Moth-ers who do this report that their weight falls off quickly after birth, since they continue to eat wisely.

Where Your Weight Goes	
weight of baby	7½ lbs.
weight of placenta	1½ lbs.
weight of uterus	3½ lbs.
weight of amniotic fluid	2½ lbs.
weight of breasts	1 lb.
weight of extra blood	
volume and fluids	8½ lbs.
	24½ lbs.

Note: These figures are just averages. Any weight over this total will be fat, a certain amount of which is healthy.

5. Extra food for extra growth. Add an extra helping from each of the five basic food groups (see page 70) for your extra nutritional needs and those of your baby.

6. A message from baby to mother: No crash diets — please! While you may want to remain trim during pregnancy, your baby needs to grow. Avoid fasting or fad diets while pregnant. It is a misconception that the fetus is a perfect parasite, that if there isn't enough nutrition to adequately nourish both persons, the baby will steal nutrients at mother's expense. Babies are nutritional parasites, but not perfect ones, and both mother and baby can suffer nutritional deficiencies if the mother doesn't eat wisely. Most pregnant women, especially in the last half of pregnancy, need about 2,500 calories a day, every day. If you wish to feel trim for your physical and mental well-being during pregnancy (and have less excess poundage to shed after birth), control excess fat by exercise, not by diet. Inadequate nutrition depletes the body of vital nutrients needed for growing tissues. Exercise, when coupled with adequate nutrition, burns off only fat, and that's the excess tissue you want to get rid of anyway. For example, one hour of sustained low-impact exercise each day (swimming, cycling, or walking briskly) can burn off three hundred to four hundred calories daily, which translates to a pound of fat lost (or not gained) every nine to twelve days. Also, avoid low-cholesterol diets, unless advised by your physician. A baby's developing brain needs cholesterol. Female hormones help synthesize cholesterol anyway; infancy and pregnancy are two times in a woman's life when she need not worry about cholesterol. Don't expect a fat-free figure during pregnancy. An overall increase in body fat is a normal part of a pregnant woman's figure.

7. Graze while you grow. Many mothers find comfort and nourishment in nibbling on nutritious foods all day long, rather than eating three big meals each day. Grazing is kinder to queasy stomachs during those mornings of sickness, nights of nausea, and hours of heartburn. In early pregnancy when eating is a challenge for some women, small carbohydrate meals, fresh fruits and vegetables, homemade soups, and eating every two to three hours will be best. The key to good grazing is finding nutrient-dense foods (see page 73), not empty calories. A snack tray full of whole-grain crackers, cheese cubes, broccoli stalks, avocado dip, veggie slices, and granola is much more body-friendly than a box of candy or a bag of potato chips. If you are too tired to prepare snacks or meals, enlist the help of a friend or your mate.

8. Pills don't replace plates. Whether or not you need prenatal vitamin and mineral supplements is a decision for you and your doctor. Theoretically, if you ate like the sample menu on page 70 suggests every day for nine months, you wouldn't need extra nutrition in a pill. In the real world, many mothers are too busy, too sick, or too tired to eat that well every day. For the health and safety of your baby the doctor may prescribe supplemental vitamins and iron during pregnancy, but taking these doesn't excuse you from eating well.

9. Keep cravings under control. During our last pregnancy, Martha craved her midnight zucchini pancakes. Occasionally, I would have to trek to an all-night supermar-

Extra Nutrition for Extra Growth

Nutrient	What You Need Daily	Sources	Comment
Iron	60 mg of elemental iron (e.g., 300 mg ferrous sulfate), more if anemic before or during pregnancy or if carrying multiples	Best diet sources: red meat, organ meat, poultry, fish, oysters, iron-fortified cereals, blackstrap molasses; supplemental iron tablets	It's nearly impossible to get enough extra iron (especially in the last half of pregnancy) from food alone without overeating. Iron supplements are usually necessary, but may be constipating. Eating or drinking extra vitamin C with meals increases the amount of iron absorbed from food. Milk, tea, or coffee with meals decreases absorption of iron; best to drink these between meals.
Calcium	1,200 mg	Dairy products (milk, yogurt, cheese); sardines, rhubarb, chickpeas, spinach, kale, salmon, refried beans, blackstrap molasses, figs, almond butter, dried beans, or calcium tablets	Calcium deficiency is uncommon because your body contains high reserves and there is calcium in nearly every food. The daily requirement for calcium can be met by drinking one quart of milk, or dairy equivalent, but no more. Milk's high phosphorous content can interfere with calcium absorption. Calcium carbonate is best absorbed.
Protein	75–100 grams	Seafood, eggs, dairy products, legumes, meat and poultry, nuts and seeds, grains, vegetables	Grains and legumes are incomplete proteins. When combined with each other, they make a complete protein. One serving equals 20–25 grams of protein. Since most American diets are high in protein, chances are good that you are getting enough protein without analyzing every bite you eat.
Vitamins	Increased need for all vitamins	All additional vitamins and minerals (except iron) can be obtained by eating a balanced diet (see sample menu on page 70). Supplements needed only if nutrition is erratic, processed, or if you have special needs.	Blood concentrations of many vitamins, especially A, B_6, B_{12}, C, A, and folate decline during pregnancy so that supplements or extra foods containing these vitamins are necessary.
Calories	300 extra calories per day	Best is a balanced source from five basic food groups (see page 70), not two extra doughnuts daily.	Best nutrition breakdown of calorie sources daily: 30–35 percent from fats, 50–55 percent from carbohydrates, and 10–15 percent from protein.

ket. Once, as I paraded through the check-out line carrying a two-foot-long zucchini, a clerk concluded, "Your wife must be pregnant." There is a principle called the *wisdom of the body* — a person craves what the body needs. Did the zucchini have what Martha's body needed — was it a comfort food that helped her feel better physically and emotionally? — or was this just a whim of a pregnant person with an indulgent husband? Try to find comfort foods that are nutritious as well as comforting. Perhaps the common craving for pickles is a reflection of a need for a little extra salt. Salads and vegetables are "free" foods during pregnancy, meaning you can indulge in these nutritious foods to your body's content.

10. Pass the salt. Excess salt was once blamed for the swelling nearly all pregnant women experience to some degree. Now we know that added water in your system has a purpose, and abnormal swelling is more the result of internal mechanisms that regulate salt and water balance rather than of eating too much salt. Salt your food to taste but not to excess.

11. Drink while you grow. As you eat for two during pregnancy, you should also drink for two. At least eight eight-ounce glasses of fluid a day should keep your body and your baby well hydrated. A lot of fluid is needed to increase your blood volume by 40–50 percent and to keep refilling the pool for your little swimmer inside. Use extra-large cups and glasses, or keep a quart bottle filled with juice or water in the refrigerator. Avoid alcohol, especially during the first trimester. Drinking juices high in vitamin C with meals increases the absorption of much-needed extra iron from foods. Drinking enough water is one of the simplest remedies for constipation. It is wise to dilute fruit juices with equal parts of water, especially if you depend on juice for a lot of your fluid intake. You can add seltzer water for a nice change — this is much better for you than drinking sugar- or sweetener-laden soft drinks. Current research is not conclusive on whether or how much caffeine is safe in pregnancy, so limiting tea and coffee to one or two cups a day seems wise. Caffeine does interfere with the absorption of certain nutrients.

Proper "dieting" during pregnancy means eating more, not less. Be selective; pay more attention to *what* you eat than how much.

Tests, Technology, and Other Interventions That Happen on the Way to Birth

THERE ONCE WAS a time when the uterus was a private place for the infant to dwell. Now, modern tests and technology provide windows to the womb that aid the obstetrician in managing pregnancy and birth. We believe the improvements in maternal and infant health over the last several decades have more to do with the childbirth reform movement than with the perfection of technology. Yet technology has found its place in the delivery room. Technology at birth is a mixed blessing, and there continues to be a conflict between women and machines in the birth place. We want to equip you to know which tests and technology are helpful, which are harmful, and what is unknown. Participate in the decision to have a test or to use technology. Ask: Is it safe for you and your baby? Is it necessary? Are there better alternatives?

One problem with tests is that you are obliged to do something with the results. By being informed about the most common tests and technology to which you are likely to be exposed during your pregnancy and birth, you are better able to participate in the decision of whether or not to undergo the test and, even more important, you are part of the decision to act on the result. The more information you bring to birth, the more likely tests and technology will be an asset to you rather than a liability.

Remember, historically in obstetrics, interventions have become common practice long before their usefulness or their safety has been proven. Witness twilight sleep (see page 19), which was used for forty years before it was judged to be unsafe. Another example is the custom of pubic shaving, which was thought to lessen infection. This humiliating practice was discontinued after it was proven to be not only useless but also a factor in increasing the chance of infection. There needs to be an ongoing system of checks and balances that keeps the technology used at birth in perspective: reform-minded women questioning machine-minded doctors. As long as this partnership continues, women are likely to have better births and doctors are likely to practice better obstetrics.

ELECTRONIC FETAL MONITORING (EFM)

How can such a small bedside box cause so much controversy? Proponents of electronic fetal monitoring (EFM) claim that it saves babies; opponents disagree. Proponents say it's safe, opponents claim it's harmful. When offered this new technology, what's a mother to say?

What Is EFM?

A briefcase-size box sits at your bedside spitting out a ticker tape–like printout. The printout shows two graphs: your baby's heartbeat and your uterine contractions. You are connected to this box by two wires called electrodes, which may be attached in two ways. With *external fetal monitoring,* two large straps are placed around your abdomen over your uterus. One strap contains an ultrasound sensor that detects your baby's heartbeat, and the other contains a pressure-sensor gauge that picks up tension in your abdomen reflecting uterine contractions. These external straps and their recording devices may be put on and removed as needed, yet they must be positioned precisely. With *internal fetal monitoring,* a catheter and wire are placed up through your vagina after your membranes have naturally ruptured or have been broken by your birth attendant. The wire, to record your baby's heartbeat like an electrocardiogram, is passed through your cervix and attached to your baby's scalp (or buttock in the case of breech presentation). A soft tube (the catheter) is threaded up inside your uterus to record the time and strength of your contractions. Internal fetal monitoring is more accurate than external, but it is also more invasive. Penetrating baby's skin with the electrode clips creates an entry point for germs. For this reason, doctors avoid internal fetal monitoring if mother has active herpes or HIV infection. If precise information is needed about baby's heart-rate patterns, your doctor may prefer

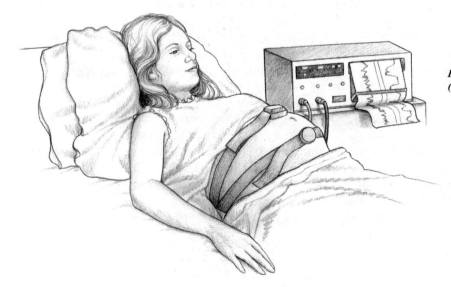

Electronic fetal monitoring (EFM) (external)

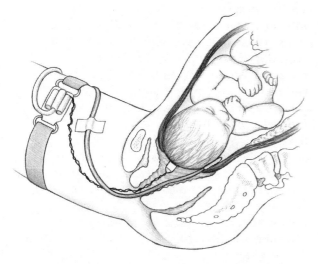

Electronic fetal monitoring (EFM) (internal)

to use internal fetal monitoring. For inter-mittent or routine checks on the baby's condition, external monitoring is sufficient.

Electronic fetal monitoring is used to evaluate the response of your baby's heartbeat to his or her own movement and to your uterine contractions. Normally baby's heart rate accelerates with movement and stays stable or goes down slightly during contractions, but recovers quickly afterward if baby is tolerating labor well and is getting enough oxygen. This is because there is a temporary decrease in oxygen delivery to the baby during contractions. Baby has enough reserve oxygen from a healthy placenta to tide him or her through the contraction, and the heart rate can bounce back to its normal pattern when the contraction is over. If the heart rate does not have normal changes (called "variability") or does not recover by the end of the contraction, there may be reason for concern. The benefit of electronic fetal monitoring is that suspicious patterns can be traced over a period of time and can alert the doctor that a baby is not tolerating labor well or is not getting sufficient oxygen. In this case intervention may be necessary. Having visual patterns on a printout ready for analysis is the main advantage of electronic fetal monitoring over the nurse-and-stethoscope method.

Why Do Babies Need Monitoring?

At first electronic fetal monitoring may sound like a good idea; if the monitor could pick up problems early, the doctor could intervene to correct the problem or get the baby out quickly before there is any lasting damage. But the problem is that what the monitor says and what's going on with the baby are not necessarily correlated. Technical problems may cause false alarms, such as the sensors shifting if the mother changes position. Moreover not everyone is equally skilled at interpreting the monitor recordings nor is there uniform agreement as to what different patterns mean. To further muddy the monitoring waters, recent research suggests that damage to a baby's brain (e.g., that which later causes cerebral palsy) occurs mainly before labor begins and is usually not due to insufficient oxygen during the final passage.

When the EFM cries wolf, the doctor has to do something, and that's the crucial question underlying the use of all medical technology — what to do with the findings. Is this just an unusual pattern, or is baby really in trouble? Not being sure and not wanting to take chances, the hospital path from delivery room to operating room has become a road frequently traveled. Shortly after EFM became part of the hospital birth package, cesarean-section rates doubled, yet babies didn't turn out any better.

By the 1980s, EFM had become standard obstetrical practice in nearly all deliveries. But it became immensely popular long before its usefulness or its safety had been proven. Never mind that for centuries babies safely lived in and exited from their homes without electronic surveillance. Now they needed monitoring. Obstetricians welcomed this electronic watchdog as a sort of "labor insurance" that all was going right. Like a home security system, mothers embraced the box as added protection for their babies. One of our patients described her feelings: "I found the monitor annoying but reassuring."

Then another factor entered the birth scene to cloud the already hazy use of technology further — the malpractice attorney, who saw there was money to be made from this bedside ticker tape. If the monitor goes off, indicating that baby may be in distress, the doctor's malpractice anxiety goes up unless he or she takes action, and that usually means a cesarean section for "fetal distress" — or possibly obstetrician distress. Even though there is no proven cause-and-effect relationship between what the monitor records and what's happening to the baby, courts still assume the monitor tells all, and they place blame based on what they perceive as fact. The use of electronic fetal monitoring peaked in the mid-eighties; but in the nineties its use is being reconsidered. Here's why.

Does EFM Do Any Good?

This question divides the birthing world. Twenty years of experience and nine randomized prospective studies (the most respected kind) have all concluded that electronic fetal monitoring has, in most cases, been of no benefit to mothers and babies. After studying thousands of births and babies, researchers concluded that electronic fetal monitoring offered no benefits to mother or baby compared to periodic listening to heart tones with a Doptone (a hand-held ultrasound device) or the old-fashioned fetoscope (a stethoscope designed to be placed on the abdomen to hear the baby's heartbeat). Overwhelmed by the research showing the non-usefulness of EFM, in 1989 the American College of Obstetricians and Gynecologists announced its position statement concerning routine EFM: "It has been shown in well-controlled research studies that intermittent auscultation of the fetal heart at intervals of fifteen minutes during the first stage of labor and five minutes during the second stage is equivalent to continuous electronic fetal monitoring in the assessment of fetal condition." In other words, a specially trained nurse listening to the fetal heart tones with a hand-held device and recording her findings is as useful as continuous electronic fetal monitoring, even with the printout. So after twenty years of tethering mothers to these machines and basing important decisions on their printouts, this wiry device has been proven to be no more useful (in uncomplicated labors) than human ears.

Does EFM Do Any Harm?

The same studies that show no benefits from EFM confirm the risks. Continuous electronic fetal monitoring is responsible for the following unnecessary trauma:

- more cesarean births, as obstetricians react to the results
- more forceps deliveries, as obstetricians attempt to get the baby out quickly
- more maternal and fetal infections from

insertion and constant presence of the internal monitoring tubing and wires, which provide easy access for bacteria to travel up into the mother's body, putting her and the baby at risk for infection

• infection of baby's scalp from electrode placement

Besides these measurable risks, there are more subtle ones. Most of the time, EFM means mother is tethered to a machine and is not free to walk during labor or encouraged to change positions. This lack of freedom often results in a more painful labor that progresses slower. Also, the mother's lying on her back (so that the electrodes can be placed more precisely) can itself cause abnormal tracings. The machine is not a labor-friendly companion. The constant clicking is annoying, and the discomfort and worrying about what the blips on the paper mean don't really help relax a laboring mother. Maternal stress can decrease uterine blood flow and compromise the baby. In fact, studies show that mothers having electronic fetal monitoring have significantly higher levels of stress hormones in their blood than mothers not electronically monitored. Some mothers find that the belt around their abdomen or the wires in their vagina interfere with their ability to cope with labor. As one mother complained, "I was doing okay until they made me lie down and put that thing on me."

Why Is EFM Still Used?

With all the studies questioning its usefulness, is it time to turn off this machine? Maybe. But that may be harder than it sounds. Doctors and nurses have become attached to these machines, and it will take time for them to get over their dependence. We have watched doctors and nurses enter a room and check the monitor before greeting the mother. One woman complained, "I felt like the nurse was so busy checking the monitor she didn't have time to check me." In superelectronic maternity wards, a nurse can stay at her station and observe the fetal heart tracings of several patients at one time without even going into the mother's room. This efficiency saves staff and money. The hospital can charge for electronic fetal monitoring, but there is no billing code for a nurse with a Doptone or fetoscope. Also, most obstetricians have one treasured anecdote about the time they think "the monitor saved the baby's life." It is these anecdotal success stories that keep physicians faithful to their machines.

Intermittent EFM is useful to assess fetal well-being during complicated labors. It can be a reassuring tool allowing the mother and birth attendant to let the labor proceed without intervention, or to help decision making should intervention be needed. On the other hand, while most obstetricians concede that routine continuous electronic fetal monitoring is unnecessary for low-risk mothers, they cling to its use for high-risk patients. While there is some truth to this, consider that high-risk mothers especially need the mobility and freedom to help their bodies labor in the best way possible. Remember Obstetrics 101: what's bad for the mother is bad for the baby. By restricting her mobility during labor, could EFM push a high-risk mother into a higher risk status?

Using EFM Wisely

So what's a mother to do? For starters, you can just say no; unless, of course, you have a specific obstetrical indication for EFM (see "Are You 'High-Risk'?" page 81). But saying no to sacred cows won't win you any friends in the delivery room. And what mother can resist a guilt-producing remark that she might be jeopardizing her baby's health? Try this change of tactics: "Doctor, I want fetal monitoring!" After you pick your obstetrician up off the floor, you clarify: "Human monitoring!" You are asking for the nurse to monitor your baby's heart rate with periodic listening. After all, this is standard practice as sanctioned by the American College of Obstetricians and Gynecologists. Who could argue with that?

If EFM proves to be nonnegotiable, ask for *telemetry* — space-age technology that allows you to roam at will without being tethered to a bedside machine. A belt and transducers to transmit baby's heart rate are still needed on your abdomen; but like the remote control on your television, telemetry transmits tracings through the air to a central receiver at the nurses' station. Many hospitals have telemetry monitors that are collecting dust because nobody knows to ask for them. Unless you have a specific obstetrical situation requiring continuous EFM, most obstetricians are happy to settle for a few twenty-minute tracings spaced throughout your labor — called *intermittent EFM.* The nurse then uses fetoscope evaluation the rest of the time.

EFM can actually be used to your advantage in prolonged labor. Long second-stage labors make obstetricians nervous because they fear that too prolonged a squeeze in the birth canal may not be good for your baby. A periodic tracing that shows the fetal heart tones bouncing back to normal following each contraction helps everyone breathe easier and your obstetrician is less likely to intervene. Above all, don't let the monitor interfere with your labor. *Insist that the machine be made to accommodate you.*

You can try all the usual position changes during your labor even with the monitor, although it will be more awkward to do so than without it. Be insistent in changing positions to your desired comfort. The moves may take a bit more work, attention, and creativity from your nurse, but that is part of her job. Try to ignore the little bleeping beast or turn down the volume. Concentrate on your work at hand, and let the medical staff worry about the monitor. There is no need to worry about a few irregularities in baby's heartbeat. If the monitor signals trouble, don't panic. It may be a technical problem or it could be a positional problem. You may simply need to change positions; shifting will encourage baby to change his position, too. Sometimes your attendant may give you a whiff of oxygen to see if the fetal heart tracings return to normal. Or if you are receiving a pitocin drip (see below) your nurse may adjust the dosage. If the monitor continues to show a worrisome pattern, your doctor may choose to perform a *fetal-scalp sample,* taking a drop or two of blood from your baby's scalp by means of a tiny tube inserted through your birth canal. Fetal-scalp sampling checks what the monitor patterns mean. (See Fetal-Scalp Blood Sampling," page 100.) If you hear the term *acidosis* — meaning the baby's biochemistry is abnormal due to not getting enough oxygen — there would be cause for intervention. If your baby's blood chemistry is okay, there is less urgency to intervene.

ULTRASOUND

Like EFM, ultrasound has stirred controversy both about its usefulness and its safety. And, like EFM, its use has become firmly entrenched in obstetrical practice before its

Are You "High-Risk"?

Being labeled "high-risk" is stressful enough to put a woman into that category. Despite its ominous sound, this term describes mothers or babies who have a higher than average risk of having health problems during pregnancy or birth. For example, if you have high blood pressure or high blood sugar (diabetes), you have a higher probability of having complications during pregnancy and delivery, and your baby has a greater chance of needing special care before and after delivery. Remember, the high-risk label reflects only statistical probability; it is not an absolute sentence. Which mothers should be included in the high-risk category is controversial, but the list is getting longer: too old, too young, too heavy, too light, and so on. Soon there will be no such thing as a mother who is low-risk.

Being "high-risk" means more than using high-priced medical care and a high-tech hospital. It means that you must take greater responsibility for your own care

and birth decisions, and your birth attendant must be more attentive. Perhaps a more accurate, less demeaning, and less scary term for this "condition" would be "high-responsibility" pregnancy. If you merit this tag, wear it wisely. Being high-risk doesn't mean that you must check into the nearest university hospital and follow rigid protocols. Instead of becoming a passive patient and neglecting your own role in your birth, put more effort into having a satisfying birth experience. Take even greater care in choosing your doctors and your birth team. Ask questions and make your own needs known. This birth partnership must operate at a higher level than if you were low-risk. Take care of yourself. Ask your doctor to give you specific guidelines as to what you can do to lower your risk. For example, can you control your high blood pressure with diet? Read all the suggestions in this book, and be responsible for figuring out what will work in your situation.

---

safety has been proven. Most mothers will knowingly, or unknowingly, be exposed to ultrasound in three ways during their pregnancy. First, the Doptone used to listen to baby's heartbeat during routine prenatal visits is a type of ultrasound. Second, the doctor may order an ultrasound exam to date the pregnancy, check on the position and growth of the baby and placenta, and incidentally take a picture of your baby in the womb. Third, electronic fetal monitoring uses ultrasound to detect the baby's heart-

beat. Prudent obstetricians — and informed consumers — use the risk-benefit principle when deciding to perform a test or use technology. The risk of the procedure must be weighed against the benefits. Because of the popularity of ultrasound, it is important to understand its risks and benefits.

How Ultrasound Works

The ultrasound transmitter, as its name implies, produces sound waves at frequencies higher than humans can hear. These sound waves strike their target, such as baby's heart, and the echoes bounce back to a receiver, which can translate these signals either into a picture of the baby or the sound of the baby's heartbeat. Sonogram, Doppler, scan, echo, external electronic fetal monitoring, and Doptone are all different names for ultrasound technology.

Is Ultrasound Safe?

How I answer this question depends upon what hat I am wearing. The doctor in me wants to offer a reassuring "yes, probably" (because ultrasound is a very useful diagnostic tool), but the scientist in me says, "nobody knows for sure." The problem lies in what happens when energy-containing sound waves strike growing fetal tissues. Could these waves shake up the cells so much as to produce subtle damage? Or do they bounce right off the tissues causing no harm? Scientists are divided on this issue. Some studies, done in test tubes, not on humans, show microscopic changes at the cellular levels. Some even suggest genetic changes at the intracellular level. Other studies refute these findings. Some studies on animals show that ultrasound stunts the growth and diminishes the performance of offspring, while others find no harmful effects of ultrasound. The concern lies in a basic observation that when sound waves bombard tissues at high-energy frequencies, they shake up the molecules making them hot, and produce microscopic gas bubbles in the cell, called "cavitation." Whether this heat or these bubbles damage the cell is unknown. The current attitude toward ultrasound research is comparable to concern about cancer in rats, the kind that always

makes headlines: If you give high enough doses of any chemical to enough rodents, some will get tumors.

Proponents of ultrasound reassure recipients that there are enough studies validating its safety to indicate that it is not dangerous to use as a diagnostic and monitoring tool in obstetrics. Opponents counter that because of the conflicting research, ultrasound should be used with caution. X rays were once thought to be safe for babies in the womb but were later found to be associated with childhood leukemia (although this cause-and-effect relationship is still disputed). Second-generation studies on the safety of ultrasound are not yet available, although twelve- to twenty-year follow-up studies in thousands of patients have shown no perceptible harmful effects. We may have to wait for our grandchildren to tell us if ultrasound is safe or not. In our review of the available ultrasound studies we found that the only thing that researchers seem to agree upon is that we need more research.

Is Ultrasound Useful?

Unlike electronic fetal monitoring, where the benefits are questionable, ultrasound has clearly improved the practice of obstetrics. As a diagnostic tool, ultrasound is apparently safer than X rays, gives more precise dating of baby's gestational age in early pregnancy, and detects potential risks for delivery (e.g., placenta abnormalities, multiple births, and abnormal fetal growth) that could influence how the pregnancy is managed. But there has never been a study, nor is there ever likely to be, that confirms that ultrasound improves the overall outcome of mothers and babies. Perhaps we may follow the counsel of Dr. Fredrick Frigoletto, Professor

Indications for Ultrasound

- to estimate gestational age when the mother is unsure of the date of her last menstrual period
- to evaluate a problem with fetal growth
- to determine the cause of unexplained bleeding
- to confirm the presentation (e.g., breech, transverse, vertex) of the fetus
- to confirm suspected multiples
- to assist medical or surgical procedures in correcting or detecting a fetal defect: amniocentesis, external version of breech baby, fetoscopy, intrauterine transfusion, or chorionic villi sampling
- when there is a discrepancy between uterine size and dates
- when uterine abnormalities are expected
- to detect suspected abnormalities of the placenta
- to look for spinal bifida if prenatal tests raise this worry

of Obstetrics and Gynecology at Harvard Medical School, and chairman of a 1984 National Institute of Health Task Force on diagnostic ultrasound: "We could find no evidence to justify the recommendation that every pregnancy be screened by ultrasound. In the face of even theoretical risks, where there is no benefit, then the theoretical risks cannot be justified."

Using Ultrasound Wisely

Here's what happened at our daughter-in-law's four-month visit to her obstetrician. As the doctor was about to place the Doptone (a device that uses ultrasound to record baby's heartbeat) on her abdomen to obtain fetal heart tones, she asked, "Is ultrasound safe?" "Yes," assured the doctor. "Can you guarantee it won't harm my baby?" she persisted. "Well, no I can't guarantee that, but studies seem to indicate . . ." "Then I don't want it," she said adamantly, but respectfully. In this client-doctor dialogue the mother expressed a feeling shared by all mothers — a wariness of tests that no one can guarantee are safe. Undergoing an unproven test seemed particularly unnecessary in this case, when the reason for using a Doptone was simply that it was more expedient for the doctor than the fetal stethoscope. Mothers may not realize that the Doptone used in the obstetrician's office to detect fetal heart tones emits a more concentrated beam of sound energy waves than the ultrasound scan that gives a picture of the whole baby even though the exposure to the whole baby is less.

In electronic fetal monitoring, ultrasound waves can be focused continuously on one spot on the baby for many hours at a time. While no one knows the answer to the worries about ultrasound, parents can be somewhat reassured by the fact that during an ultrasound procedure only around 1 percent of the sound waves are transmitted into your body. The other 99 percent of the energy is involved in picking up the sound waves that echo back. In Europe and Scandinavia, ultrasound is a required part of prenatal care. But in the United States nearly every lay and professional birth organization and the FDA have come out against the routine use of ultrasound without clear indications. Some doctors feel that it's good obstetrical care to do at least one ultrasound during pregnancy to avoid surprises during labor. Other obstetricians prefer to do an ultrasound only when there are signs of a problem, such as bleeding or uterine growth different from the usual pattern. In our opinion, knowing the sex of your baby or having a photo to pass around at your childbirth class is not a good enough reason to expose your baby to ultrasound, nor is the desire for "prenatal bonding" a valid indication. Commercial ultrasound "photographers" even offer color pictures of the baby in the womb. Avoid these as a curiosity. Color exposes the baby to much more ultrasound wave energy and is an example where the risk is clearly greater than the benefits. Also, if you don't want to know your baby's sex, be sure to tell your doctor or the ultrasound technician in case the photo reveals all. Oftentimes both parents and obstetricians welcome an ultrasound so they can enter the delivery room with no surprises. If the doctor advises an ultrasound and mother decides to accept one, it's important to remember that this is a partnership. The doctor should thoroughly inform the mother about why an ultrasound is necessary. The mother should understand the reasons and participate in the decision. Demand no less for yourself and your baby.

PITOCIN (Oxytocin)

Sometimes known as "pit," this labor-stimulating drug can be a help or a hindrance. As with all obstetrical interventions, ask these questions about pitocin: Is it safe for you and your baby? Is it necessary? Are there better alternatives?

The Purpose of Pit

During labor your body naturally produces a contraction-enhancing hormone called oxy-tocin. The fetus also secretes oxytocin, which passes through the placenta and contributes to the pool of hormones circulating through the mother's body. Pitocin, a synthetic version of oxytocin, is used to induce contractions or speed up a labor that is dragging. In theory, pitocin is used only when it is necessary to induce labor or stimulate stronger contractions for the sake of mother or baby's health. In practice, however, pit is used liberally as a sort of labor tonic, even though its usefulness and its safety are open to question.

The Problem with Pit

There is a time and place for everything. During natural labor your body produces oxytocin on an as-needed basis — the right dose at the right time. Oxytocin is normally produced in spurts, and both the amount of oxytocin secreted and the sensitivity of the uterus to its effects increase during labor. Artificial oxytocin — also known as a *pit drip* — is administered intravenously through an automatic infusion pump at a steady rate. Because the way the uterus receives its hormonal boost is unnatural, the contractions pit produces are different from the ones the body would produce on its own. Pit-produced contractions are stronger, longer, and closer together. This different type of contraction can be intolerable for the mother and unsafe for the baby.

Consider the effects on the baby. With normal contractions, the uterine muscle briefly constricts the blood vessels carrying oxygenated blood to the placenta, but the blood-rich reservoirs within the placenta continue to deliver oxygen to the baby during these periods of decreased uterine blood flow. During natural contractions the oxygen supply to baby may be diminished briefly, but the time when baby, in effect, holds her breath is short because the contractions are short and the interval between them is long enough for the baby to catch up on the oxygen she needs. With pit-produced contractions, however, the increased force of the contraction may decrease uterine blood flow even more, and the time between contractions may be too short to allow the reservoirs in the placenta to refill with blood. Pit-produced contractions may, therefore, result in lower delivery of oxygen to the baby. In fact, fetal distress, as detected by electronic fetal monitoring, is more common during pitocin infusion. Pit may also continue to affect the baby after birth. Jaundice, for example, has been found to occur more frequently in newborns whose mothers received pitocin during labor. Why aren't these potential problems recognized? you may wonder. They are. Why do you think labors where pitocin is used require continuous fetal monitoring?

Pitocin is also unkind to the mother. Witness the domino effect. Being attached to an intravenous line and an infusion pump confines a mother to bed. Pitocin-induced contractions are more painful, so an epidural is usually required, further limiting mother's freedom of movement. And because of the risks associated with these two interventions, a third intervention is needed to monitor the effects of the first two — continuous electronic fetal monitoring. Now mother is wired, numb, and stationary. She has lost the freedom of movement that can stimulate the release of her own natural oxytocin. Her labor stalls and the dose of pit is increased to treat the problem that should never have occurred in the first place. With increasing doses, the risks increase, and pretty soon the

---

Pit Pains

Studies show that 80 percent of laboring women found their "pit pains" were much more intense than the sensations they felt with their natural contractions. Many mothers cannot handle pitocin-induced contractions with their natural pain-easing mechanisms. Most require epidural anesthesia, as one intervention leads to another. Contractions produced by a mother's naturally occurring oxytocin come on gradually, with a slow buildup allowing mother to prepare for the contractions and muster her own coping mechanisms, which she comes to trust as the intensity of the contractions increases. On the other hand, pitocin-induced contractions may come on without warning and quickly overwhelm the mother and her ability to cope. Most women surveyed stated they would rather try alternatives to pit with their next labor.

---

mother has been "pitted" all the way to the operating room.

Alternatives to Pit

Want to avoid this pitiful scene? Consider natural ways to increase your own oxytocin. Nipple stimulation (use only with your birth attendant's advice; see page 99) and walking and moving freely during labor are do-it-yourself oxytocin inducers. Eating and drinking lightly, avoiding exhaustion, and employing a labor-support person also help set the conditions for your body's natural hormones to work. In fact, studies show that nipple stimulation and walking during labor may work as well as, or even better than, the synthetic stuff. This is where a midwife's approach to birth can help. Because midwives are not licensed to use drugs, they have learned more alternatives to pitocin. Because most obstetricians are not wise to the ways of midwifery, they are quicker to intervene with drugs. This is another situation where birthing would be better if obstetricians and midwives could labor together.

When Pit Helps

Pitocin can be helpful in some labors (approximately 5 percent), but only when safer alternatives have been tried and have failed, and when the body is not forced to handle an artificial substance for which it isn't ready. Proponents of pit have shown that it works best if you give it before the mother and her uterus are exhausted. Pitocin-users believe that there is a critical window of opportunity during which a mother's labor can effectively be set back on track with pitocin; after that, stress and exhaustion take over, and both the mother and the doctor are likely to abandon further intervention and proceed to a cesarean.

When inducing labor, pitocin works best when the uterus is ready to receive it. Throughout the pregnancy the growing uterus has been growing receptor sites — microscopic areas that become increasingly sensitive to the contraction-producing effects of oxytocin. This uterine readiness is thought to be the physiological basis for when labor is ready to begin. Giving pitocin before the uterus is sensitive enough or before the cervix is ripe enough (sometimes

a cervical softener such as prostaglandin gel is applied to an unripe cervix) is likely to produce a long drawn-out ineffective labor resulting in a cesarean birth. This scene sometimes occurs when pitocin is used for a postterm induction when the calendar says it's time for baby to come out but the uterus doesn't agree.

For a safe and satisfying birth, rather than reaching for the artificial oxytocin, it is better to create a labor environment that helps the mother make her own.

ACTIVE MANAGEMENT OF LABOR (AML)

Every birth is a managed birth, but who is doing the managing? Birth can be managed primarily by the mother by empowering her with the tools to do so (which is our philosophy in this book) or by a trusted knowledgeable birth attendant in partnership with the mother. While doing your birthing homework, you are likely to hear the term *active management of labor* (AML). You may be confused about its meaning and uncertain about how it fits in to your birth plan. Because, as some birthing experts believe, AML seems to be the obstetrical offering of the nineties, it's important that parents understand the pros and cons of this new way of birthing.

What Is an Actively Managed Labor?

In AML the obstetrician, nurses, midwife, and mother work together determinedly as a team, with the goal of helping mother's labor progress efficiently. Active management means that if a mother's labor is not progressing at a "normal" rate (the established criteria is 1- to 2-centimeter dilation per hour), rather than patiently allowing the mother's labor to set its own pace, and risk exhaustion and failure to progress, the obstetrician intervenes with artificial rupture of membranes, pitocin augmentation, and often epidural anesthesia. This concept was initiated by the National Maternity Hospital in Dublin, Ireland, in 1968 (which we recently visited), and it is becoming an increasingly popular way of handling birth.

Benefits of AML

The goal of active management is to lower the cesarean-section rate. Here is the rationale: if the uterus becomes fatigued (as any muscle can), it can stop working efficiently. When this happens, a mother's labor can stall, and she will be labeled "failure to progress." Once the uterus and the whole mother are fatigued, pitocin augmentation of labor won't work as well and mother will receive a surgical birth. Advocates of AML reason that, since augmentation of labor works better if offered early rather than when mother is already exhausted, early intervention could help a mother progress to a vaginal birth.

Proponents of this way of birth cite these advantages observed in first-time mothers in Ireland:

- shorter labors — 98 percent delivered within twelve hours of beginning AML, 40 percent within four hours (These quicker deliveries could be due to the fact that the Irish don't define a woman as actually in labor until labor is well advanced by our standards.)
- a cesarean-section rate of 5 percent
- no apparent difference in the condition of the baby

When a hospital in Houston, Texas, tried this Irish system, the average duration of labor was shortened from twelve to seven hours. Their cesarean-section rate fell from 23 percent to 10 percent. The number of cesareans for "failure to progress" was reduced by half. Fifteen percent of mothers in the Dublin study and 66 percent of mothers in the Houston study had epidurals. Large-scale experience with AML has been reported from six cities around the world, and all reports show shortened labors and fewer cesarean sections.

Risks of AML

Opponents of AML come from two sides. Studies show that AML doesn't work in American hospitals as well as it does in Ireland. Natural-birth enthusiasts dub AML a "Trojan Horse," a gift that opens the door for too much intervention and takes management of birth away from the mother. These criticisms stem from a misuse and misunderstanding of the term *active management.* AML should not be synonymous with aggressive, physician-in-control, high-tech, low-touch birthing. Nor is there any biological reason why it should work better for Irish than American women.

Ireland's system and attitude about birth are different from the prevailing ones in America. In the Dublin hospital that has the most experience and best results with AML, birth is a women-run show. In this "organized labor," all the obstetrical nurses are midwives, and most of the uncomplicated deliveries are attended by midwives with obstetricians used as consultants. This midwife-obstetrician team offers the mother the best of both professions. In addition, these mothers receive thorough prenatal education and specific preparation; they have a labor-support person continuously available to them throughout labor, and they participate fully in their birthing decisions.

We are concerned that the we-do-it-all-for-you attitude may become the "modern" way of birth, and may devalue a woman's power and trust in her body. We also fear that the so-called "stalled labors" — actually a normal, temporary plateau that many first-time mothers encounter — will be redefined as "abnormal" and in need of active management. (See "If Your Labor Stalls," page 204.) While AML is neither necessary nor desirable for most laboring mothers, it may be an alternative for mothers who might otherwise become exhausted and go on to have a cesarean for failure to progress. But ideally, the mother should be given the time, energy, and resources to keep from becoming exhausted in the first place.

Our hope is that doctor-directed births will be limited to women with special needs, and that obstetricians will focus on nourishing the natural rather than orchestrating the artificial.

EPISIOTOMY

Want to be able to sit comfortably after birth? By understanding the latest research on episiotomy (an incision made in the perineum to enlarge the vaginal opening for birth), you can protect your perineum from this unkind and usually unnecessary cut.

How Is an Episiotomy Performed?

Following injection of a local anesthetic, the stretched skin of the vagina and underlying tissues are cut approximately two inches. This cut is usually made just before crown-

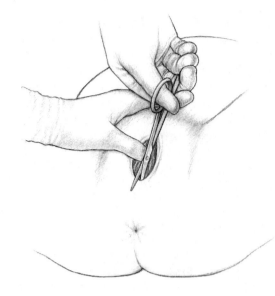

Median episiotomy

ing of the baby's head, allowing it to apply pressure on the bleeding. There are two types of incisions: In the *median incision* (see figure on this page), the preferred method in the United States, the cut is made through the connective tissue of the perineum between the vagina and the rectum. The preferred method in Europe is the *mediolateral incision,* which is made diagonally through muscle. There is less bleeding and less scar tissue formation with the median incision, and it is easier to repair, but there is more likelihood of extension of the cut into the anal tissue. This complication can be minimized by easing baby's head out and supporting the perineum just as if no episiotomy had been performed. In some situations (e.g., breech delivery and forceps rotation), the obstetrician may need to make the mediolateral incision. No matter how the incision is done, this cut is made in a type of tissue and an area of the body that is not known for easy healing.

Why Do an Episiotomy?

An episiotomy is a procedure left over from the days when women were heavily drugged and immobile during labor. They couldn't help push their babies out, and physicians often used forceps to get babies out. The episiotomy was done in order to get the forceps inside (into a place where they don't belong in the first place). Also, when women gave birth with their legs up in stirrups and speedy deliveries were the goal, the perineal tissues were more likely to tear because the perineum was not allowed to stretch gradually and evenly around the baby's head, and because the legs up in stirrups kept the perineum from relaxing. This

---

Easing Post-Episiotomy Pain

Cold packs to your perineum numb the pain and reduce swelling for the first day. The hospital nurse will then supply pads containing a soothing remedy. Also, your birth attendant or nurse will instruct you on "peri-care": squirting warm water onto the episiotomy site after urinating and sitz baths (sitting in a warm bath). Sit squarely on a soft seat. Leaning to one side puts tension on the stitches. Report increasing pain to your doctor. And keep yourself from getting constipated by drinking lots of fluids and eating well. Wait until the wound is healed to have intercourse (at least three weeks) and then go easy, use a lubricant such as K-Y Jelly, and adopt a position that lessens direct pressure from the penis on the wound. If discomfort persists, notify your health-care provider.

---

operation has become a routine part of the total birth package, even though a better understanding of how women give birth should have made it unnecessary. Consider for a moment that women's birth canals have been adequate for delivering babies since the beginning of womankind. Why should they now be too small and need surgical enlarging? As you travel east from the United States to England and on to the Netherlands, the incidence of routine episiotomy gets lower and lower, but it is unlikely that birth canals are larger in Europe.

Why, then, are episiotomies still commonly performed in the United States? The birth practices that ushered in this questionable cut still remain, and today's obstetricians concentrate more effort on improving their episiotomy technique than they do in learning ways to avoid it. And, of course, episiotomy is a surgical skill. If women didn't need episiotomies, they might not need the surgeon either.

Obstetricians justify the continued use of episiotomy by claiming that it helps mothers heal better and is safer for the baby. Too many women have accepted this surgical decision with blind faith. Here are the most common reasons given to support routine episiotomies and the latest research that counters these claims.

What You May Hear vs. What Research Shows

1. A neat straight incision heals better, and it's easier to repair than a jagged tear. The belief that a cut made by scissors heals better than a natural tear has failed the research test. It is true that a surgical cut is easier to repair than a jagged tear, but since many women suffer no tears and need no stitches at all, why cut? And any smaller tears that do occur heal more quickly and better (sometimes without any stitching) than the larger episiotomy incisions, which include more layers of muscle than most tears. In midwife language, what nature cuts, nature heals. Midwives call these little tears "skid marks." In fact, research suggests that it's better to allow a few little tears than to make one big incision. But even natural tears sometimes require stitches. Women usually heal more quickly and experience less discomfort with their own tears than with an episiotomy.

2. Without an episiotomy you run the risk of the tear extending into and damaging the rectum. There is no research supporting this worry. On the contrary, some obstetricians we have interviewed feel that episiotomies are more likely than natural tears to extend into the rectum. Even though currently available studies suffer from some design problems, which makes it difficult to draw conclusions, they do seem to suggest that episiotomy incisions are likely to tear even further and extend into the rectum, causing more long-term problems than naturally occurring tears. This makes good sense. A piece of cloth will tear more easily where it has already been cut. Experienced labor and delivery nurses and midwives can attest to the fact that most natural tears that occur are confined to a first-degree classification (involving the skin only) or occasionally extend into a second-degree classification (extending through the skin and into perineal muscle). Rarely is a third-degree tear (extending into the anal muscle) seen without an episiotomy. And a fourth-degree tear (extending through the anal muscle) is almost unheard of. In contrast, an episiotomy by definition is a second-degree cut, which frequently extends to

a third-degree and even sometimes to a fourth-degree when instruments are used on a large baby.

3. Episiotomy shortens the pushing stage of labor and this reduces the risk for your baby. True, in some mothers, episiotomies may shorten the second stage of labor by five to twenty minutes. But a shortened second stage of labor makes little difference to baby. Large studies have shown no difference in the condition of babies whether or not an episiotomy was done.

4. Episiotomy lessens your chances of long-term pelvic floor problems, such as bladder incontinence. Around 15 percent of mothers may experience some urinary incontinence following birth, but a three-year follow-up study showed no difference in problems with incontinence, whether or not the mothers had had an episiotomy. Here's where postpartum Kegel exercises can help.

5. It keeps your vagina from stretching out of shape. Nonsense. The vagina has already been stretched to its utmost. It is unlikely that cutting a few minutes off the total stretching time will make any long-term difference. If the purpose of an episiotomy is to prevent vaginal stretching, it would be done much earlier. (It is not done earlier because of the danger from excessive bleeding.) It is a myth that the doctor can cut and sew and return the vagina to "like-new" condition. But your birth attendant's management of the second stage of labor can influence your postpartum vaginal function, as can doing Kegel exercises faithfully postpartum.

6. We can't do much to keep you from tearing, so you might as well tear properly. False. The birth canal used to be viewed as a passage that was traumatized doing its job and needed fixing. When a deliberate attempt is made by the birth attendant to minimize tearing and prevent episiotomy (e.g., encouraging laboring in a vertical position, using perineal massage and support, easing out the head and shoulders, and encouraging instinctive rather than forced pushing), episiotomy is found necessary in only 10 percent of mothers. The incidence of both tearing and episiotomy has always been much lower in midwife-attended births, where more attention is paid to supporting and protecting the perineum.

In 1992 researchers published a study of seven hundred women who delivered at three university hospitals in Montreal. These mothers were randomly selected and divided into two groups. Physicians in one group were instructed to use episiotomy liberally to avoid perineal tears. Doctors in the second group were told to restrict use of episiotomy unless there was a clear medical indication, such as fetal distress. The incidence of severe tearing was much higher in the group that liberally used episiotomies. The researchers concluded that the routine use of episiotomy should be abandoned and used only when specifically indicated, such as with fetal distress. They also advised that even the use of forceps and vacuum extraction should not be absolute indications for episiotomy.

Risks of an Episiotomy

It seems that there are no benefits to routine episiotomies, but only risks. The obvious complication of this controversial cut is postpartum discomfort. Many mothers experience severe postepisiotomy pain. Mothers who were unable to sit for weeks have told us, "The episiotomy was worse than the birth!" We have noticed that even postoperative cesarean patients sometimes move around better than women who had episiotomies. There may also be problems with infection such as an abscess around the stitches or even extension of the abscess into the rectum resulting in rectal-vaginal fistula (an opening forming between the rectum and vagina). Hemorrhage is another possible complication, and a collection of blood under the suture site, called a "hematoma," may be very painful for a long time. If the episiotomy tears into the rectal muscle, the result may be dysfunction of the muscles involved in defecation. This type of tear is much less likely to occur in women whose perineum was left uncut. Finally, consider that many women report painful intercourse up to three months following an episiotomy, and a few for as long as a year. Recent studies show that women who give birth without episiotomies are able to resume sex more quickly, experience less pain during sex, and report greater sexual satisfaction.

Besides the risks to mother, an episiotomy may also be unkind to baby. Women who have postepisiotomy pain may be distracted from bonding with their newborn. This may result in a mother who doesn't look too kindly on the little person who "caused" her to be unable to sit comfortably or enjoy sex. At least knowing all these facts will help you be angry at the appropriate party.

Remember that an episiotomy is not just a little cut into trivial tissue. Many women experience pain and sexual dysfunction for several months or more after this operation. The good news is that there are ways that you can lessen your need for an episiotomy.

Negotiate with Your Obstetrician Before Birth

Perhaps you are thinking, "I'll just leave the decision up to my doctor at the moment of birth. After all, he or she should know best whether I need an episiotomy." Yes and no! Ideally, your obstetrician is the best person to make a last-minute judgment call on whether or not you need an episiotomy. But in reality, most of the time the obstetrician can't predict whether his cut or your tear will turn out better. The doctor may assume it's no big deal to you and go ahead with the cut, especially if this is your first baby and you haven't voiced a scissors-off preference ahead of time. The American College of Obstetricians and Gynecologists now discourages "routine" episiotomies. Many doctors regard episiotomy as necessary only when the baby is in distress (baby's heart rate is falling and not bouncing back to normal) and must be delivered quickly, when there is a need to use forceps, or to ease the passage of a very large baby.

Be aware that simply announcing "I don't want an unnecessary episiotomy" is not enough to keep you from having a cut. You must do your part by using the episiotomy-sparing suggestions mentioned below and by discussing the subject with your birth attendant ahead of time. The issue is not just episiotomy — it's the management of the whole second stage of labor. If, as part of your birth plan negotiation with your doctor, you specify an ambulatory first stage, a squatting second stage, a vertical position for the birth, patient-controlled pushing (with instructions from your birth attendant on when to stop pushing), and no stirrups, you are less likely to end up with an episiotomy.

Be Kind to Your Perineum

Normally, with patient-controlled instinctive pushing, the birth canal tissues fan out in response to baby's slowly descending head. But pushing too often and too hard (because the attendants are urgently shouting "push, *push*") is likely to jam the head against these tissues before they are ready. In our classes we use the coat sleeve analogy. Before putting your arm through a lined coat sleeve, if you take the time to straighten the sleeve, smooth the lining, and ease your arm through gently, you meet less resistance. But if you try to shove your arm through, you're likely to meet more resistance from the puckered-up lining. And if you persist forcefully, you are likely to tear the lining. Specifically, there are three ways you can lower your chances of needing an episiotomy:

- Use all the birth tools discussed in chapters 9 and 10 to help your birth progress normally, namely, relaxation techniques, ambulatory labor, squatting, and vertical or side-lying birthing. These measures lessen your need for instrument assistance and therefore an episiotomy. You'll put less strain on the perineal tissues at the critical moments of maximum stretching if you avoid the "legs up in stirrups" position.

- Perineal massage before labor and during the second stage prepares the tissues, making them more likely to stretch without injury. (See "Perineal Massage," page 93.) Rather than sitting with scissors in hand,

Perineal Massage

The better you prepare your perineal tissues for the stretching of birth, the less they will tear, and the better they will heal. Like training muscles to perform at their best in an athletic event, conditioning the tissues around the vaginal opening with massage prepares the perineum to perform. Midwives report that women who practice perineal massage daily in the last six weeks of pregnancy experience less stinging sensation during crowning. Mothers with a more conditioned perineum are less likely to tear or get an episiotomy. An added value of perineal massage is that it familiarizes a woman with stretching sensations in this area so she will more easily relax these stretching muscles when stinging occurs just before the moment of birth.

Try this technique:

- Scrub your hands and trim your thumb nails. Sit in a warm comfortable area, spreading your legs apart in a semisitting birthing position. To become familiar with your perineal area use a mirror for the first few massages (a floor-to-ceiling mirror works best). Use a massage oil, such as pure vegetable oil, or a water-soluble lubricant, such as K-Y Jelly (not a petroleum-based oil) on your fingers and thumbs and around your perineum.

- Insert your thumbs as deeply as you can inside your vagina and spread your legs. Press the perineal area down toward the rectum and toward the sides. Gently continue to stretch this opening until you feel a slight burning or tingling.

- Hold this stretch until the tingling subsides and gently massage the lower part of the vaginal canal back and forth.

- While massaging, hook your thumbs onto the sides of the vaginal canal and gently pull these tissues forward, as your baby's head will do during delivery.

- Finally, massage the tissues between thumb and forefinger back and forth for about a minute.

- Being too vigorous could cause bruising or swelling in these sensitive tissues. During the massage avoid pressure on the urethra as this could induce irritation or infection.

- As you become adept with this procedure, add Kegel exercises (see page 62) to your routine to help you get a feel for your pelvic muscles. Do this ritual daily beginning around week 34 of pregnancy.

- Many midwives and obstetricians believe that perineal massage is neither useful nor necessary as long as the mother's perineum is properly supported during crowning, her pushing is properly timed, and baby's head and shoulders are slowly eased out. Discuss the value of perineal massage with your birth attendant.

birth attendants can assist the perineum's stretching by a kind of sweeping movement with fingers, gently pulling the tissues, drawing the perineum outward as the baby's head approaches, a maneuver called "ironing."

- Controlling your pushing is the best tool you have to prevent an episiotomy. Long, hard, straining pushes ("purple pushing") are likely to tear the muscles; shorter, more gradual, gentler bearing down will stretch them. Pushing the way it comes naturally to you rather than pushing on command is easier on the perineum. And it's important to know when not to push. Once you feel the burning sensation that goes along with crowning, let up on your bearing down. Obstetricians who don't push pushing, instruct the labor staff not to say "push," and tell the mother when to blow or pant with her mouth open to keep from pushing have well-reduced episiotomy rates. Doing Kegel exercises consistently (page 62) may add to your control in easing the baby out.

- Do not accept a local anesthetic in your perineum "just in case I need to cut." Doctors, thinking they are sparing you potential discomfort, will inject local anesthesia between the various layers of tissue in your perineum before, or as, your baby crowns. This fluid in the tissue interferes with the natural stretching process, so that when the head stretches the tissue, it splits like a watermelon does when it's dropped. Even if a last-second episiotomy is done, the pressure of the head against the perineum renders it numb, so it is not painful to the mother.

SCREENING TESTS FOR BIRTH DEFECTS

Sometime between fourteen and eighteen weeks of your pregnancy your doctor may suggest that you have a blood test to screen for possible birth defects. The purpose of prenatal screening tests is to give you information so that you could terminate the pregnancy if there is a problem, if this choice is acceptable to you. If it isn't, there may be no need to have the test.

The Alpha-Feto Protein (AFP) Screen

The AFP screen is the most frequently used prenatal test. The main problem with it is that there is a high incidence of false positives, meaning the test suggests a problem when there actually isn't one. There may also be some false negatives, meaning that the test misses defects that may be present. And women spend weeks of needless anxiety waiting for the results instead of enjoying this precious time of pregnancy. Because of these concerns, here is what a wise consumer should know about AFP.

What's it for? AFP is a natural chemical produced by the baby's liver. It enters the mother's bloodstream via the amniotic fluid and placenta. The amount of AFP in the blood increases as the baby grows. AFP levels are elevated in babies with neural tube defects (NTD), because this substance leaks out of an open spinal cord. They are also high in multiple pregnancies. AFP levels are low in babies with Down syndrome. This test is most accurate if performed between sixteen and eighteen weeks. Results of the test are available within one week. The AFP detects only open neural tube defects in which spinal fluid leaks out. AFP is not elevated in closed spinal defects (e.g., meningomyelocele or hydrocephaly). A newer test, called the *triple screen* (also known as the prenatal risk profile) measures AFP, HCG (human chorionic gonadotropin), and estriol. It is more accurate in detecting Down syndrome than the AFP alone, which detects about one in five babies with Down syndrome. Even the triple screen may miss 20–30 percent of Down syndrome babies in women over age thirty-five, and 40 percent in women under thirty-five. Some states require that the AFP test be offered to pregnant women. We in no way endorse this kind of testing and include it only to be complete. Our seventh child, Stephen, has Down syndrome (which we did not know about because we did not have AFP or triple screen). He is a wonderful child, accepted by all who know him, and responsible for much personal growth and maturity in each member of our family. As with any challenge, our lives have become richer because of the birth of Stephen.

What to consider. We believe that there are a lot of problems with the AFP. Spinal defects are rare (1–2 per 1,000 births); many babies with a spinal defect miscarry. A meaningful AFP result depends on accurate dating of the pregnancy. Not only is the AFP seldom useful, but it also may lead to more unnecessary and expensive tests. An abnormal AFP usually requires further investigation by ultrasound and/or amniocentesis, and 98 percent of "positive high" or "positive low" AFPs turn out to be false positive (the baby has neither Down syndrome nor a spinal defect).

Consider the following example: One thousand mothers have the AFP screening test to detect one or two babies with NTD. Around 3 percent (thirty) of these mothers show high AFP. All thirty of these women are subjected to an ultrasound test to establish whether or not their babies have a spinal cord defect or if there is another

explanation for the elevated AFP, such as twins or incorrect dates. But in approximately half of these women, ultrasound does not provide enough information, so fifteen of these mothers have to have amniocentesis, which may finally detect one baby with NTD. But what about the risk of the amniocentesis to the fourteen normal babies? Amniocentesis carries a risk of miscarriage of approximately one in two hundred. This translates into the concerning fact that approximately one normal baby could be killed in the process of detecting thirteen babies with a spinal defect. The AFP test is a classic example of the search-and-destroy bureaucrats going too far. Prenatal screening programs are the product of bureaucratic board rooms where decisions are made with regard to their overall impact on society, not on their risk or benefit to the individual woman. We question the wisdom of the AFP test.

The following are some other common tests that you are likely to encounter during your pregnancy and birth. Try to avoid being overtested, lest you spend more time waiting for the outcome of the tests than anticipating your baby. Participate in the decision to have a specific test. Ask why this test is necessary for *your* pregnancy. "It's routine" is not an acceptable answer. Also, inquire whether the same information could be obtained in a less invasive way. Remember the big three questions: Is it safe for you and your baby? Is it necessary? Are there alternatives?

Test (Pregnancy Stage)	What It's For	Considerations
Chorionic Villus Sampling (CVS) (8–11 weeks)	Using ultrasound guidance, a catheter is inserted through the vagina and cervix and into the uterus near where the placenta is forming. A tiny sample of tissue is taken from the chorionic villi, which are fingerlike projections of tissue that surround the baby in the early weeks and ultimately form the placenta.	This sample provides the same information as obtained with amniocentesis. CVS has advantages over amniocentesis: it can be performed earlier in pregnancy (8–11 weeks) and the results are available in 1–2 weeks. Although providing information earlier in pregnancy, CVS carries a much higher risk of damage to the baby than amniocentesis. Depending on the expertise of the physician, CVS has a miscarriage risk 2–4 times that of amniocentesis, and studies suggest a possible increased risk of limb deformities. There is also a risk that CVS may cause a decrease in amniotic fluid production. These risks vary with the level of skill of the individual specialist. Also, false positives are more likely with CVS (suggesting the baby is not normal when in fact he or she is), because the cells in the chorionic villi may not contain the same material as those in the baby. Considering these added risks and added expense, most parents and physicians do not choose CVS over amniocentesis.
Amniocentesis (12–16 weeks)	After a local anesthetic numbs the skin and under guidance by ultrasound, the doctor inserts a long needle through the abdomen into the uterus and obtains some amniotic fluid, which contains fetal urine, cells from baby's skin, and some metabolic chemicals. Usually performed 12–16 weeks after gestation, this fluid can provide genetic and biochemical information about the baby. Results are available in 2–4 weeks. Amniocentesis is used to determine the sex of the baby, detect chromosomal abnormalities such as Down syndrome, and some hereditary diseases. Later in pregnancy it is also used to monitor severity of Rh-blood disease; it is valuable in assessing maturity of fetal lungs by measuring the amount of the special chemicals that keep baby's lungs open for breathing. This measurement determines whether or not baby's lungs are mature enough to survive a preterm delivery.	Amniocentesis is generally safe but it is not without risk. Ultrasound guidance reduces the risk of injury to the placenta or baby. There is a 0.5 percent chance of causing a miscarriage by this procedure. For women under age 35, the risk of miscarriage from the amniocentesis may be greater than the chance of having a baby with Down syndrome. Ask your doctor what his or her rate of postamniocentesis miscarriage is. If the doctor seems vague in answering this question, ask if he or she does enough "amnios" to be skillful, or ask to be referred to a specialist. Don't be offended if your doctor advises an amniocentesis. If you will be 35 years of age or older at your due date, the doctor is legally obligated to offer this procedure.

Test (Pregnancy Stage) (cont.)	What It's For (cont.)	Considerations (cont.)
Glucose Tolerance Test (GTT) (24–28 weeks)	The hormones of pregnancy normally suppress insulin release, allowing a mother's blood sugar to be higher during pregnancy, thus providing more glucose to nourish her fetus. This is why many women normally spill some sugar into their urine occasionally during pregnancy. In a small percentage of pregnant women (2–10 percent) the blood sugar is too high throughout part of pregnancy — a temporary condition called *gestational glucose intolerance* (a less alarming and more accurate term than *gestational diabetes*). Long exposure to this high blood sugar causes the infant to grow excessively large, resulting in more birth complications, such as prematurity and respiratory problems. Or, in response to the high blood sugar, baby may manufacture too much of his or her own insulin, causing the baby's blood sugar to drop quickly and dangerously immediately after birth. By identifying this condition during pregnancy, the mother can alter her diet to keep her blood sugar from getting too high. Gestational glucose intolerance is more common in obese women, older mothers, those with a family history of diabetes, or women who have previously delivered a baby weighing more than 9 pounds.	The GTT is usually recommended at 24–28 weeks and repeated around 32–34 weeks in high-risk mothers. The woman drinks a sweet liquid called *glucola*, and her blood sugar is checked 1 hour later. If the 1-hour screening test turns out to be positive, the doctor may recommend a more accurate 3-hour test. Only around 15 percent of women with an abnormal 1-hour GTT will have an abnormal 3-hour test. If the 3-hour test is abnormal, the doctor may recommend a diabetic diet throughout the rest of pregnancy. An alternative is to measure the blood sugar 1–2 hours after a heavy meal. The results of the GTT should be available within a few hours. After ingesting the test "meal," stay active (walking, moving about the place, etc.) so your body has a better chance of metabolizing the sugar load than if you just sit there waiting to have your blood drawn. New research questions the value of routine screening for gestational glucose intolerance. A 1990 study of 1,307 women (533 of whom were not screened and 774 who were screened) showed that screening resulted in more tests and worry during pregnancy and a significantly higher cesarean rate in the screened mothers, but it did not decrease the rate of large infants. We question the physiologic wisdom of the GTT. Pregnant women seldom drink a 50-gram slug of glucose solution on an empty stomach. This is unnatural eating; therefore, would the test show unnatural results?
Fetal Movement Counting (late pregnancy–early labor)	This simple exercise is a do-it-yourself test of fetal well-being sometimes advised in high-risk pregnancies. Also known as the "kick count," this test is based on the belief that an active baby is a healthy baby. Set aside a few minutes at the same time each day to count your baby's movements. A good time is after the evening meal when you are relaxed. Keep a daily record, beginning timing with the first	Counting fetal movements is a way to help you get a feel for your baby in the womb. It helps you get to know your baby's normal activity patterns. However, because babies' movements in the womb are as variable as their personalities, changes in fetal activity levels may be normal, and the test may be only a cause of needless anxiety. Remember, a kick count is only a screening test, and definitive tests

Test (Pregnancy Stage) (cont.)	What It's For (cont.)	Considerations (cont.)
Fetal Movement Counting (late pregnancy–early labor) (cont.)	movement and recording how long it takes to feel ten movements (hiccups don't count). Notify your doctor if each day you notice less and less fetal movement, if your baby is taking progressively longer to reach ten moves, if there is a sudden burst of fetal movements, or if you have not noticed fetal activity for twelve hours.	are needed before intervention is indicated. **Sample chart of fetal movements** Date: Starting Time: Movements: Time of Tenth Movement: Total Time:
Nonstress Test (NST) (at or near term)	Despite its name, no test is without stress to a pregnant mother. But this test is without risk, and, with the exception of the kick count, it is the simplest and least expensive of all tests of fetal well-being. The NST is based on the observation that the heart rate of a healthy baby accelerates by about fifteen beats per minute for fifteen seconds when the baby moves unless he or she is being deprived of oxygen. While mother is sitting, an ultrasound electronic fetal monitor is placed across her abdomen, and the baby's heart rate is recorded. The doctor asks the mother to signal when she feels the baby move, and the change in fetal heart rate during movement is observed on the monitor. When two increases in fetal heart-rate patterns are noticed during a 20-minute test period, the NST is considered normal or reactive. When no significant increase in heart rate is noted during a 40-minute test period the NST is considered abnormal or nonreactive.	The NST is most accurate when the pregnancy is near term and is most often used either in a high-risk pregnancy or to assess fetal well-being postterm. A reactive NST correlates well with a healthy infant, but more than 75 percent of the time a nonreactive NST is a false alarm. Baby may be sleeping, and more often than not, when the test is repeated later in the day, it is normal or reactive. If the NST is nonreactive on repeated testing, the obstetrician may wish to perform a CST (see below) to assess further fetal well-being.
Biophysical Profile (BPP) (at or near term)	This 40-minute procedure performed in the doctor's office combines the nonstress test with other ultrasound assessments of fetal well-being: reactive heartbeat, breathing movements, muscle tone of limbs, movement of body, and quantity of amniotic fluid. As in an Apgar score, the baby gets 0–2 points for each of these five components. A high score (8–10) suggests the baby is all right, and the doctor may monitor baby by repeating the BPP once or twice weekly. A low score (0–2) suggests baby's intrauterine well-being is in jeopardy, and the doctor will advise immediate delivery.	The BPP is used to monitor high-risk mothers (e.g., mothers with insulin-dependent diabetes or high blood pressure) during the last few weeks of pregnancy. It is also used for monitoring postterm pregnancies. High scores and low scores are relatively accurate predictors of the health of the baby. But intermediate scores (3–6) are more difficult to interpret. While the BPP is open to some subjective interpretation, it is a relatively risk-free and useful test for monitoring the sufficiency of baby's intrauterine environment.

Test (Pregnancy Stage) (cont.)	What It's For (cont.)	Considerations (cont.)
Contraction Stress Test (CST) (at or near term)	The CST is a tiny test dose of labor that assesses whether or not the baby is able to tolerate the stress of contractions. While the baby's heartbeat is electronically monitored by ultrasound, uterine contractions are stimulated, either artificially by intravenous pitocin or naturally by nipple stimulation. A negative, or reassuring, CST means that during three normal contractions baby's heart-rate patterns remained normal on the electronic fetal monitor. A positive, or nonreassuring, CST means that baby's heart-rate patterns were abnormal during or following a contraction. The infant may not be receiving adequate oxygen during contractions, and it may be dangerous to expose the infant to the prolonged contractions of real labor. The CST usually takes several hours to complete, is usually done in a hospital, and is reliable only in the last few weeks of pregnancy.	This test is usually done if the nonstress test is abnormal. The obstetrican uses the CST to determine if it is in the best interest of mother and baby to continue the pregnancy to term or if it would be wiser to deliver the baby surgically before labor begins. Because the CST may trigger labor, it is not done in situations in which induction of labor could cause problems, such as preterm, placenta previa, prematurely ruptured membranes, or multiple pregnancies. Mothers may prefer to use nipple stimulation to release their own natural oxytocin rather than submit their baby to the stress of artificial contractions from intravenous pitocin. One study showed that applying a warm towel to both breasts for 5 minutes or massaging one nipple for 10 minutes achieved adequate uterine contractions in 30 minutes or less in 76 percent of 300 patients tested. The study also showed that nipple stimulation and pitocin were equally reliable. Nipple stimulation is easier, less expensive, and faster than pitocin. Instead of continuous nipple stimulation, a mother can stimulate her nipples intermittently by gently stroking the nipple of one breast with the pads of her fingertips through her clothing for 2 minutes and then stopping for 5 minutes. CST has a high incidence of "equivocals" and false positives (the test suggests that the baby is jeopardized during contractions when he or she really is not). For this reason, a positive CST does not always mean a baby must be delivered immediately by cesarean section. Rather, it alerts the birth attendant to monitor baby more closely during labor and intervene if there are definite signs of fetal distress.
X-ray Pelvimetry and/or Fetal-Pelvic Index (prelabor or labor)	Using a series of X rays the radiologist measures various dimensions of the pelvic passage to determine if it is large enough for baby to pass through safely. These measurements are compared with tables of "normals." Pelvimetry studies are often performed on a	X-ray pelvimetry is gradually being used less frequently because of concerns about its safety and accuracy. There are studies linking exposure of the fetus to X rays with increased odds of developing childhood cancers. Because the methodology of the studies showing

Test (Pregnancy Stage) (cont.)	What It's For (cont.)	Considerations (cont.)
X-ray Pelvimetry and/or Fetal-Pelvic Index (prelabor or labor) (cont.)	mother whose baby is failing to descend during labor, if vaginal delivery is being contemplated for a baby in a breech position, or if the mother has had a previous history of difficult birth because of presumed cephalopelvic disproportion (CPD). A newer technique, called a *fetal-pelvic index* (FPI), measures both the size of the pelvis by X ray and the size of the baby by ultrasound. And it considers the size of the whole baby, not just the head. The FPI is very useful in screening mothers desiring a VBAC but who have had a previous diagnosis of CPD based on X rays. This test is also helpful in screening for the advisability of attempting a vaginal breech delivery.	a possible link is flawed and conflicting studies exist, the question of whether or not exposure to X rays increases a baby's risk of cancer later in childhood is still unanswered. Not only is the safety of X-ray pelvimetry open to question, so is its accuracy. X-ray pelvimetry is done when a mother is lying still. Labor is a dynamic process, and studies have shown that in certain positions, such as squatting, the size of the pelvic outlet may increase as much as 20 percent. Also, there are two variables to consider: the passage and the passenger. X-ray pelvimetry measures only the passage. A large baby may not fit through a small passage, but a smaller baby might. Also, the baby twists and turns so many ways during the pelvic journey that it is impossible to measure every possible angle that the baby will have to pass through. Consider the analogy of trying to fit a table through a doorway. If you measured the dimensions of the doorway and the table, you might conclude that it would be impossible to fit the table through. But if you experimented and turned the table this way and that, it might pass through quite safely, especially if the doorway and the table could change sizes. Recent studies claim that the FPI is 90 percent accurate in predicting whether or not a vaginal delivery would be successful. But don't lose confidence in your pelvis and schedule cesarean delivery based on test numbers alone. Both your pelvis and your baby's head change contour during birth, a biologic fact that machines don't account for. Remember, cesarean birth has its own set of risks.
Fetal-Scalp Blood Sampling (during labor)	Sometimes it is uncertain whether a concerning pattern on the electronic fetal monitor is a false alarm or if the baby truly is not getting enough oxygen. Taking a sample of baby's blood answers this question. After the membranes have ruptured, the doctor inserts a thin tube through the vagina and cervix and places it	Sampling baby's blood takes the guesswork out of interpreting the EFM printout and keeps the doctor from jumping to conclusions and intervening unnecessarily on the basis of an EFM pattern only. Some obstetric departments have a blood-oxygen analyzer right near the labor room so that a result is available

Test (Pregnancy Stage) (cont.)	What It's For (cont.)	Considerations (cont.)
Fetal-Scalp Blood Sampling (during labor) (cont.)	against the baby's scalp. A tiny incision is made in the scalp, and a blood sample is drawn. If the oxygen concentration in this sample is normal everyone can be reassured that the baby is all right.	within a few minutes; otherwise it may take as long as 20 minutes to obtain the result. The longer the time span between sampling and getting the result, the less valuable the test in deciding whether or not to intervene.
Amniotic Fluid Volume (AFV) (prelabor or labor)	Amniotic fluid in intact membranes is useful to provide a cushion for baby, allow fetal movement, help the lungs develop, stabilize baby's temperature, and provide a barrier against infection. This fluid comes from two sources: mother and baby. Some comes from mother's serum and baby contributes to the fluid by the secretions from kidneys and lungs. Much of the amniotic fluid is actually fetal urine. In the last month of pregnancy, fetal urine may contribute as much as one ounce per hour to the amniotic fluid. In the final weeks of pregnancy, the amniotic fluid volume normally diminishes.	The volume of amniotic fluid is kept in balance by constant production and absorption. If this balance is upset, either excessive fluid (polyhydramnios) or insufficient fluid (oligohydramnios) results. Either of these conditions means a possible problem in fetal well-being. For example, too little fluid may mean baby's kidneys are not working to produce enough urine. A rapidly falling AFV may be a worry near term, alerting the obstetrician to consider induction if other indications of fetal well-being are also compromised. However, since AFV determination by ultrasound is not precise, and because there are so many factors affecting AFV, this test alone should not influence obstetrical intervention.
Amnioinfusion (prelabor or labor)	In situations in which the membranes have ruptured and/or the amniotic fluid volume is insufficient to maintain the health of the baby, the doctor can inject normal saline into the amniotic cavity in a technique similar to amniocentesis (see above). The purpose of intrauterine saline amnioinfusion is to correct the insufficient volume of amniotic fluid — a condition that makes the cord more vulnerable to compression during uterine contractions. This procedure is used for a variety of obstetrical reasons, such as fetal distress during labor, premature rupture of membranes, meconium aspiration, insufficient amniotic fluid volume (called oligohydramnios), and intrauterine growth retardation complicated by low amniotic fluid volume.	Amnioinfusion is an alternative to immediate cesarean section for fetal distress. Studies have shown that using amnioinfusion in labors exhibiting fetal distress dramatically lowers the incidence of fetal distress as detected by electronic fetal monitoring and lowers the C-section rate for fetal distress.

Cesarean Births

LEGEND HAS IT THAT Julius Caesar came into the world through an abdominal incision, giving rise to the term *cesarean*. But since no mother in those days survived this operation, yet history shows that Mrs. Caesar lived on after the birth of her son, any connection between the term and Julius must be false. More likely the term came from the 715 B.C. Roman *lex caesarea,* a law that required abdominal surgery to remove the baby from a dead or dying mother. Another possible explanation is that the word "cesarean" derives from two Latin words, *caedere* and *secare,* both meaning "to cut." Since in the United States currently around one in four babies is born by cesarean, it's important for a pregnant woman to learn how to avoid an unnecessary surgical birth.

WHY SO MANY CESAREANS?

Is there a cesarean epidemic? Yes! Can it be stopped? Yes! In 1970 5 percent of American births were surgical, and the rate has been climbing in surges at an average of 1 percent a year each year since. By 1990 it reached 25–30 percent as nearly one million mothers birthed their babies through an abdominal incision. The United States leads all industrialized countries in the rate of abdominal births. We cannot medically justify these technological "improvements on nature." The increase in cesarean births has not yielded a corresponding improvement in mortality rates for mothers and babies, nor has there been an improvement in the health of new mothers and babies. The women most likely to have a surgical birth are private, rather than clinic, patients, have private insurance, have higher levels of education, and are married, older, and richer — just the group one would imagine would be healthier and better prepared for birth.

In most European countries the cesarean rate is 5–10 percent. It is unlikely that the uteruses of European women work better than their American counterparts. Are European women more birth-savvy than American women? Probably not, since prepared-childbirth classes are an indispensable part of the American birth package (although much of what is taught is superficial). There's only one factor that determines the high rate of U.S. surgical births: *our birthing practices.* Fortunately, that's the one factor that is most within women's power to change.

Interference with nature is the most common and most correctable malady to infect American birth practices. American hospitals make use of I.V.s and monitors, which require stationary laboring, drugs that speed labor up and drugs that slow it down, and epidurals, which promise a pain-free birth but make it difficult for the mother to take an active role. While this new obstetrics may be baby-saving in a few instances, mothers often pay a high surgical price.

The notion of the "premium baby" is another factor leading physicians to advise and parents to agree to a surgical birth. Several decades ago obstetrics was recognized as a science of risks. While nature is satisfactory, it is not perfect, and both doctors and parents accepted the uncomfortable fact that occasionally a birth would have a less-than-perfect outcome. There was no guarantee of a perfect baby. While there are still no guarantees, physicians and parents now share the belief that the more you intervene, the better for the baby. We test, measure, invade, monitor, and try to control every aspect of pregnancy and delivery, and we intervene if birth doesn't go exactly according to a predetermined timetable. Also, with parents having fewer babies and having them later in life, they don't want to take any chances that something might go wrong. Besides, everyone regards a C-section as a safe procedure, so why take chances? Many doctors and parents seem comfortable with this attitude.

Fear of malpractice is another contributing factor to the cesarean epidemic. A 1993 study showed that the greater the number of malpractice suits in a given area, the greater the number of C-sections in that area. If a doctor "did everything," including

a section, and the baby was still less than perfect, the jury is less likely to find the doctor at fault than if he or she claims to have "acted in my best medical judgment" and not done a section. Obstetricians we have interviewed believe that the number of surgical births could be cut in half if this courtroom cloud were not hanging over every obstetrician attending a laboring mother. The fear that "the only cesarean I'll be sued for is the one I don't do" is a powerful force that scars women's bodies and memories and drives up the cost of medical care.

Could making more money be a factor in devaluing vaginal birth? Having been around the surgical birth scene for a long time, we honestly believe that financial incentives play a minor role, if any, in most surgical birth decisions. It is a tempting thought, especially if you consider that "time is money." Consider these two births. A mother desiring a VBAC enters the hospital at 3:00 A.M. following a call to her doctor. After a series of checks by her doctor, several management decisions, and multiple phone calls she is still laboring. It's 2:00 A.M. the following morning and she finally delivers, after 24 hours of intense labor on her part and labor-intensive care from her doctor. This same mom could have had a scheduled cesarean at 8:00 A.M. According to this scenario, the doctor is finished at 9:00 A.M., no sleep is lost, and he is in time for his office appointments. Or they could have decided to do the section midway through labor, perhaps because of "failure to progress." This action saves the doctor many hours of hanging around the hospital. It means less wear and tear on the doctor. Plus, the doctor is $500 and the hospital $3,000 richer with no questions asked by the insurance company.

The savior complex may be a final reason

for the rising number of cesareans. Normal, uncomplicated labors can be long, tedious, inconvenient, and possibly downright boring — not at all worth the long, grueling years of honing one's surgical skills. After the birth is over, what credit can the doctor take? The mother did the work and she gets the glory, rightfully so. The doctor gets a handshake, possibly a cigar. But when there's a glimmer of something going wrong, the doctor feels needed and powerful. The baby is snatched from the brink of damage within minutes after the monitor sounds the alarm. Another baby saved! All those skills used and justified. After birth, while a drugged, numb mother is in the recovery

---

Labor For a While Before Your Cesarean

You may think, "Why should I go through all that work and pain if I'm going to have a cesarean anyway?" While it may be inconvenient for the hospital or the doctor, it is often medically beneficial for your baby if you labor as long as possible before an elective cesarean. Besides indicating that baby is ready to be born, some precesarean contractions let the baby benefit from the natural hormones of labor (see "Endorphins, the Body's Natural Narcotic," page 138). Studies show that babies delivered by cesarean after mothers labor a while have fewer breathing problems in the first few days after birth than babies whose mothers were not in labor. Labor prepares baby for changes that are coming rather than being snatched from his nest without warning.

---

room, without the immediate reward of her baby, the doctor gets a hearty round of congratulations and thanks.

WHAT HAPPENS IN A SURGICAL BIRTH?

It's best to enter birth prepared for surprises; often you'll get them. Be prepared to do everything possible to deliver your baby vaginally, but also be well informed about what to expect should a cesarean birth be medically necessary. The more you understand surgical procedures, the less you will fear them, and, though you may not have the birth you wanted, there are ways to make the best of it. This is why in our section on birth plans (see chapter 13) we advise parents to work out an alternative plan for a surgical birth, in case you are part of the 6 percent who truly need one.

Before the Birth

Depending on the urgency of the situation, expect the following procedures to occur prior to your surgery. The obstetrician will explain to you why he or she thinks a cesarean is necessary. Parents should participate in the decision making in order to be assured in their own minds that a surgical birth is necessary for the health of the mother or baby. Be sure that a vaginal birth is either impossible or unsafe and that there are no other alternatives still to be tried; knowing that the cesarean is necessary increases your chances of having no regrets later. Next the nurse will shave your abdomen and the upper pubic hair. An intravenous line will be placed in your arm to keep you adequately hydrated prior to and during the surgery and as a site to give medications that may be needed. To keep your bladder empty so that it is not injured during surgery, a urinary catheter will be inserted. Because of the possibility of nausea, vomiting, or the sudden need for a general anesthetic, you will not be allowed to eat or drink for a few hours before surgery. Also expect some preoperative medications that diminish the likelihood of complications from the anesthetic. It may be routine to leave an external or internal fetal monitor running during the preoperative period until the surgeon is ready to make the incision.

Choosing Your Anesthesia

Two kinds of anesthesia are available to you: *general anesthesia,* in which inhaled gas puts you quickly to sleep; and *regional anesthesia,* either spinal or epidural, in which the doctor injects an anesthetic around your spinal column numbing you from lower ribs to toes. (See pages 170–181 for a description of the procedure and for feelings associated with epidural anesthesia.) You will have an opportunity to discuss these choices and their potential risks with the anesthesiologist before surgery. Be sure to alert this doctor to any allergies you have to medications, previous reactions to anesthetics, or any other medical problems. He or she should ask you about these issues.

General anesthesia, usually reserved for emergency cesarean, has disadvantages for you and your baby. You are asleep during one of the high points of your life, and the same medication that puts you to sleep may depress baby, necessitating some temporary breathing assistance after delivery. Compared with an epidural, spinal anesthesia is technically easier, takes effect quicker, and may give more complete anesthesia, but complications such as headache and

decrease in blood pressure are more frequent.

A benefit of epidural analgesia is that you can have regional pain control immediately postpartum. Before you leave the operating room, the anesthesiologist can inject a long-acting morphine pain reliever into your epidural tubing. This analgesic lasts 24 hours and relieves postoperative pain without the groggy, drugged feeling you get from pain medications injected intravenously or into your muscles. Feeling less pain helps you get moving and into mothering sooner. After the epidural analgesic wears off, you can take pain pills that won't interfere with breastfeeding.

Except in emergencies, epidural anesthesia is the anesthetic of choice. You will be awake during the procedure and aware of what's happening as you see your baby being lifted out. Expect to sense the pulling and tugging of delivery but not to feel the cutting.

A cesarean delivery is an operation, but it is also a birth, and it should be attended to not just with safety and efficiency, but also with dignity and wonder. By going over your surgical birth plan with your doctor prior to delivery you can help to make it this way.

Expect five professionals around your delivery table: two surgeons, a pediatrician, a surgical nurse, and an anesthesiologist. Other people present at the birth will be the circulating nurse and a nurse who helps the pediatrician care for the newborn. The circulating nurse scrubs your abdomen with an antiseptic solution and covers you with sterile drapes. The baby's father usually sits alongside the anesthesiologist at the head of the table holding your hand during delivery and giving emotional support. Before the incision is made, your surgeon will do a few test pokes and ask if you feel anything. It is common to shiver and feel nauseated and anxious for a few minutes as the anesthetic takes effect. Communicate your feelings to the anesthesiologist, who can administer remedies for your discomfort.

During the Birth

By now you and your partner may not only be worried about your baby, but also may be feeling overwhelmed with all the theatrics surrounding a surgical birth. Try to focus more on the birth and the baby than on the operation. Don't be dismayed by the casual atmosphere and the joking that helps to keep all players in the drama relaxed. As one surgeon reassured a curious father, "When we're *not* joking is when you need to worry." Underneath this banter, there is a serious side, and an aura of surgical efficiency prevails. This is the time to relax and anticipate the big moment to come. The surgeon makes a horizontal incision, called a "bikini cut," just above your pubic bone, and a similar incision into the lower part of your uterus. This type of incision leaves a scar that is often hidden in a skin crease or partially covered by pubic hair, and the low transverse incision heals well, with a strong scar safe for future vaginal births. In addition to a scalpel, much of the cutting is done with an electric knife, which zaps its way through the skin, producing a buzzing sound. As your uterus is opened, expect to hear a swooshing sound as the amniotic fluid is suctioned.

You may request it or the doctor may offer to lower (but not remove entirely) the drape placed between you and the operating area so that you can view your baby's birth directly or through a mirror. Here you may sense pushing and tugging as the doctors ease baby from his or her home. Baby is lifted out and up so that you can see your newborn held above the mound of blue-green drapes and surrounded by the crowd of capped, gowned, and masked persons. The entire procedure from first incision to baby-viewing takes only five to ten minutes. After the obstetrician suctions excess mucus from baby's mouth and nose, the doctor hands baby to the pediatrician, who whisks the infant onto a warming table. More suctioning of mucus, a whiff of oxygen, and a vigorous back massage may be needed to jump-start baby's breathing since he did not have the stimulation of squeezing through the birth canal. Some babies already release their first protest cry as they are being lifted out of the uterus.

After "all systems are working" and baby is warm, the pediatrician or nurse will wrap your baby snugly and bring him or her over to you to hold. Though it may feel clumsy, you can put one arm around your baby and nestle cheek to cheek while your partner lays a supporting hand on both of you. At this point the anesthesiologist usually turns photographer and snaps shots of parents and baby. After a brief time for you and baby to be together, the nurse ushers baby, and many times daddy, into the observation nursery while the doctors sew up the incisions and you doze. Expect another fifteen to thirty minutes for removal of the placenta and repair of the incisions. Afterward, you go either to the recovery room or, in some hospitals, immediately back to your LDR room, where a nurse checks your vital signs, and helps ease your physical and possibly emotional discomfort. Fathers may feel confused about whether to go with their baby or stay with their mate. A sensitive dad once said to me, "It's hard for me to enjoy my baby while my wife is still undergoing surgery." However, we encourage dad to go with his baby to the nursery and begin father-baby bonding. As soon as baby is stable and mother is able (which may be a few minutes or several hours), you can all be reunited in the recovery area.

After the Birth

Both baby and mother need some recovery time. Cesarean-birthed babies often have more mucus the first day. Some may take a day or two to clear excess fluid from their lungs and may require extra oxygen and observation in the special-care nursery. Oth-

Easing Postoperative Pain

In addition to the usual "afterpains" as your uterus contracts back to its prepregnant size, expect pain at the incision site, especially when coughing or laughing. The best postoperative pain relief is the long-acting morphine given in the epidural (see page 170). Second best is do-it-yourself analgesia, called *patient-controlled analgesia* (PCA). You administer your own medication through your I.V. by way of a pump that you can turn on and off as you need relief. Research has shown that when using this innovative method, mothers use less medication but get more consistent pain relief than if given scheduled doses by nurses.

Pillows will be a cesarean mother's best friend. During coughing or a gas pain, place a pillow over your lower abdomen and press your hands on each side of the pillow. Try lying on your side with extra pillows between your legs and under your abdomen. Intestines often go on strike after any surgical invasion of their privacy, so expect gas pains and constipation. Your doctor will prescribe remedies for these upsets. Walking will also assist the passage of gas.

First steps may be painful ones, and you will be tempted to walk bending over to ease tension on your incision, a movement dubbed the "cesarean shuffle." Try to stand as upright as possible while walking. Support your abdomen with your hands as you did prenatally, and have someone assist you in those first few post-op days when walking is painful and you feel lightheaded. You don't need to shun pain relief after birth. A hurting patient does not make for a relaxed mother. Pain-relief drugs, especially short-acting ones, will not affect your baby through your milk. In fact, not enough pain relief can inhibit your milk flow. Above all, don't forget to use baby to help mommy. As we have previously advised, frequent doses of a cuddly baby in the arms of a recovering mother are proven pain relievers or at least pain diverters. One mother, who was not about to let the physical and emotional pain of a cesarean dampen her entry into motherhood mused, "It's not so bad after all! At least I can both enjoy sex and sit a lot sooner than my friends could with episiotomies!"

ers seem not to care how they got out. They're just happy to be here and eager to get going with the things newborns do. If baby is healthy and you're awake in the recovery room and experiencing the normal longing-for-baby feelings, ask for your baby to be brought to you as soon and as often as possible after birth. If baby is not brought within ten minutes, ask again — you may have to insist. Nursery nurses tend to get attached to brand-new babies and may sometimes have to be reminded who the mother is! "We're too busy" is not an acceptable explanation. If baby is healthy, you can have your baby room in after a cesarean birth if your partner or a support person is with you at all times. In our experience, the best postoperative pain reliever is frequent doses of seeing, holding, and feeding your baby.

Despite the safety and efficiency of modern surgical births, recovery time varies greatly among mothers. Some rally quickly and are able to feed and care for their babies within six hours after birth. Others feel incapacitated for days. Depending on what type of pain-relieving medications you are given, expect to feel groggy for a day or two. Pain at the incision site may lessen your mobility for a few days, but the nurses will assist you in caring for yourself and your baby.

WHEN CESAREANS ARE NECESSARY

In a variety of circumstances, cesarean births can be lifesaving for the mother and, more often, for the baby. Experts believe that around 6 percent (10 percent at most) of mothers really do need cesarean births.

"Hard" Indications for a Cesarean

The following conditions virtually always indicate the need for a cesarean delivery: health problems in the mother (e.g., severe toxemia, uncontrolled diabetes), active genital herpes at the time of delivery, placenta previa, abruption of the placenta, prolapsed cord, or transverse position of baby (baby lies horizontally across the pelvic outlet). See pages 48–49 for a description of these conditions.

"Soft" Indications for a Cesarean

The following are indications that mothers can, given proper advice and support, often circumvent.

- Failure to progress. Also called *uterine dystocia*, this situation accounts for nearly 30 percent of all cesarean sections. Approximately one in four American babies is delivered surgically, but does it make sense that 25 percent of women's delivery systems can go wrong? We believe in most cases it's the failure of the obstetrical system to progress, not the mother's. We tackle this problem in the section on how to avoid a cesarean (see below).

- CPD (cephalopelvic disproportion). Accounting for around 5 percent of cesareans, CPD means the baby's head or body (also called "macrosomia") is too large to pass through mother's pelvis. Many OBs believe that true CPD is unusual, and many of these cases really fall into the category of "failure to progress." Some experts also believe that in many mothers, true CPD is a diagnosis that can be made only after some time spent in labor. Prenatal ultrasound and X-ray pelvimetry are not always accurate (see pages 96 and 99). If no progress is being made once baby's head enters the birth canal (the second stage of labor), a cesarean is considered not only because the baby's head may get stuck but also because the head may descend and the shoulders may get stuck ("shoulder dystocia"), an emergency complication that can seriously harm the baby.

- Fetal distress. Accounting for about 16 percent of surgical births, fetal distress is the most imprecise of all the indications for a cesarean section. By experience, doctors know that certain patterns on the electronic fetal monitor (EFM) strip suggest (but don't prove) that baby may not be getting enough oxygen. Whether or not a particular tracing means real distress in this particular baby or if the baby is really all right and the monitor is crying wolf is impossible to judge correctly all the time. Certain tracings on the monitor trigger "OB distress." The doctor cannot (and perhaps should not) gamble on their being a false alarm.

- Repeat cesarean births. These account for nearly 30 percent of all cesareans, but, as we point out in chapter 7, thorough research has shown that 70–90 percent of women who have had a previous surgical birth can safely deliver their next baby vaginally.

- Breech presentation accounts for 4–5 percent of cesareans and various other conditions (e.g., multiple pregnancies, eclampsia, diabetes) account for the rest.

Now for the surgery-saving statistics. If mothers, using the methods suggested in chapter 7, can increase VBACs from a national average of 20 percent (in 1990) to at least 70 percent, there would be a 20 percent overall decrease in the number of cesarean sections. In addition, if the number of mothers who fail to progress could be cut in half, another 15 percent of babies would come out the way they were designed to. Knock off another 5 percent with more accurate diagnosis of fetal distress, and we have a 40 percent reduction in cesareans. This translates into 400,000 American women each year avoiding surgery (and saving over one billion dollars).

TEN WAYS TO AVOID A CESAREAN

While a cesarean section may be lifesaving surgery in certain circumstances, we believe that at least half of cesarean surgeries could be prevented by parents taking responsibility for their births. Specifically, here's what you can do:

1. Choose your birth attendants and birth place wisely. Reread chapter 3. After examining your own obstetrical needs, ask yourself which people and what facilities are most likely to give you the best and safest birth. Because of the lack of an organized medical backup system, we do not advocate home birth for everyone, but remember that of the three birth-place options (home birth, birth centers, hospitals), the choice of a hospital is most likely to result in a cesarean. For information and support on avoiding a cesarean, attend ICAN meetings (see "Cesarean Resources," page 123).

Interview your prospective obstetrician to make sure he or she is not stuck on the horizontal birthing position. If so, this OB is not for you. What is his or her point of view about walking during labor and vertical birthing? Would he or she accommodate a squatting or side-lying position? Determine his or her birth philosophy. Is there a relaxed attitude, or is the doctor's mind preoccupied with a lot of "what if"s? What is the obstetrician's VBAC success rate? Insist on at least 70 percent. What is the obstetrician's personal cesarean-section rate? Anything over 15 percent is suspect and suggests a predominantly surgical mind-set about birth. Ask about "routines." Does he or she routinely use continuous electronic fetal monitoring? What percentage of his or her clients "need" fetal monitors?

2. Bring a birth buddy. If you choose the obstetrician-hospital birth system, as most mothers do, your chances of having a surgical birth go way down when you employ a professional labor assistant. (See the benefits of a labor-support person, page 35.)

3. Think upright. Scratch out the picture of a laboring woman lying on her back, feet up in stirrups, with the doctor sitting comfortably at the foot of the delivery bed. Back-lying is the position for a cesarean. The more time you spend in the cesarean position during labor, the more likely you are to need one. Research has shown that laboring upright increases uterine efficiency, shortens labor, dilates the cervix better, and allows your labor to progress more comfortably and efficiently. As more mothers and their doctors overcome the horizontal mind-set and start thinking vertical, more babies will come out the way they were designed to. Stand up for your birth. Insistence on horizontal deliveries ranks as the number-one reason for long, agonizing labors that pro-gress to the operating room. The horizontal position is a carryover from the days of anesthetized births and forceps delivery when women who were drugged during delivery couldn't stand up or help push their babies out. The upright squatting position, for example, widens the pelvic outlet and makes good use of gravity. Thinking vertical does not mean that you must not rest horizontally during labor. Many women are able to lie on their sides periodically, supported by pillows and attended to by a back-rubbing and face-caressing partner. If you try this and it is too uncomfortable, you can choose to do your resting in a tub (see page 152). Freedom of choice in laboring positions is your best ticket to a vaginal birth. (See chapter 11 for information on positioning during labor and delivery.)

4. Take a walk. Once you're thinking vertical, get moving. Research has shown that walking helps labor progress and is good for the baby.

5. Use electronic fetal monitoring and interventions wisely. Advocates of routine electronic fetal monitoring claim that it reduces the number of stillborn and brain-damaged babies by alerting physicians to early signs of trouble. Before its usefulness was proven, electronic fetal monitoring became standard obstetrical practice, and physicians now hesitate to deviate from that standard for fear of a lawsuit. But numerous controlled studies of low-risk mothers have shown no difference in infant outcome whether electronic fetal monitoring or a person monitoring the baby's heartbeat with a fetoscope is used. Furthermore, these studies found that mothers who had the "benefit" of this new technology were twice as likely to have a surgical birth. Besides, recent studies have shown that most cases of cerebral palsy are due to mishaps to the developing baby before labor begins. The accumulated evidence should be enough to cut the wires on routine use of electronic fetal monitoring. Remember, as soon as any monitor is placed around your abdomen, the chances of having a cesarean go up. In some cases, however, EFM can spare mother a cesarean. If your doctor suspects a complication (e.g., your labor is not progressing), but the EFM suggests baby is not bothered by this long labor, your doctor may be inclined to let you labor longer instead of rushing to a cesarean. Technology can be your friend if appropriately used; your foe if misused. (See chapter 5.)

6. Consider the epidural carefully. Like electronic fetal monitoring, epidurals are a part of the friend-vs.-foe dilemma. In a study of five hundred first-time mothers, those who received elective epidurals were more likely to require a cesarean for failure to progress. Other studies suggest that epidurals do not increase the chances of a surgical birth. We have witnessed labors where a well-timed epidural relaxed an anxious mother and actually improved her progress toward a vaginal birth. On the other hand, overuse of this "blessing from heaven" (as some of the mothers in our practice refer to epidurals) can interfere with uterine efficiency; when you receive an epidural, you lose a valuable birth friend — gravity. You're flat on your back and possibly on your way to the operating room. (See "Epidural Anesthesia," page 170.)

7. Take your time. Birth, like sex, shouldn't be rushed. Don't feel pressured to give birth in a hurry because of others' convenience or timetables. You're the star and everyone else is the supporting cast. Birth is a life event too important to operate on time limits. Often a mother's "failure to progress" is really the obstetrician's "failure to wait." There is no evidence that a long labor in and of itself is harmful to a baby. There are no absolute time limits on individual labors. While there are charts of "normal" labors indicating at what stage the average woman is after a given number of hours of labor, these give only averages and you are an individual. Your uterus hasn't seen these charts. The worry about long labors is based upon the belief that with each contraction the uterus delivers less oxygen to the baby, and therefore the more and longer the contractions, the less oxygen the baby gets. This occurrence has never been scientifically documented.

Also, be mindful of economic pressures on today's hospitalized women to push their babies out quickly — in what has been labeled a "take-out delivery." Some insurance plans restrict the amount of time a woman may spend in the hospital. A hospital administrator recently confided to us, "We can no longer afford a long, drawn-out vaginal birth." For those planning a hospital birth, it is best to labor as long as possible at home, deliver in the hospital, and quickly return home.

8. Use discernment about managed births. While there is a back-to-basics trend toward nonintervention at birth, an opposite force is attracting women toward what are called managed births: A pregnant woman, screened for normalcy and certified by ultrasound to be near term, books her birth near her due date. She enters the hospital in the morning, gets a pitocin drip to get things going and an epidural to keep from hurting. Her labor is chemically stimulated, electronically monitored, and technically managed. Parents and baby are back home that evening, apparently none the worse for the wear. Before you sign up for this new way of birthing, consider the probability that a disproportionate number of these births will be *mis*-managed and will wind up in the operating room.

Proponents of managed births claim that they sometimes lessen the likelihood of a cesarean delivery. In one study, researchers intervened early in labors that did not seem to be progressing satisfactorily. By giving the mothers pitocin and pain relief before labor exhaustion set in, the researchers reduced their cesarean rate from 20 to 6 percent. Waiting too long to intervene — after fear and exhaustion took over — increased the likelihood that both mother and doctor would abandon the vaginal birth and sign up for operative relief. A mother who is well prepared for birth, who knows how to relax and what her body's signals mean, is better able to handle a long, drawn-out labor. She knows how to avoid exhaustion; she is able to stay with her original plan rather than getting scared and opting for a cesarean. Before you rush to sign up for a managed birth, keep in mind two facts: (1) Pitocin-stimulated contractions are often much more painful than the ones induced by the natural hormones of labor since they seem to peak faster and sharper than the mother can adjust to them, and (2) the American birthing system is not geared toward providing the midwife support needed for this kind of birth. (For more information about managed births see "Active Management of Labor," page 86.)

9. Lobby for legal letups. Doctors need pain relief, too! Obstetricians believe, and we agree, that the number of surgical births is not likely to decrease significantly until the cloud of courtroom fear is lifted. Obstetricians we interviewed believe the cesarean rate could be cut from 25 percent (30 percent or more in some areas) to less than 10 percent if there was no fear of being sued. There once was a time in medicine when the obstetrician was able to make decisions based only on what was in the best interest of mother and baby, without taking into account what a jury might believe. But, burned by a multitude of court cases, doctors don't think like that anymore. While some indications for cesarean birth are absolutely black-and-white, others are shades of gray, requiring a judgment call by the physician. The fear of a lawsuit is likely to cloud a physician's judgment and lead him or her into a "take-no-chances" mind-set, which leads to the operating room. It often takes more discernment to decide *not* to perform a cesarean than it does to go ahead and cut. It also requires commitment to helping the mother through a difficult birth and a confident understanding of the natural birth process. Pilot programs have successfully demonstrated that there are better alternatives to the current climate, such as a no-fault insurance fund that compensates for poor obstetrical outcomes. Until such a change, obstetricians aren't going to do any risky vaginal deliveries. Doctors aren't going to lower cesarean rates; women must.

10. Remember your vulnerability. Plan ahead. When offered a surgical birth as an alternative to "two more hours of hell," you are often in no condition to make a wise choice. Part of your prenatal preparation should be learning about the indications for a cesarean birth; which ones are absolute and which are judgment calls that can go either way. Also, be sure you understand the risks and benefits of interventions and are aware of alternative ways of handling your birth should things not be going along as you planned. Here is where having a professional labor assistant helps. If you have exhausted all the alternatives in your birth plan, you can participate in the decision about surgery with no blame, no regrets, and no permanent scars in your birth memories. (For more information on avoiding a cesarean, see related section "Improving your Chances," page 118.)

MUST BREECH BABIES BE DELIVERED SURGICALLY?

The Problem

Around 4–5 percent of all cesareans are done to deliver a breech baby. The surgical rationale for this innovation is, again, "take no chances." The new obstetrics, with some statistical research to support it, says that babies in a breech position (bottom down) are more likely to be damaged in a vaginal

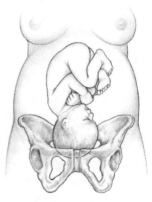
Vertex presentation (head down)

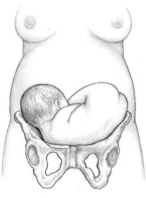
Transverse lie

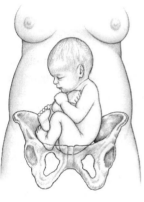
Complete breech

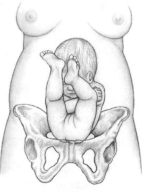
Frank breech

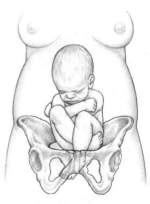
Footling breech

birth than if they had been rescued from the womb by cesarean. In 1970 only 12 percent of breech babies were born by cesarean section. By 1987, 85 percent of these bottom-first babies were surgically born. Opinions vary on what is best for mother and baby. At one extreme, in some areas of the country (usually those with high litigation fears), all breech babies are born surgically. In others, some "brave souls" attempt to select which breech babies can be safely delivered vaginally.

Once the standards in a community accept cesarean as the way of birth for all breech babies, any deviation from this standard puts the doctor at risk for a court case if things don't go well. Even though the American College of Obstetricians and Gynecologists has officially sanctioned vaginal birth for breech babies in selective situations, the expert hands available to maneuver a breech delivery may be either unable, unwilling, or retired. If a new obstetrician trains in a medical center where all breeches are delivered surgically, it is conceivable that he or she may enter practice never having delivered a breech vaginally — or never even having seen it done.

The Solution

Women have two choices. If you are near term and your baby is in a breech position, you may be able to avoid surgery. Try the following alternatives:

A Turn for the Better

Remember that nearly half of all babies start out breech early in pregnancy and the majority of them turn head down by themselves before term (usually by thirty-two weeks). However, 3–4 percent of babies remain breech.

If baby doesn't turn himself, an obstetrician may attempt a maneuver called *external version.* Usually doctors wait until around thirty-seven weeks to attempt this procedure because some babies do turn themselves eventually, and the procedure, not without risks, may trigger premature labor. With the help of ultrasound, electronic fetal monitoring, and intravenous medicines to relax the uterus, the doctor manipulates mother's abdomen and tries to turn baby into the head-down position. In skilled hands, 60–70 percent of babies turn. Some of these turn back and require a second version, and a few simply revert to breech position regardless of attempts at version.

Search for a Breech-Friendly Birth Attendant

This person is not likely to be found in the yellow pages. Be prepared for most obstetricians to approach a breech with an "I don't do vaginals" mind-set. One mother, surprised at how matter-of-fact her doctor was about vaginal births being too risky for breech babies, told us, "He scheduled my cesarean like he would his golf game." Before you let your doctor determine your mode of breech birth, do your homework and look for a physician experienced in vaginal breech births. Consider this paradox: doctors who dare to try something different are the ones responsible for new advances in medicine, but in some circles being different is equated with being less competent. It's likely that most physicians skilled in breech deliveries have some gray hair and that they learned their skills in the days when breech babies were usually delivered vaginally. You might try a university hospital that has responsible criteria for attempting breech deliveries vaginally, such as babies weighing less than nine pounds and being a frank or a complete breech.

Find a Breech-Experienced Midwife

Another option is to find a midwife experienced in breech deliveries, preferably in a hospital. In some states, it's against accepted practice for a certified nurse-midwife to deliver a breech baby at home. Check the legal protocols in your state. You might first want to consult an obstetrician experienced in delivering breeches. Even if he or she is unwilling to attend the birth, this physician may be willing to give you an opinion on the safety of attempting a vaginal birth, based on an ultrasound and a review of your situation. Then if you get the go-ahead, have your birth attended by a breech-experienced midwife.

Steps Toward a Safe Vaginal Delivery of a Breech Baby

Here are the safe and often successful steps a breech-experienced obstetrician takes. Purists may argue with this high-tech approach, but the risks associated with vaginal breech deliveries make taking these precautions prudent.

Before labor begins. An external version is tried first. If it is unsuccessful, a prenatal assessment of mother and baby follows. Is the mother's pelvis adequate (evaluated by pelvimetry or often by a new technique called a Fetal Pelvic Index; see page 99)? Is the placenta well located and are there any structural abnormalities of the uterus (evaluated by ultrasound)? Is the pregnancy healthy (e.g., no diabetes or hypertension)? Is baby's position a frank or a complete

breech? Is baby's estimated weight less than nine pounds? Footling breeches and those weighing over nine pounds are usually delivered by cesarean. Also is baby's head not hyperextended? If these criteria for safety are met, some obstetricians will support a trial of labor with a view toward vaginal birth.

When labor begins. Electronic fetal monitoring is advised, but not so that it interferes with mother's freedom to walk and change positions. If labor progresses normally (around 1 centimeter dilatation per hour — but breech labor may be slower) and EFM is normal, no intervention is needed. If progress is unsatisfactory, pitocin augmentation is considered. A professional labor assistant is a must in breech vaginal births.

During the second stage. If labor progress continues normally and EFM suggests baby and mother are handling labor well, there is no need for intervention. Meanwhile, precautions are taken during first and second stages to watch for the cord coming down through the cervix and being squeezed. Also, to help the cervix dilate, the membranes are not ruptured artificially until toward the end of labor. If epidural analgesia is needed or desired, it is turned off during the second stage to allow the mother to be upright and to push naturally. The obstetrician often asks a neonatologist or pediatrician to be present at delivery in case baby needs some temporary assistance after birth.

It is important to find a birth attendant who has a proven record of breech deliveries because he or she will be confident in the procedure and that confidence will be transferred to you. The fear factor becomes crucial in a breech birth because once the cervix has dilated to allow the shoulders to pass, the possibility of a tense cervix trapping the head is very real. This condition would be caused by fear.

Part of taking responsibility for your birth is being informed of all the choices and weighing the risks. All births have risks, but some are less risky than others. Some obstetricians still believe that in selected mothers, with skillful hands in attendance, a vaginal delivery is less risky to mother and breech baby than surgery.

7

VBAC — Yes, You Can!
(Vaginal Birth After Cesarean)

THERE'S GOOD NEWS FOR women who have had a previous surgical birth: the rule "once a cesarean, always a cesarean" is no longer true. Most mothers who had a previous cesarean birth can now deliver their next baby vaginally.

WHY THE WORRY?

The old rule was based on the worry that a previously operated-on uterus couldn't withstand the stress of contractions and might rupture during labor, and if the uterus ruptured, mother and baby could die. But here are the facts on this unwarranted worry. Twenty or more years ago cesarean sections were performed with a vertical incision made in the upper part of the uterus — the area most prone to rupture. Today the incision is usually made horizontally in the lower part of the uterus. Called a "low-transverse incision" or "bikini cut," this type of incision is highly unlikely to rupture. If a mother had a low-transverse incision, VBAC authorities now estimate the risk of uterine rupture in subsequent labors to be around 0.2 percent, which means that a VBAC woman has at least a 99.8 percent chance of going through labor without rupturing her uterus. In a survey of thirty-six thousand women attempting VBAC, no mothers died from uterine rupture, *regardless of type of prior uterine incision.* And researchers studying the medical literature on VBAC over the last forty years found that not a single mother died from rupture of a scarred uterus. (But mothers have died due to complications of repeat cesarean sections.) In a study of seventeen thousand women attempting VBACs, no infants died as a result of uterine rupture. And uterine "rupture" doesn't mean a mother will suddenly explode. Instead, in the rare cases that a scar does pull apart, it does so gradually and incompletely. Considering that the estimated risk of death from cesarean section is around one in one thousand (two to four times that of a vaginal birth), there is no reason to advise a mother to have a repeat cesarean section because of the risk of uterine rupture. According to the numbers game, the risk of death or damage to mother or baby is higher with a cesarean birth than during a VBAC labor. Experts in VBAC, backed up by thorough medical research, don't consider VBAC high-risk, so neither should you.

WHAT ARE YOUR CHANCES?

At present VBAC success rates are around 20 percent nationwide. However, mothers who are supported by knowledgeable VBAC birth attendants have a 75–90 percent chance of having a successful vaginal birth after a cesarean — an encouraging statistic. A successful VBAC depends not only on the reason for your previous cesarean, but also on your attitude, attendants, and preparation for this birth.

The reasons for your previous cesarean may have no bearing on what happens this time around. Many of the reasons for a first cesarean may have been chance happenings that will not occur again, such as a baby in breech position, an active herpes infection, eclampsia, or true fetal distress. Though long believed to be the main indication for the "once a cesarean, always a cesarean" myth, cephalopelvic disproportion (CPD) — where the baby's head is said to be too big to go through the mother's pelvis — is no longer considered a valid reason. Studies report a 65–70 percent chance of having a VBAC even though the previous reason was CPD. In one study one-third of VBAC mothers delivered a larger infant vaginally than they had by cesarean. Also, some obstetricians believe that the mother's pelvic outlet becomes more stretchable with each delivery. Also, realize that true CPD is uncommon; this casual label is often a needless source of "my body doesn't work" anxiety.

Some cesarean births that were supposedly done for CPD reasons may in reality be "failure to progress" during labor. In fact, it was very likely the failure of the birth attendants to have patience, to support the mother during labor, and to provide an environment conducive to birthing. Given this

new knowledge about an old problem, vaginal birth after cesarean need no longer be considered "high-risk," and it is an option available to a great majority of women who do not wish to repeat their previous surgical birth. It is amazing to us how few women take the time to research thoroughly whether or not they truly need elective major surgery. Some doctors still operate under the rule of "once a cesarean, always a cesarean." And even if they have ventured forth and now and then allowed a client to "give it a try," they practically guarantee that the VBAC attempt will fail by treating these women as high-risk. The list of precautions taken includes no use of LDR room or birth center, continuous monitoring, and I.V.

Improving Your Chances

Now that you know you can do it, here are ways to increase your chances of having the vaginal birth you want.

Select birth attendants supportive of VBAC. Find out your doctor's mind-set about VBAC. Is he or she up on the latest figures regarding VBAC? If you have to bring in books and articles to educate your obstetrician on VBAC, chances are this doctor is not for you. Look for a doctor who is willing to comanage your present birth as if you never had a cesarean. Unless an obstetrician truly believes in the wisdom and safety of VBACs, he or she is likely to become anxious and start thinking cesarean at the first irregularity on the fetal monitor. Anxiety is contagious in the labor room. Do you sense that your doctor is as enthusiastic as you are? Or is he or she uneasy about VBACs, conveying an "It's dangerous" attitude — one that makes you uneasy? When labor grows especially uncomfortable or when nothing much is happening, it is easy to replay the record of your previous C-section and start thinking negative thoughts: "I didn't dilate last time, so I guess I won't this time." You need a birth attendant to inject periodic "Yes, you can" pep talks. Find out what your prospective doctor's VBAC success rate is. It should be at least 70 percent. Be sure to be specific about your question. The receptionist at one of my colleague's offices was asked, "What is Dr. Smith's C-section rate?" She answered, "Twenty-five hundred dollars." It may not be easy to find a doctor who will give VBAC more than lip service, an amazing fact, considering the many professional books and journal articles written in support of VBAC. For help with finding a VBAC-supportive obstetrician or midwife, talk to friends, childbirth educators, or local cesarean-awareness groups. You need birth attendants who believe you can give birth vaginally.

Choose a VBAC-friendly birth place. Find out what your hospital's policies are about VBAC. Are they restrictive? Do they label you "high-risk"? Shun hospitals that have inflexible policies regarding VBACs, such as insisting on continuous fetal monitoring or regarding you as "too risky" to deliver in an LDR setting. These restrictive policies cause a VBAC mother to begin labor with two strikes already against her. VBAC mothers used to be considered *Very Brave And Courageous*. Now they're considered very motivated and informed. Experts experienced in VBAC believe that, except in unusual circumstances, a mother with a previous cesarean birth should be handled with no more "precautions" than one who has never had a cesarean.

One mother who read all the VBAC books but failed to drill her doctor and her hospital about their attitudes knew she was in the wrong hands and the wrong place the moment she entered the hospital. "When I walked into the delivery area, I felt like my doctor was already sharpening his knife. I barely got my shoes off and I was hooked up to continuous fetal monitoring and an intravenous line, and I, or at least my uterus, was viewed by the nursing staff as a disaster waiting to happen. As a final blow to my confidence, the lab technician came in to blood-type me 'in case I needed blood' during an emergency operation. I was made to feel that I was doing something unnatural to myself and risky to my baby — a feeling that did nothing to help my labor progress."

Employ a professional labor assistant. A professional labor-support person who empowers a woman is helpful in all births; in a VBAC she is a must. Surround yourself with birth attendants who believe you can deliver vaginally. You need people around you who are experienced at guiding you toward your goal, and who will believe in you to help you better believe in yourself. Discuss with your labor assistant those factors that you feel contributed to your previous cesarean so that she'll know which of these factors you will need help with during this labor (see "Choosing a Labor-Support Person," page 35).

Join a support group. Get involved in a cesarean-awareness support group, such as ICAN or C-SEC (see page 123 for information on these resources). Take a childbirth class that emphasizes ways to cope with pain in labor and body positions to help labor progress (see "Choosing a Childbirth

Class," page 50). Attend several meetings of your support group to hear the testimonies of VBAC women. Listen carefully to what these women did to increase their chances of VBAC. Soak up tips from mothers who have been there before. A room full of "yes, you can" mothers empowers you to feel likewise. Also, these group discussions are helpful to learn the coping strategies of women who did need to have another cesarean birth.

Learn from your past cesarean. While one of the roads to a VBAC is to avoid dwelling on what happened before, it is helpful to critique your cesarean experience and sort out what factors contributed to it, and what you would like to do differently this time. For example, did you spend a lot of time in bed on your back and end up diagnosed as "failure to progress"? This time you will want to move around more during labor. Do you believe that interventions slowed your progress or contributed to "fetal distress"? If so, become more knowledgeable about alternatives to intervention so that you are better equipped to participate in your birthing decisions. Be careful not to get bogged down in self-reproach ("if only I had done this"). These feelings, though normal, can escalate into a counterproductive guilt that clouds your next birth. Each birth is different, and what you might have done differently is only speculative. You were doing the best you could at the time, and that's all you can expect of yourself. Your past birthing experiences are lessons that will help future births, and learning from them can prevent history from repeating itself. If you find that you are tied in knots emotionally (anger, guilt, fear, depression), seek counseling from a professional experienced in this area so you can

approach your next birth with a healthy set of emotions and self-esteem, able to trust your body.

Prepare a birth plan. Read chapter 13, "Composing Your Birth Plan." It's wise to make a two-way plan: one for the VBAC you expect and a contingency plan should you have another cesarean birth. (We recommend this for all births.) Having a cesarean birth plan is not being defeatist; it's being realistic and flexible. The two-way birth plan helps you do everything you can to increase your chances of having a vaginal birth, but not feel guilty if circumstances beyond your control necessitate another cesarean. You'll be able to walk away without regrets, knowing you planned and prepared and did everything you could. Plus you have a strategy laid out that can make that surgical birth as close as possible to your first choice (see sample, page 236). Discussing your birth plan with your birth attendant is a valuable way to find out his or her attitude toward your VBAC. If you sense insensitivity to your reasonable requests, consider changing doctors. Consider your doctor your partner in birth, and together work out a birth plan that gives you the best odds for a VBAC and the best chance for remaining a healthy mother and delivering a healthy baby.

After discussing your birth plan with your doctor, have him or her sign it to document approval. If your doctor is part of a group, have the other members preview and sign it as well. In case an on-call doctor attends your birth, one who is less understanding of VBAC, you have your own doctor's support in writing, defending your choices. Insist that your birth plan be made part of your medical chart that your doctor sends to the hospital prior to your expected date of delivery. Take along another copy when you go to the hospital. It's wise for birthing attendants (i.e., nurses) who may not have previously met you to get an overall view of your expectations before you arrive at the hospital. It's especially helpful for the nurses and a substitute obstetrician to preview the plan before delivery. This avoids last-minute bedside negotiations. A well–thought out birth plan conveys to all the birth attendants that you have done your homework and are sharing responsibility for your birth decisions; that you are neither fanatic nor inflexible, but you want the best for yourself and your baby; that you have put your best efforts into this birth; and that you expect the same from everyone else.

Prepare for flashbacks. Expect vulnerable moments. Events such as an irregularity on the electronic fetal monitor can trigger the fear that the same thing's happening again. Relax and remember that this is not the same labor as before, and even if it seems similar you are now better equipped to handle setbacks. Rather than clicking into an "oh no, not again" mind-set, stay in the present, know why this is happening, and know what to do.

Get over the hurdle. Besides flashbacks to your previous labor, be prepared for other obstacles that may shake your confidence and slow your progress, such as: "You're *still* only at four centimeters," from a well-meaning but counterproductive nurse. You may have periods in your labor when "nothing's happening." Patience and determination are needed to get over the physical and emotional hurdles, and to get on with the desire to take on the next hurdle and round the turn toward a VBAC.

Other things to consider. Resist any suggestion to have your labor induced unless it is medically absolutely necessary. Inducing labor decreases your chances of a vaginal delivery and implies your body can't be trusted to start labor naturally. If your body is not ready to labor, you will face either a failure-to-progress situation or a very long, hard labor. Also, current fetal-dating methods, as advanced as they are, are not always accurate. Artificially inducing labor before the baby is ready increases your chance of a surgical birth and a premature baby. On the other hand, occasionally a managed birth (pitocin augmentation and epidural analgesia) may help some mothers progress to a vaginal birth (see "Active Management of Labor," page 86, and "Epidural Anesthesia," page 170).

Review the ten ways to avoid a cesarean (page 109), and study the chapters corresponding to these tips, especially the chapters on pain relief (chapter 10) and best birthing positions (chapter 11). You want to have everything possible going for you during your labor.

Questions You May Have

I want a VBAC — at home. Is a home birth safe in this situation?

Yes, depending on several factors. Many obstetricians discourage home birth in this situation because of the possibility of uterine rupture — remote as that may be. Midwives and mothers counter that in many instances the circumstances that led to the previous cesarean are more likely to be found in a hospital than at home. Obstetricians feel that fetal distress is less likely to be detected at home; midwives argue that fetal distress is less likely to happen at home. Many mothers whose previous cesar-

Avoiding Pelvic Prejudice

Don't let your birth attendant plant a "too-small pelvis" fear in your mind. Many petite mothers have successfully pushed out big babies. Estimates of pelvic size are inaccurate. Due to the hormones and the forces of birth, your pelvic outlet enlarges during labor, and your baby's head changes shape to accommodate the passage. Mechanical measurements don't account for these biological changes.

ean was due to failure to progress have their best odds of progressing normally during this labor at home. Just as "once a cesarean, always a cesarean" is a myth, "once a cesarean, never a home birth" is equally untrue. If you follow the guidelines listed on page 46, home-birthing is a safe alternative for most mothers desiring a VBAC.

I've already had two cesarean births. Should I still consider a VBAC?

Yes, depending on the reasons for your previous cesarean. Studies show that mothers with two and three previous cesarean births have a 70 percent success rate with VBAC. Also, studies conclude that the risk of separation or rupture of the uterus does not increase with the number of incisions, especially with the modern low-transverse incision.

By ultrasound my doctor estimates that my baby will weigh around nine pounds at birth. Could I still have a VBAC?

Yes. Conventional medical wisdom discourages women from having a VBAC if the baby

is over 8¾ pounds, but there is nothing scientific about this figure — just a fear that as the size of the baby increases so does the risk of uterine rupture. Recent studies fail to show any correlation between the size of the baby and the chances of scar separation. However, the accuracy of fetal weight estimates obtained by ultrasound are not always reliable, especially as babies get larger. In general, a large baby is not sufficient reason not to attempt a VBAC. Many mothers have birthed larger babies in a VBAC than they previously had by cesarean.

My last baby was delivered by cesarean because of failure to progress. I want a VBAC, but as I tour my hospital and speak to my doctor, I get the feeling they think I'm some kind of nut. How can I persuade them?

Hospitals who plan to stay in the baby business have become more accepting of VBAC patients, especially in view of the recent studies confirming VBAC's safety. You no longer have to feel like you are "courageous" or a "pioneer" to have a VBAC. You shouldn't have to persuade your medical attendants. It sounds like *they* are the ones who are failing to progress, but attempts to change someone's mind-set single-handedly are likely to fail. Consider changing doctors and hospitals. For a successful VBAC you need people teaching and supporting you, not vice versa. Research on the wisdom and safety of VBAC is on your side. You never have to apologize for asking for good medicine.

I want to have a VBAC but I also want an epidural. Can I have both?

Yes. VBAC mothers are not "high-risk" and can avail themselves of all the options of noncesarean mothers. Research shows that epidurals are no less safe for a VBAC, but some studies suggest a mother is more likely to have a cesarean if she has an epidural. Other studies show no such correlation. In fact, occasionally an epidural anesthesia breaks the fear–tension–pain cycle and enables the mother to progress to a VBAC (see "Using Narcotics Wisely During Labor," page 169). If you absolutely wish an epidural, yet you want a VBAC, try to progress as far into your labor as possible before the epidural. By having muscle tone, movement, and gravity to help you, baby is able to turn and adjust to better progress through your pelvis.

I'm afraid to have a hospital VBAC because I don't want to be treated as a high-risk patient. I am considering delivering in a birth center. Is this safe?

Yes. According to the policies of the National Association of Childbearing Centers (NACC), a VBAC delivery in a birthing center is considered just as safe as a delivery where mother has not had a previous cesarean — as long as the uterine incision was the low-transverse type, there is an obstetrician assigned to back up the birthing center, and the particular birthing center you are considering meets standards of safety (see page 40). For more motivation to have a VBAC, see "I Witnessed Myself Become a Woman—VBAC Water Birth," page 242.

DIFFERENT BIRTHS — DIFFERENT FEELINGS

Birth is a life-changing experience for a woman. For many women, how they give birth is intimately tied to how they approach life. One evening at an Interna-

> ### Cesarean Resources
>
> **Cesarean Support Education and Concern (C-SEC)**
> 22 Forest Road
> Framingham, MA 01701
> (617) 877-8266
>
> **International Cesarean Awareness Network (ICAN)**
> P.O. Box 152
> Syracuse, NY 13210
> (315) 424-1942
>
> **Once a Cesarean** (a 35-minute video about VBAC)
> Nick Kaufman Productions
> 14 Clyde Street
> Newtonville, MA 02160
> (617) 964-4466

tional Cesarean Awareness Network (ICAN) meeting, we asked several mothers to compare their feelings about their cesarean and their vaginal births. We were struck by how these women healed themselves of their traumatic birth memories. Perhaps these women spoke so intensely about their feelings because they weren't convinced that they had needed a cesarean with their first birth. We have noticed that women who know that they really needed to have a cesarean, and who participated in the decision, are better able to handle their disappointment.

A Life-Changing Experience

"My first birth was an 'emergency' C-section due to fetal distress — a bit of a puzzling emergency considering it took forty-five minutes from the time I signed the consent form to get the baby out. The anesthesiologist said that the epidural took much longer than usual because I had a very difficult back. I was extremely scared and traumatized because I thought somehow my body was hurting my baby. At the moment of truth, I remember hearing my son cry frantically, and I cried lying there flat on the table, unable to move or see him, and feeling relief that he was safely out of my body and alive.

"My second was a VBAC — home birth. I remember everything about the birth of my daughter — how I felt at each moment physically and emotionally as she was coming through my body, for *I* was truly bringing forth this life into the world. When she was born, my midwife guided her up to my chest where she nursed while I easily birthed my placenta. At the moment of birth, I remember holding her in my arms and saying, 'Oh my baby, my baby, I would do anything for you, my baby.' I was completely devoted to her, and felt a strong love for her, and there was nothing done to us to interfere with those precious moments after birth. The whole experience of researching for this birth, preparing emotionally for this birth, and the actual birth itself has been completely empowering for me and this continues to translate into my life on a daily basis."

The Incredible High of a Natural Birth

"The natural 'high' that I experienced when I delivered my daughter naturally was *the* best experience of my life! When my son was born by cesarean, I remember crying tears of joy also, but nothing compared to the feeling I had during my VBAC. I think there must be a 'chemical' reason that caused the difference in the two feelings.

After being blessed by experiencing the natural delivery, I feel sorry for those women who have had only cesareans and will never know what they missed. And for those who are expecting, I *beg* them not to let anyone or anything rob them of the 'high' of a natural delivery."

A More Fulfilled Beginning

"After my C-section with my first daughter, I felt emotionally and physically vanquished. Everything was taken from me — my dignity, my husband, and my baby. *They* did everything that *I* was supposed to do — birth, feed, and comfort my new baby. I felt completely emotionally detached by the time I saw Chelsea four hours later. I had to ask for her, and then they propped her next to me since I couldn't hold her across my tummy. I wondered if she knew who I was. I had to persevere in order to establish breastfeeding. Everything felt stilted and awkward.

"My VBAC, on the other hand, was an exhilarating experience of total mind-and-body harmony. After birth, my daughter was placed gently into my loving arms. We just gazed at each other in amazement. She immediately wanted to breastfeed, and did so. I felt so emotionally validated that she instinctively knew I was her mother."

Determined to Have a VBAC

"After a troubling cesarean 4½ years ago, I was determined to have a VBAC with my second child. I selected a supportive doctor this time, hired not one but two labor-support people, and read, read, read. I did not expect my VBAC to be easy. My first child weighed nine pounds one ounce, and I was sectioned after he had a brief period of fetal distress caused, my former obstetrician said,

Westfield Memorial Library
16 AUG 2010 05:34pm
Phone: 908-789-4090

Dillaway, Maura

When the duke returns /
39520040207865   Due: 13 SEP 2010 *

Dead over heels /
39520025521579   Due: 13 SEP 2010 *

Breastfeeding /
39520040305451   Due: 13 SEP 2010 *

The birth book : everything you
39520022210671   Due: 13 SEP 2010 *

For 24/7 access to all that
your library offers, visit
www.wmlnj.org. Have your
library card available.

by CPD. All indications were that this second baby would be as large or larger.

"It's hard to say when my labor began, but it went on with only brief respites for three days. My labor assistant for laboring at home came over on the second day. Anne was great, using imagery and massage to help me through my contractions. But I remained stuck at 2 centimeters. We walked, squatted, rested, even went people-watching at John Wayne Airport for a change of scenery (and turned down several offers of a wheelchair from concerned airport staff). But although the contractions would get fast, strong, and regular after walking, they would ease off, time and again. I had another sleepless night full of contractions, and when Anne left Monday morning, I was less than 3 centimeters dilated, and my cervix was still not fully effaced. I was exhausted and getting demoralized, but more than anything, I feared getting to the hospital too soon, which I was convinced would lead to unnecessary interventions. Apprehensive, I kept my doctor's appointment Tuesday morning, when I learned I had dilated now to 4 centimeters, and was fully effaced. Bone-tired I reluctantly agreed to check in to the hospital, where Sherri, my other labor assistant, met me. Sherri was terrific, her massages were heavenly, and as we walked the halls I felt more encouraged than I had in days. We managed to talk the doctor out of an I.V. when the baby's heart rate went up. We brought it down instead with a shower and Jacuzzi.

"But my spirits were suddenly dashed about 9:00 P.M. when the doctor 'dropped the bomb.' I was stuck at 4 centimeters, and the baby's head was very high. The doctor said she had read my birth plan and knew I had my heart set on a VBAC, but she said,

'You can't always get everything you want.' Given my history of CPD and the knowledge that this was a big baby, she said, 'We're looking at a C-section.' My jaw must have dropped. 'I'm not ready for that,' was all I could manage to say. Sherri suggested the doctor break my bag of waters, but the doctor feared the cord would prolapse. Instead, she agreed to do a slow leak, while she held the head and eased it down into place. But first she wanted me to have an epidural so that the muscles around my pelvis would relax and allow the baby to progress downward more easily. Also, in case the cord did prolapse during the leak, I would not have to have general anesthesia during the emergency cesarean that would follow. It was difficult for me to agree to the epidural; I felt it was wimping out. But Sherri was terrific and helped me see that the epidural was called for, that it could help me, and that I had been no wimp during a very difficult labor. Besides, the doctor seemed convinced I was cesarean-bound, and if that happened, the last thing I wanted was to be unconscious for my baby's birth.

"The slow leak took twenty-five minutes to complete. But this still did not help the dilation, so I agreed to a Pitocin drip. An hour or so later, there still was no progress, so the Pitocin was cranked up; I was starting to get worried.

"By midnight, I was only at 5 centimeters. And now I was definitely discouraged. I sadly came to terms with the prospect of having a repeat cesarean. We had tried everything, and my body was not responding. Perhaps I really was one of those few who truly needed a surgical birth.

"Imagine my surprise when shortly after 3:00 A.M. the nurse checked me and casually said, 'You're fully dilated. You can start pushing.' I was so happy, I expected bells to ring! The epidural was decreased, so I had good control over my legs and pushes, and pushing went incredibly fast. In no time we saw the top of the head. It was great to see such rapid progress, after days of snail-paced dilation.

"At 4:36 A.M. my baby son, Alexander, easily slipped out and into the world. Such exhilaration! My husband, Sherri, and I all gasped and laughed when the nurse announced his weight — ten pounds one ounce, a full pound heavier than my first son, who was born by cesarean 'because of CPD.'

"I had no episiotomy and, thanks to Sherri's warm compresses, had only a small tear — smaller than if I had been cut. Recovery, both physical and emotional, was a breeze, compared to the cesarean.

"What a sense of accomplishment and joy I have from this birth. Now, when people admire my big, strapping baby and hear how much he weighed at birth, they often say, 'I hope you had a cesarean.' And I proudly respond, 'Absolutely not!'"

Our comments: The keys to Mary's success were her determination, preparation, and the wise use of all support resources — social and medical. This was birthing partnership at its best. Mary trusted her body and pushed it to its maximum. She did all she could do and when her natural resources became exhausted she used medical assistance to complement her work. This happy mother told us that the single most important factor in getting the birth she wanted was the continuous support of a professional assistant throughout labor.

This story also underlines the fact that sometimes dilation of the cervix departs from the usual pace. This departure does not indicate surgical intervention but rather a respect for this difference and a willingness to support calmly and monitor carefully this type of birth as long as it takes and as long as mother and baby are healthy. This requires a system of care that recognizes the importance of how a baby is born.

II

EASING PAIN IN LABOR — WHAT YOU CAN DO

Easing the discomforts of labor is a partnership between you and your birth attendants. Relying only on medical pain relief is likely to yield a less-than-satisfying birth experience. You will be amazed at the overwhelming sensations of labor and delivery, and equally amazed at the power of your mind and body to muster up your own pain-management system.

Why Birth Hurts — Why It Doesn't Have To

PAIN IS NOT INTRINSIC to normal labor — sensation is. Labor involves many new sensations for the first-time mother, but no woman should have to suffer while giving birth. Contractions (pressures in the abdominal and pelvic area during labor) and stretching and burning sensations of the perineum as birth nears are just some of the many sensations. In this chapter we will teach you skills that will help you prevent pain and manage it if it occurs, and help you find out what medical pain relief is available to you. Then you can look forward to a labor that is bearable and even a positive experience. To aim for a childbirth free of all discomfort is unrealistic. But to preplan an anesthetized birth for fear of pain may rob you of a valuable experience and wonderful birth memories.

Women are led to believe the goal of managing labor discomfort is to achieve control over labor. The very word *control* implies you can master its progress, including any pain that might occur, and suggests that your goal is to keep your mind in control over your body. This belief could be the downfall of many strong-minded, capable women who have everything in their lives scheduled and "under control." Birth is not such a controllable event. Birth by its very nature is unpredictable. That's part of the miracle of it. We believe that a laboring mother's true goal must be understanding how to relinquish control to her body, which already knows how to birth. This is a conscious decision. The knowledge you gain by understanding the process of birth and your options surrounding birth allow you to be prepared mentally to let go. And the techniques you learn from this book, classes, other mothers, and your health-care team will make it easier to surrender physically to your body's workings, making the birth process both more efficient and less uncomfortable. Rather than striving for control, which implies working against your body, we encourage *release,* which implies understanding your body's signals and working with them. We will describe well-researched and proven techniques for childbirth that will help you create your own labor-management strategy. While no amount of preparation or number of classes will guarantee you a pain-free childbirth, in general, the more you can relax, the less it will hurt.

Pain — A Useful Signal

Pain has a purpose. This unwelcome alarm sounds to make us aware that something unphysiologic is going on in our body and serves notice that we need to make a change. So it is with pain during labor. It is a signal that implies the woman needs to relax. When a woman is relaxed, the sensations of her contractions signal that labor is progressing normally and she can simply let it happen. When this relaxed woman feels pain, she is being signaled to make a change. For example, back pain during transition would urge her into some creative positions to deal with the pain. Besides making the contractions more bearable, her new position helps her baby also change positions, rotating to find an easier way out.

Because women have been so conditioned to expect pain in childbirth, they often discount its significance as a signal. If the pain is ignored, its value as a signal to make changes is lost. Another problem with the "pain in childbirth is normal" belief is that women automatically opt for anesthesia, or they bite the bullet and go natural "for the sake of the baby," not knowing they could make changes in their labor that would alleviate the pain.

Unmanageable pain during birth is not normal. Even in athletic training, the old axiom "no pain — no gain" has been disproven. When a muscle hurts, its function is compromised, and it is more prone to injury. In labor, the less the pain, the more gain. Pain in labor stimulates release of hormones that inhibit labor (see page 138). You do not have to hurt to deliver a baby. Pain, properly understood and sensitively managed, is a valuable labor assistant. Listen to its signals.

WHY BIRTH CAN HURT

By understanding where pain in labor might come from, what you can do, and how others can help, you are more likely to have a satisfying birth experience.

Discomfort goes with the territory. Until nine months ago your organs fit nicely inside your abdominal and pelvic cavities. Each one had a place; it had been there for years. Your bones and muscles were used to supporting a certain amount of weight. Then came a rapidly growing baby and her environment, which soon became the size and weight of a watermelon. Like an oversized guest in an already crowded elevator, this extra person forced everything else to make room. Just as your body began to adapt, this space-occupying person began to push her weight around and now she wants to get out, forcing everything else to move around to make way.

Tension contributes to pain in labor. The stretching of the lower uterine segment and the intensely contracting muscles of the upper uterus are commonly thought to be the primary source of pain in labor. The uterine muscles, however, like those of the stomach and intestines, have few pain receptors. These muscles all contract and relax without causing pain unless these muscles are forced to work in a way they weren't designed to.

Pain from contractions is felt in the tissues around the uterus if a woman is tense and fearful. In this case, the pressure from the contracting uterus is felt in the abdomen, throughout the pelvic area, and across the lower back because the uterus is fastened to the lower-back structures. All of these areas are liberally supplied with pain receptors. There is a direct relationship between the amount of discomfort or pain a laboring woman feels during contractions, and the amount of muscle tension she has.

Martha notes: This tension-muscle pain principle is why I tell the women in my childbirth class: "During a contraction, let go of all your abdominal muscles to look like you are eleven months pregnant instead of maintaining the eight-month look you get by pulling them in."

Fatigue contributes to pain in labor. Stretched muscles hurt when overworked. One theory about pain in labor is that the uterus simply "runs out of gas." The womb muscles work harder and faster and the circulatory system can't keep up with the demand for fuel, especially oxygen. This is especially true if the mother is not relaxed and the uterus has to work harder and less efficiently against tense muscles. Just as depriving the heart muscles of oxygen results in angina pains, the oxygen-deprived uterus also hurts. The key to avoiding pain in the uterus and surrounding tissues is to keep the uterus from running out of gas by keeping the surrounding tissues relaxed and

out of its way. Don't create a "brick wall" (tense muscles) for your baby-laden uterus to have to push through!

Martha notes: With Erin's birth, my fifth, I learned that simply letting my uterus "hang out" by releasing all of my abdominal muscles as a contraction started made a big difference in how it felt. When I braced for a contraction, pulling in my abdominals, I was hurting and miserable, hanging on like I was biting the proverbial bullet. Letting go lessened the pain considerably and it also sent a message back to my brain that I didn't have to be afraid. After trying it both ways several times, I learned to stay in the release mode and then the pain subsided entirely.

Tired and tense muscles hurt. Here's why. Biological systems, especially muscles, have an optimal physiological environment, which, if disturbed, is registered as pain. When a muscle is tired, the biochemistry in the muscle tissues gets out of balance. When it's tense, its electrical activity increases. These physiological changes lower the point at which the muscle begins to hurt. This principle applies to all the muscles surrounding the uterus and to some extent the uterus itself.

The passenger won't fit through the passage. If baby is too big or mother's pelvis small, pain results. If baby is in an unusual position (e.g., transverse — lying across the pelvic outlet instead of head down) or if mother is in an unphysiologic position (horizontal instead of upright), pain results. These abnormal sensations signal that something is going wrong and a change is needed, such as mother needs to change

---

A Rite of Passage

Can there be a correlation between how you birth and how you parent? Just as women have different views on what makes a positive birth experience, there are also different answers to this question. Having satisfying birth memories gets most women off on the right foot as mothers. But what constitutes a satisfying birth memory? One woman may view a managed, medicated birth as the best start to her mothering career. Unlike the mother who feels victimized by an agonizing labor and is consciously or unconsciously angry at her baby for "doing this *to* me," the medicated mother at least doesn't have negative feelings about her birth that translate into a negative attitude toward her baby.

Mothers who believe in unmedicated childbirth are likely to view birth and having a baby as a challenge and an opportunity for growth. They believe that the effort required to birth the baby helps a woman make the transition into motherhood and to value it more highly. The tremendous sensations of labor and birth make them pay attention to birth, to see it as an enormous event that needs to be reckoned with, a high point of female sexuality that a woman shouldn't miss. Martha instructs her childbirth class, "If birth were as easy as falling off a log, women might tend to minimize the importance of birth. The effort in childbirth prepares a woman for the great changes ahead and the commitment demanded of her as she cares for this new child."

---

positions until the pain subsides or obstetrical intervention is needed (see "Pain — A Useful Signal," page 130).

UNDERSTANDING PAIN MANAGEMENT

One key to managing pain is in understanding how your body perceives it. Let's follow a typical pain impulse from a pinched finger to the moment the brain says "ouch."

The Gate-Control Theory of Pain

Throughout nearly every organ of the body there are microscopic bundles of nerves that transmit pain. When these bundles are dis-turbed (for example, when you pinch your finger), they send lightning-fast impulses up the nerves in your finger, hand, arm, and eventually into the spinal cord. Here they meet a bit of resistance, a sort of checkpoint or gate (hence the term *gate-control theory*). The gate allows some impulses to reach the brain and stops others. There are two types of nerve impulses: lifesaving reflex responses, which cause a quick, automatic motor response ("Quick! Move your finger from the pincher!"), and slower impulses, which are under your control. These slower impulses travel to the higher brain centers and cause you to think and make judgments about what you did and how to stop your finger from hurting so much.

How a person perceives pain plays a role in how he or she deals with it. If a mother, by preparation and study, understands what different sensations mean, she undergoes a sort of cognitive rehearsal that lessens the surprise and therefore the intensity of the sensation. Let's take as an example the burning sensation in the perineum as baby's head crowns. If a laboring mother perceives this signal as dangerous (she fears that she is coming apart), she triggers a stress response that magnifies the feeling into pain. If, however, she perceives the sensation as normal (stretching skin naturally smarts), and understands the meaning of the message (elastic tissue is designed to stretch to let baby get through), she perceives the sensation as merely uncomfortable and, being without fear, she knows to stop pushing.

Managing the Pain Gate

To understand how the pain pathway works and how you can influence it, picture pain impulses as miniature race cars sprinting from the pain site on the hurt finger to microscopic pain receptors, like parking places, on the nerve cells of the brain and spinal cord. There are many ways you can alleviate pain. First, you could prevent or reduce the painful stimulus: "Don't let your finger keep being pinched!" or "Get into the tub of water and relax before the next contraction." If, however, the painful stimulus has already begun (the cars are running), to manage these pain-carrying cars you could do the following: close the gate in the spinal cord so that the cars can't get through (stimuli such as massage send impulses that inhibit the transmission of pain impulses); and gridlock the gate by sending a large variety of competing impulses (touch, music, imagery, hot or cold counterpressure) so that the pain-carrying cars are stalled; finally, you could fill up the parking spaces in the brain (receptor sites) so that the cars have no place to park. (By attaching

to these receptor sites medication can do this artificially; so can the body's own pain-killing substances, endorphins; see page 138.) People use these methods subconsciously: the sprinter focused on the finish line doesn't realize she was hurting until the race is over; a headache goes away during a distracting event. Pain-management techniques for labor employ all of these strategies, and you can make them work for you.

Martha notes: In our early childbirth experiences I had learned and tried to use distraction techniques such as trancelike fixing of my eyes on a focal point combined with patterned breathing or tapping out a tune. When my labor became so demanding that these techniques no longer worked, I intuitively began to do what did work: I learned to let my body take over and do what it had to do. In our experience, distraction techniques seldom relieve the pain of labor for long, and can increase tension in labor. Focusing on a distraction requires mental strain, which tends to keep your body on edge. Experience has shown that neither mind nor muscles relax when a person tries to concentrate on something else to escape from pain. Pain during labor requires relaxation of mind and muscles.

The Psychology of Pain

Probably the biggest factor in your ability to deal with pain in labor will be your mental and emotional attitude toward it. For most women there will be some point during labor (specifically late active labor and transition) where efforts at distraction and even relaxation may seem inadequate. This is when the woman's birth value system and mental preparation will come into play. If she values not only the outcome of the birth, but the life experience of the process as well — with all the emotion, struggle, and victory involved — she will find it within herself (with a little encouragement from those around her) to go on, work with the pain, and give birth to her baby with little or no medical pain relief. If she places little value on experiencing the process itself, the pain she would endure feels "not worth it." She will choose medical pain relief to assist her. This does not mean that one woman is better than another. It's simply a value choice. Both women can look back at their birth experiences with satisfaction because they made decisions for themselves based on who they are and what they want from birth.

If a woman gives birth in a way that satisfies her needs in becoming a mother, so that she can in turn satisfy her baby's needs as that baby adjusts to life outside the womb, she has done well. Surgery is the hard way to be initiated into motherhood, as is a birth fraught with fear and unbearable pain. Make choices that give you and your baby the best chance at a smooth start together. Keep in mind that high-tech solutions to pain often take away much more than just the pain. And when "high-tech" leads to surgery, you wind up with pain after the birth instead of before.

FEAR — LABOR'S FOE

It's no wonder women are afraid of childbirth. Instead of learning about birth as a high point of female sexuality, young women hear horror stories of half-drugged mothers strapped to delivery tables surrounded by masked strangers and metal machines. Television and movies portray the pain of birth but seldom the pleasure. Because birth has been moved out of the home into the hospital, most first-time mothers have never been around someone in labor or seen a birth. (Our daughter-in-law wanted to be at the birth of our seventh baby for this reason.) Birth is surrounded with mystery, and people fear what they don't understand. Women who know more about birth fear it less.

The Fear-Tension-Pain Cycle

In his classic book *Childbirth Without Fear,* British obstetrician Grantly Dick-Read describes how fear tightens the cervix. When examining a woman in labor he noticed that when she was relaxed in between contractions, her cervix was softened and dilated. But when she reacted to contractions with uncontrollable fear, the previously relaxed cervix tightened and closed. Observations like this prompted Dr. Dick-Read to study the connection between mind and body during labor, and led him to describe the fear-tension-pain cycle that makes an otherwise manageable labor unbearable. By breaking this cycle at any one of several points, women can lessen or avoid the pain of childbirth. Learning how their bodies work in labor, why they feel the way they do, and working *with,* rather than against, their bodies reduces the tension in muscles and the mind produced by fear, and thus lessens the pain. In the era when twilight sleep took away some of the pain but also much of the pleasure of birth, Dr. Dick-Read proved to the obstetrical world that most women do not have to suffer or be heavily drugged to give birth.

How Fear Frightens the Uterus

The uterus is not just an automatic pump that pushes a baby out. The workings of this magnificent muscle are affected, for better or for worse, by a neurohormonal pathway that connects the brain, the circulatory system, and the uterus. Fear alters this pathway, reducing the blood flow and oxygen supply to the uterus (and, if prolonged, oxygen to the baby). As a result, the cervix tightens instead of relaxes. Pushing a baby against an unwilling cervix during intense contractions can cause unbearable pain. As she anticipates and fears the agony of the next contraction, a woman becomes more tense, so does her cervix, and the pain grows. Eventually, in birth attendant jargon, "she loses it!" She no longer feels she can handle what is happening to her. Fear has robbed this woman of a satisfying birth experience. Rather than blame the resistant cervix and administer drugs to help it dilate, the mother could be helped to identify her emotional stress and fear and be shown how to deepen her muscular relaxation so that her sympathetic nervous system would loosen its grip on her cervix.

Fear upsets the balance of birth hormones, allowing the labor-inhibiting hormones to overtake the labor-enhancing hormones, resulting in increased pain and length of labor. The surge of stress hormones (see page 138) is the fight-or-flight mechanism seen in humans and also witnessed in the animal kingdom. When confronted with danger, animals use this fear reflex to stop labor, allowing them time to move to a safer birth place. To obtain a deeper understanding of the physiological basis of fear, consider what happens during normal contractions. The pathways affected most by fear influence the workings of the lower uterine muscles. Normally, the upper and lower uterine muscles work in harmony with each other to push the baby out. Fear causes the lower uterine muscles to tighten instead of relax, while the upper uterine muscles (the muscles not so affected by the fear pathway) automatically keep on contracting, in effect pushing baby against a resistance. Remember, pain is often a body's signal that something is not working right and that a change is needed. Pain is also produced when muscles are working unnaturally. The mother perceives this pain as abnormal (which it is) and panics that something is going wrong, which increases the effects of fear and the fear-tension-pain cycle intensifies.

Rx for Healing Fears

The good news is that you can control your fear. Besides altering the conditions that produce pain, you can change your perception of pain. After all, if you are afraid something will hurt, it usually does — maybe even more. Knowing what to expect and understanding the sensations of birth help banish the fear. Here are some tips for preventing fear from depriving you of the birth experience you desire.

Know when normal fears become abnormal. It's normal to be apprehensive during pregnancy about your birth and the responsibilities that go with motherhood. What will my labor and delivery feel like? How am I going to manage labor? Am I going to "lose it" or stay in charge? Will my baby be healthy? Will I be a good mother? These are normal concerns that come and go. But if they persist and dominate your thoughts about the upcoming birth so that you feel really scared, they are no longer normal fears. Recognize this fear factor and deal with it honestly.

Consult the experts. No one can predict or fully describe what your labor will be like. But if the unknown makes you uptight, talk to veteran mothers who overcame their labor fears, and ask them what they did. While descriptions and perceptions of what contractions feel like are as variable as how women would describe the sensations of lovemaking, you can get a sense of what labor sensations would be like. One experienced mother counseled a novice, "I wouldn't describe contractions so negatively. They weren't awful, but were more like incredible rushes throughout my body."

Information helps. Throughout your labor new and intense feelings are bound to trigger thoughts such as "Is baby okay?" or "Is this normal?" The more informed you are, the less you fear. While there are no guarantees that you will go through labor with no surprises, the more you prepare for and understand what will happen and what you can do about it, the less afraid of birth you will be.

Identify your fears. Try this exercise in fear-busting. List all the aspects of labor that you are afraid of. Ask yourself why you have this fear, then decide what you can do about it now, and what you will do if it resurfaces during labor. For example, say your fear is of being cut, either with a cesarean or an episiotomy. To help yourself address that fear, read about what you can do to prevent a cesarean and say "no" to an episiotomy. And, so there are no surprises, read all about what will happen if you do need a cesarean

(page 104). Be prepared to participate in the decision about these procedures so that you will feel in control of what is happening to you and have no regrets later. Remember that the odds of avoiding a cesarean or episiotomy are much in your favor (at least 90 percent) if you are prepared to speak up for yourself.

Another way to release the fear that binds you is to tackle the subject of fear in general. Are you a fearful person? If so, pick out your favorite fear and work through it. For example, Martha had a fear of water. Her father drowned when she was an impressionable four-year-old, and the association between water and her father's death in the past caused her to have an unreasonable fear of water in the present. Replaying the tragic incident in a rational way without dwelling on it and focusing on her present enjoyment of swimming helped her break the mental connection between past and present and she gradually learned not to fear water. Going through the exercise of releasing a major fear in your life will give you the tools you need to release birth fears as well.

Heal past birth fears. If there are ghosts in your body's closet, open the door and let them out. Labor has a way of digging up memories from the past. If fear and pain predominated at your last birth and you haven't dealt with these feelings, history is likely to repeat itself. To be less fearful of the future, work on healing the past.

Who else is afraid? Fear is contagious. During pregnancy and labor surround yourself with people who do not project fear. You don't need your mother telling you how awful childbirth was for her. If your mother or a friend has a fearful mind-set about labor, better they should watch your birth video after the event than be in the birth room infecting you with their fears.

How about your partner? He may appear to be Mr. Fearless, but deep down most men get scared when women go into labor. Prepare your partner for the normal sounds laboring women make and the usual happenings during labor and delivery. The more men know about birth, the less they have to fear.

The professionals you hire (childbirth educator, midwife or doctor, support person, nursing staff) all have the potential for infecting you with fear. As you go through the interview process, specifically look for a professional who communicates trust in the birth process.

By knowing yourself and knowing your body you will have less to be afraid of at birth. Women who fear tend to look toward the "strong ones" around them (mate, birth attendants) to "fix it" for them, without any guarantee that the fix will suit them. We believe that an informed woman fears less, and a mother who participates in her labor and in the decisions accompanying it has less pain and a more satisfying birth experience.

STRATEGIES FOR A MORE COMFORTABLE LABOR

Childbirth has always been hard work, and babies haven't changed the way they negotiate their way out. What has changed, for better and for worse, is the approach to pain in childbirth. For better, today's laboring mother has more options for pain prevention and/or relief than ever before. No longer is it deemed desirable or necessary

to suffer unbearably through birth. For worse, with modern medicine, a mother may wind up handing over all responsibility for whatever pain relief she needs to her doctors and responsibility for the birth along with it. The responsibility for pain relief must remain with the laboring woman. To choose medication automatically, without first exploring other options is seldom best for mother or baby. The motto of the International Childbirth Education Association says it well: "Freedom of choice through knowledge of alternatives." To make a wise choice, you must first explore all the alternatives. Educate yourself about all the pain-relieving options in birth, along with their risks and benefits. Select what best fits your desires for a birth experience and your obstetrical situation. Then, create your own birth strategy.

Heal your past. Birth has a way of replaying past experiences and long-held feelings, some constructive, some not. Pregnancy is a time for exploring and healing, and for freeing yourself from blocks that stand between you, your baby, and a happy life ahead. In a satisfying birth you must surrender to your body, yield to your urges, tune in to yourself, open up, and let baby out. This may be difficult to do for a woman who carries baggage from her past that competes with her ability to free herself and allow her body to work. For some women, birth pushes buttons from the past. A woman who has a past history of sexual abuse, for example, may understandably have trouble mustering up all the stuff needed for birth: being assertive, trusting, and surrendering to her body or to the suggestions of caregivers. Having a "tense up" button pushed in the middle of contractions is a setup for an unbearable birth. Therapists term digging up

Endorphins — The Body's Natural Narcotic

Circulating throughout your body are natural hormones that relax you when stressed and relieve pain when you hurt. Most mothers don't even know these biologic labor assistants exist and, more important, that they can influence when and how these hormones are released. In the 1970s researchers studying drug addiction stumbled upon the presence of specialized areas in the brain, called receptor sites, for morphinelike substances. They discovered endorphins (from *endogenous,* meaning "produced in the body," and *morphine*-like substances), chemical pain relievers produced in the nerve cell that attach to receptor sites on the cell blunting the sensation of pain in these cells. Here's what we know about these natural remedies and how they can work for you.

- Endorphin levels go up during contractions in active labor (especially during the second stage of labor), are highest just after birth, and return to prelabor levels by two weeks postpartum.

- Endorphin levels were found to be highest during vaginal deliveries, less high in cesarean births in which the mother had also labored, and lowest in cesarean births performed before mother's labor had begun.

- Endorphin levels are elevated in newborns who had signs of fetal distress during delivery. The baby also receives these natural pain relievers during birth.

- Endorphin levels are increased during strenuous exercise, and there is no activity in the world that is more strenuous than labor.

- As an added benefit, endorphins stimulate the secretion of prolactin, the relaxing "mothering" hormone that regulates milk production and gives a woman a boost in interacting with her baby. Researchers believe that it is a combination of these hormones that contribute to the "birth high."

- Endorphins may account for the "high" mothers experience after a birth when sleep eludes them. Also, it seems possible that a mother having a surgical birth without going through labor may experience lower hormone levels after birth, which could account for the sometimes observed delay in milk supply after a cesarean birth.

- Endorphins are tied to a person's emotions. Unresolved stress and anxiety may increase the body's stress hormones (catecholamines), which counteract the relaxing effects of the endorphins.

- Like commercially produced narcotics, endorphins behave differently from woman to woman. This may be why some women are more sensitive to pain than others.

- Instead of the periodic "blast" you get with injectable narcotics (often making you groggy), your endorphins give you steady assistance throughout labor.

Laboring mothers who are aware of these hormonal effects describe their feeling as "naturally drugged." Set the birthing conditions that let these labor helpers work for you.

memories "having flashbacks." If your past is littered with flashbacks that are likely to surface during birth, don't wait until your first contraction to explore these issues. Take a psychological inventory of possible past problems that may hinder your birth, work through them, and seek professional help if necessary. If there are problems from your past or problems in the present that keep you from relaxing, ideally you should explore them before the pregnancy. If you're pregnant, seek professional help *well before* the day of the big event.

Plant good birth memories. Women carry their childbirth memories with them for the rest of their lives. For many women how they give birth affects the very heart of their identity as a woman, and is part of their sense of self-worth. For today's women, a successful birth is more than just bringing home a baby. Women also want to bring home a "positive birth experience."

A mother recalls the birth of her children in vivid detail — where she was when her water broke, a kind nurse who rubbed her back, even the pattern on the doctor's tie. All the nice little things that birth attendants do are imprinted in mother's memories. Positive words, such as "Everything's going as expected," "You're doing really well," and "What a beautiful baby" mean a lot. "I love you" are three little words from your partner that will be imprinted forever. Since you will carry around this treasure chest of birth memories forever, be sure to store up all the pleasant things that happen. The best way to prevent filling your mind with disturbing reruns is to make the episode right in the first place.

Heal bad memories. It's okay to be happy about your healthy baby but sad about your birth. Unresolved birth memories have a way of gnawing at your insides, affecting your sense of who you are. What happened at your baby's birth can influence your feelings about yourself during the postpartum period and for the rest of your life. Unpleasant memories from past births often resurface to infect subsequent births. It's healthy to confront the fact that you failed to have the birth you wanted rather than pretending

it doesn't matter, so that you can deal openly with the feelings of loss. You can then realistically examine what happened, see where you went wrong, and make changes to keep it from happening next time. By coming to terms with the past ("I did the best I could at the time, and I know better now"), you can avoid a replay of your previous birth.

Prepare for a no-fault birth. If you have high but rigid expectations, where anything less than an unmedicated, intervention-free delivery is considered a failure, you will set yourself up for an unsatisfying birth. Any deviation from perfection may make you feel that your body failed you, and these flashbacks of "failure" crop up for a long time. If, however, you confidently participate in all the decisions made during your labor and delivery — even those that weren't in your original birth plan — you are likely to look on your birth with no blame and no regrets. Even when things don't go as planned, you can have positive memories of your participation in the decision making. You can say "Yes, I failed to have a completely unmedicated birth, yet the little bit of drug I had helped me salvage the rest of my birth plan; and next time I'll know not to let myself get so exhausted that my coping level hits bottom."

Educate yourself for birth. Knowledgeable mothers experience labor differently. By understanding what's happening, and what your body's pain signals mean, you are less fearful and therefore more likely to find ways of getting more comfortable. The term *labor pains* is loaded and misleading. What used to be called labor "pains" childbirth educators now soften to the more accurate *labor contractions.* Physiologically, that is what they are — contractions. To call them "pains" implies that each and every one is inherently painful, and that simply isn't true.

We don't want to sugarcoat labor. Birth is an overwhelmingly powerful physical experience with many new sensations that can give rise to pain. Understanding the causes of pain in birth will help you accept these new sensations as a signal. Work to make changes rather than tensing up in fear, which will only make labor more painful. This will be the hardest work you will ever do in your whole life, and the rushes and waves of sensations may overwhelm you with their intensity. But try to balance these expectations with the confidence that you have the power to manage them, and equip yourself with the mental attitude that empowers you to do so. Long before delivery day practice the labor-easing tactics we suggest in chapter 9. Use your imagination to discover what will serve you best when the real work begins. Store these strategies in your birth bag of tricks to pull out when the need arises.

Moving for birth. While there are no absolute right positions for you to birth in, there is a right attitude about movement during labor. It is best to respond instinctively to your body's signals and, before the contraction becomes overwhelming, adjust your body to whatever position eases the discomfort. Add to this basic ingredient a supportive staff and the freedom to improvise and you have the recipe for a satisfying birth. The worst attitude toward movement during labor is clinging to the stereotype of birthing on your back without the freedom to move. Many women seem to be so culturally fixed in the horizontal labor position that they can't heed instinctual urges that would move them into vertical positions. Try these position-changing schemes:

- Don't look at pictures or videos of "on-your-back" labors. Scratch this birth scene from your memory. Twentieth-century women need to be deprogrammed in order to get back to basics and reclaim their birthing intuition. Studies show that women who are not culturally locked in to one birthing position tend to assume around eight different positions during the course of labor, and most of these are vertical or semiupright.

- Do look at the pictures of better birthing positions on page 189. Fix them in your memory. Photocopy them to hang on the wall by your labor bed. Think upright.

- Rehearse for birth during the last trimester of pregnancy. Practice all of these positions and devise some arrangements of your own. Practice not only accustoms your body to different moves; it also opens your mind to find your own individual approach.

The best labor position is one that helps your labor progress, and do so less painfully. Don't forget that the most comfortable position for mother is also often the most comfortable for baby.

Relaxing for Birth

MIND RELAXATION and muscle relaxation are the most helpful ways to lessen pain in labor. For birth, relaxation means to release tension so you can open up. Relaxation is a healthy part of daily living. Words for relaxing are part of our everyday vocabulary: "loosen up," "take it easy," "unwind." Relaxation is also a valuable tool for healthy birthing.

HOW RELAXATION HELPS YOUR LABOR

Relaxation helps in five ways:

- untenses birthing muscles to help them stretch more comfortably
- raises pain threshold, lessening labor discomforts
- releases natural pain-lessening hormones
- enhances mental acuity for decision making
- conserves energy, lessening exhaustion

Staying loose when the going gets tough conserves energy. Tensing all your muscles wastes energy, whereas relaxation releases tension and redirects energy to where it counts, to the big muscle that needs it — your uterus. Also, muscles send messages to each other. Clenched fists, a tight mouth, a furrowed brow, all send tension signals to the birth-passage muscles, the very ones that need to be loose. Tensing the top part of your body tenses the bottom, but opening up to relax these upper body parts opens up lower ones. A loose and relaxed mouth signals the birth canal to relax as well. This is why astute birth partners or labor-support persons spot-check the face, neck, and shoulders for signs of tension, and work on these upper areas, freeing mother to concentrate on her lower ones.

The mind–body connection. A relaxed mind mellows a tense body and vice versa. The brain and muscles communicate with each other not only by nerve impulses but through hormones — those magic substances that travel through the highways of one's body telling it how to respond. Every person produces stress hormones. You can't live or labor without them. Called catecholamines and cortisol, these helpful hormones enable the body to adapt quickly to life's sudden changes. For example, you hear a

---

Audiotape Resources to Relax By

- *Breastfeeding Your Baby and Relaxation Tips,* by William and Martha Sears and psychotherapist Dr. Lee Bewersdorf (29 min.). Available from La Leche League International ([800] LA-LECHE), or Medela, Inc., P.O. Box 386, Crystal Lake, IL ([800] 435-8316)
- *Relax for Childbirth,* by Penny Simkin (16 min.). Available from Pennypress, 110 23rd Avenue East, Seattle, WA 98112 ([206] 325-1419)

---

strange noise in the night. You awaken, and these quick-response hormones help your body cope. Suddenly you're awake and aware, your mind races with surprising clarity, and you act to protect yourself and your family. Your heart rate speeds up and you are ready for action. This is a normal and healthy stress response. But after you discover the nighttime noise was only the family cat, your mind can relax, your body resettles, and you reenter sleep. Or, you can continue to lie there in fear, your heart continuing to race, anxious and wide awake. Stress has now become *dis*tress. The hormones that helped you out before are now working against you.

Similar things happen in your body during labor. Any woman who has birthed a baby knows that birth is stressful. But in birth as in life the goal is to achieve the right balance of stress hormones — enough to get the job done but not enough to make you distressed. During a normal stress response, these hormones shunt blood from less important organs to the organs more vital to the body's well-being, such as the brain, liver, and heart. Blood can be shunted away from the uterus during prolonged and unresolved stress, depriving the uterus and its guest of vital oxygen. The result: diminished uterine efficiency, prolonged labor, and a distressed baby. Stress hormones go up during labor to help you push the baby out. But they also need to be kept in balance. Otherwise you are constantly anxious and fearful, and your body revs up and operates at a high and inefficient energy level, wearing out before the job is done. That's where relaxation can help.

Relaxing for two. Not only is the womb affected by stress hormones, but so is its resident. Besides feeling the effects of mother's changing blood chemistry, baby in utero also makes stress hormones to help adapt to the journey of birth. The electronic fetal monitor records how baby's heart rate drops during each contraction but bounces back up to normal afterward. Just the right balance of hormones helps the little person inside adapt to life in the working womb, and to all the pressure and biochemical changes that are going on around him. But, as with mother, too much stress and baby's well-being is jeopardized — fetal *dis*tress.

After birth these birth hormones, in the right balance, help baby adapt to life outside the womb. Perhaps they help stimulate the state of quiet alertness babies show after an unmedicated labor and delivery — that wide-eyed penetrating stare newborns often give their parents in the hour or so after birth. This opening look is a powerful enforcer of parent-newborn bonding. If, however, the natural birth hormones are out of balance, a baby who is exposed to a constant barrage of stressor hormones during pregnancy and delivery could be born with an overcharged nervous system resulting in fussy and agitated behavior. So, during pregnancy and labor you are relaxing for two.

The mind–pain connection. The more tension in the mind, the more pain in the laboring body. On page 131 we discussed how a relaxed muscle has a higher pain threshold and therefore hurts less. Unresolved stress upsets the body's master pain-control mechanism. Normally during labor, your body enjoys the right balance between stressor hormones and relaxer or pain-relieving hormones. If stressor hormones continually override your body's natural narcotics, pain prevails. If your mind is uptight, your cervix may be too.

Martha notes: Telling yourself the contractions you are feeling are "just prelabor" is a good way to keep stress off your back. In my labors, as soon as I realized "this is IT," my mind would switch into high gear and I would have instant tension as a labor companion. With baby number six I spent the morning thinking my contractions were just a trial run, and I did not shift out of my putter mode. Looking back on my "twenty-minute labor," I realize it was more like three or four hours. The only negative in this story is that we were too rushed before the birth to find our video camera.

The cycle of exhaustion. Your laboring body pays the price for exhaustion:

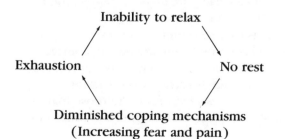

Inability to relax

Exhaustion

No rest

Diminished coping mechanisms
(Increasing fear and pain)

When you are worn out, your pain awareness increases, but your body's pain-coping mechanisms decrease. As a result, tired muscles hurt more and a tired mind perceives more pain. This is a double whammy. When you run out of steam, you also exhaust your reserves to push baby out and risk losing the motivation to improvise position changes that will help you during the second stage of labor. You just lie there and hurt and feel helpless to change your plight. Relaxation helps you conserve your energy during and between those first-stage contractions, so that when it's time to push, you are ready to go. If you don't relax and if you let yourself become too fatigued in the first stage of labor, you may feel exhausted by the second stage. It is easier to relax in early labor than in later stages. The contractions are usually not so intense and close together. As labor progresses, relaxation is more important but more challenging to achieve, especially in transition, when contractions are intense with little or no break in between.

RELEASING EXERCISES

Practice makes perfect. During your childbirth classes and birth rehearsals find out what relaxing techniques work best for you (though, admittedly, it's hard to know how you will respond to real labor). Create your own bag of mind- and muscle-loosening tricks that you will bring to birth. Enter labor equipped with a mind and body full of signal-responses that you can click on and off at will, like flipping a switch — tension off, relaxation on: "I hurt here, I do this, I feel better." Don't get stuck at the "I hurt here" phase. Some women freeze when pain hits, especially if they weren't expecting it. They never get to the "I do this, I feel bet-

Humor at Birth

Laughter is good medicine — for life and for labor. A little humor injected into a tense labor may be just what the doctor should order. Humor breaks the ice, reduces anxiety, and allows mother to refocus on her job. While birth is no comedy it doesn't have to be serious drama either. A well-timed joke raises the spirits of the whole birth team and breaks the monotony of a long, tedious labor. Laughter acts as a social lubricant, loosening up tight people.

Once I was called to attend a possibly high-risk birth. When I arrived, mother was laboring hard but making slow progress while a team of care providers stood around waiting for something to happen. Dad quipped, "This reminds me of my office. One person working hard, while everybody else stands around watching."

Not only is humor good for the mind, it's good for the body, especially in labor. Laughter increases the level of endorphins, the body's natural pain relievers and relaxers. It decreases levels of unwelcome stress hormones and relaxes muscles. Laughter is like an internal massage. As the ancient writings of Proverbs advise, "A cheerful spirit is health to the body and a strength to the soul." Bring a bit of humor to your birth.

ter" phase. Don't let pain incapacitate you. Listen to it and make changes. And remember, birth rehearsals are just that — rehearsals. They're never quite like the real thing. Don't become so attached to one set of tricks that you're unable to improvise on opening night.

The goal of releasing exercises in pregnancy is to learn to identify which muscles are tense and then to learn how to release tension from them. They also teach your birth partner to be a more astute tension-spotter. First get comfortable in the side-lying position (see figure, page 193), with your body well supported by pillows. With your partner's help, get your whole body comfortable before focusing on individual muscles. If you are practicing solo, lie before a mirror. Look for tension-telling signs (e.g., frowning forehead, tight mouth, clenched jaws, limbs straight instead of slightly

flexed). Check your whole position, then do head-to-toe spot checks of specific tight muscles: Open your mouth, drop your jaw, release your fingers. These releasing cues — open, release, loosen, unfold, ungrip — should become ingrained into your vocabulary during pregnancy. To do this well, you'll find you must relax mentally as well. Use music, dim lighting, quiet surroundings to encourage your mind to let go of all the daily pressures and distractions. Think "open!" Take a deep breath using your whole abdomen and slowly release it — a cleansing breath — to release the tension from your body.

This total-body relaxation prepares you for relaxing between and during contractions. After learning total-body release, practice contract — release exercises for individual muscles, especially those that you habitually tense under stress and those most

The Chemistry of Birth

Just as there is chemistry in love, there is chemistry in birth. Circulating throughout a laboring woman's body are chemical messengers — hormones that improve fetal growth, speed the progress of labor, and ease its discomforts. There are at least ten known birth hormones, each having its own time, place, and work to do during birth. *Endorphins* are the body's natural narcotics, which lessen pain and elevate moods, not only in the laboring mother but also in the baby. *Prolactin,* the mothering hormone, relieves tension and promotes milk production. *Oxytocin* enhances contractions. The *adrenal hormones* cortisol and catecholamines empower the mother to persevere through the stress of overwhelming sensations. *Relaxin* softens the cervix and relaxes the pelvic tissues helping form "the birth canal." *Prostaglandins* ripen the cervix and play a role in fetal maturity. Others, such as *estrogen* and *progesterone,* regulate the contractility and excitability of the uterine muscle. These hormones are automatically released during pregnancy and labor, but how much and when these biological aids play their part are somewhat under your control. You need to feel relaxed and unencumbered for this biochemistry to work best. Laboring in poor health or where fear and tension prevail may cause the release of biological substances that are counterproductive to labor. Being informed and prepared helps you flow with your body's signals and gets the right stuff working for you and your baby.

likely to tense during labor. Tense your mouth and concentrate on recognizing this tense-muscle feeling. Then relax your facial muscles and appreciate the difference. Get used to disliking the tense feeling and enjoying the relaxed one. For limb-release exercises, practice both tightening your limbs toward your body and straightening them out stiffly. For example, clench your fists and then release the tension as you unfold your fingers. Then fan out your fingers starlike and stiff, and release them as you feel your fingers fold slowly and limply toward your palms. Practice both flexing and straightening exercises since both muscle-tensing extremes occur during labor. There is no need to do these in an orderly head-to-toe progression. It's better to skip around slowly from part to part, much as you do in touch-relaxation practice (see page 157), since this is more like real labor. In the labor-embrace and dangle-squat positions (see figures on page 189), the birth partner is able to sense tension directly instead of only seeing it. Birth partners, practice watching for tension: what you see is what the laboring woman feels. During your daily activities, such as while dining, make her aware of her hot spots — muscle groups that she habitually tenses. If you notice a frowning forehead, help her release this area by identifying and letting go of the stress that caused it.

After you have become accustomed to release exercises while side-lying comfortably on the floor or bed, practice them in other birthing positions, such as kneeling, squatting, standing, and leaning. These are more realistic poses than lying on your side. Practice relaxation techniques in horizontal positions to use between contractions, and upright positions to use during contractions. This is where it gets tricky. You're asking some of your muscles to relax when others don't. During a real contraction all your other muscles may relax but your uterus certainly doesn't. And of course you can't practice for this. You can use one arm to play the part of your uterus and practice contracting your arm muscles while releasing all other muscles, including your perineal area. Much of the time in your childbirth classes will be spent focusing on specific relaxation exercises such as these. Play soothing music during your relaxation practices at home or try unwinding to a relaxation tape (see "Music to Birth By," page 147, and "Audiotape Resources to Relax By," page 142).

USING YOUR IMAGINATION

An increasingly popular relaxation technique is *mental imagery* — visualizing in your mind places, persons, or events that help you relax. These may be pleasant, memorable, real events from your past, or a fantasy that helps you unwind. Use birth-related images (riding a wave, climbing a mountain) that get you more involved with working with your labor. Sports psychologists use these techniques to help athletes perform better: "Picture yourself standing on the winners' platform holding a trophy." The rationale of this mental motivation is that if you can focus on the reward, you will muster up extra energy to achieve it. You are walking along your favorite beach, dining in your favorite restaurant with your mate, making love — whatever thoughts make you happy. Any time that your mind begins to be filled with counterproductive thoughts, immediately click on a better scene, as though you were changing channels. A marathon runner uses this mental cleansing to keep going. As soon as an "I can't go on" thought slows her down, she erases it from her mind and replaces it with more positive images that make her believe she can indeed finish the race.

During pregnancy you might find value in *meditation.* Meditation in various forms is a practice common to most religions. (The spiritual aspects of life are heightened in pregnancy and birth, so meditation is a natural.) It can be simply clearing your mind of disturbing thoughts and filling it with pleasant and calming ones. Some think of it as prayer. You've had a horrendous day at work. By day's end your mind is exploding with hundreds of life's little jabs. Instead of letting your mind overcome you, take charge. Retreat into a quiet place, turn on soothing music, and fill your innermost being with everything that's right with you and the world.

By learning these stress-releasing habits during pregnancy, you bring to birth a mind full of positive images, like having a large film library and being able to replay any scene on command. Mental imagery breaks what we call the molehill-to-mountain scenario. Little mental thorns have a way of escalating into big-time worries. Labor can quickly transform a mind full of little molehills into one filled with mountains that block your way. Mental imagery can prevent that from happening. Imagery is a relaxation tool, not a distraction gimmick. In our experience distraction is ineffective in most

Music to Birth By

Bring along your favorite sounds to birth. Music eases your mind and body, putting them into harmony with your labor. Music fills your mind with pleasant sensations that compete with the painful ones. Besides relaxing you, soothing background music also loosens up your birth attendants, mellowing your whole working environment.

Studies on the pain-relieving value of music (called *audioanalgesia*) have shown that mothers using music during labor required less pain-relieving medication. Researchers believe that the rhythm of sound may affect the rhythm of the body by stimulating release of those feel-good hormones — endorphins. It may also give the body a cue to do some rhythmic moving.

Best Birth Hits

Select your already tested favorites, rhythms that relax rather than rev up your system. Most women also prefer instrumental rather than vocal music unless it is very mellow like a lullaby. You may want to put together your own tape of selections and play this compilation during your birth rehearsals. There are even professional music therapists, who will help expectant parents create a tape to birth by. Try melodies with an ebb and flow, such as Pachelbel's Canon in D Major. Here are the Sears family's favorite birth selections:

- Harp concertos, for example: Premier Concerto, by Boieldieu
- Pachelbel's Canon in D Major
- Beethoven's Sixth Symphony
- *A Time for Peace,* by Ivory Sessions, Maranatha Music
- *Perfect Peace Instrumental,* Integrity Music
- *Winter Solstice II,* Windam Hill Records
- *Out of Africa* (original soundtrack)

Listening Tips

To use music as an imagery enhancer, associate the melody with a flashback of a pleasant event. We played harp concertos during our labors. Each time Boieldieu's Premier Concerto came on it recalled the scene where we played this piece a lot: sitting by the fire in a friend's ski chalet watching snow fall in the porchlight.

labors and we question whether or not a mother should try hard to distract herself from such important work. Distraction is actually a negative concept. It assumes labor is so terrible you must mentally escape from it. Even if you could (and some do) you are not dealing with the root cause of the pain.

Best thoughts. Visualization is not meant to make you deceive yourself but to help you free yourself from the thoughts that bind you. Search for images that will enhance your labor and not restrict it. There are no correct or incorrect thoughts, only those that work and those that don't. Let your mind run free. Don't let your creations go unrecorded. Write down the images that relax you during pregnancy. Most mothers find peace in water and beach scenes: waves rolling, waterfalls, streams meandering. Imagine: "I'm lying on a beach with water lapping at my feet. . . ." If fabricated images don't work, dwell upon real thoughts that trigger past pleasant associations: "That man walking on the beach later became my husband." Of course if imagining ocean scenes reminds you of being seasick, you may need to travel to the mountains instead. Some mothers have even recalled conception night as an image to get them through intense labor pains. Others find comfort visualizing their favorite dessert. One mother found it helpful to erase the word "pain" from her thoughts. When her contractions began, instead of anticipating a "pain," she imagined, "Here comes a *pleasant*"!

Get real! There are as many visualization and thought maneuvers as there are laboring women. During your childbirth classes you will learn several techniques. Select what works for you and fits your personality and beliefs. It is not necessary to manufacture some mystical *Star Wars*–like force that you imagine traveling in and out of your body. If you don't believe in "the force" in real life, you're not likely to believe in it in real labor. Nor is it prudent to rehearse visualizing an escape from your body. Your goal in all these pain-easing tools is to make labor manageable, not to avoid it. No matter how well you rehearse an out-of-body experience, labor will bring you back down to earth, where you need to be.

Package the pain. Few mothers using visualization are able to convince themselves that contractions are painless. But if you are a pictorial person easily swayed by the powers of suggestion, your imagination can help you relax. Here is a strategy we call "packaging the pain." Instead of trying to escape from pain, face it head on. Grab the pain like a big glob of modeling clay and massage it

down into a tiny ball. Wrap up the pain, put it in a balloon, and imagine it leaving your body, floating up into the sky. You can use the same floating-away imagery to send off the distressing stuff in your mind. Wrap the junk up in a package, put it in the balloon, and let it go. Take a deep breath and exhale, blowing the balloon away. This is a real sigh of relief.

Visualize your labor. During pregnancy practice visualizing your labor. "See" your labor progressing normally, rehearse it in your mind so when real labor begins you are prepared. Some mothers manage their contractions by visualizing what's happening in their uterus. Picture your baby inside trying to push his way through a stretchy turtlenecklike cervix. Visualize your cervix expanding as it pulls up over this adorable little head that you will soon hold. Some mothers visualize the cervix and then the vagina as a flower that is slowly opening. As your contractions build up so can the vividness, or the outrageousness, of your imagination. Big contractions require bigger thoughts.

Keep the end in mind. Focusing on your goal rather than on what you have to go through to get it helps get you through your contractions. By visualizing the finish line and the prize, the runner doesn't get hung up on the hurdles; neither does she forget they are there, lest she run into them. Picture life after labor. Envision your baby and what you will do when you see her. You'll reach down to feel her head as it emerges. Then you will hold her wet slippery body against your warm abdomen. She will open her eyes and suddenly the ordeal becomes worthwhile.

The Sexuality of Birth

While few women would equate having a baby with having sex, many feel that birth is the ultimate expression of their sexuality. We know women who said they were very aware of sexual pleasure they felt when the baby emerged. During the pushing stage a few women even claim to have had a "birth orgasm." Could it be that most women are missing something here? Consider these physical and emotional similarities between birth and sex.

Giving birth and experiencing sex share the same hormones. Oxytocin, for example, both enhances labor contractions and produces orgasm. Prolactin and endorphins account for pleasurable feelings during both sex and childbirth. Nipple stimulation, a favorite foreplay technique, also intensifies birth contractions. The release of all these mood and response regulators can be enhanced or inhibited by the emotional and physical setting.

Because birth and sex are so intimately related, a woman's sexuality and her self-worth can be affected by how she experiences birth. If, instead of controlling her own birthing, she views her experience as being controlled by others, a woman may feel devalued and violated. With time and some emotional effort, she may come to terms with this loss and compensate for it in other ways.

Or she may feel that her body failed her, a feeling that may carry over into her view of herself as a woman and as a mother, and how she regards sex.

Birth pushes buttons that release sexual feelings from the past. If a woman's sexual memories are scarred with molestation, for example, she may have trouble surrendering to herself during birth, or take on a victim mentality, setting herself up for an intervention-filled birth (see also birth memories, page 139). How a woman experiences sex is a clue to how she may experience birth. A woman who is comfortable with her body (and her environment) and is able to surrender to her instinctual self during sex is more likely to do so during birth. A woman's mind-set about sex may also affect how she views birth. If she views sex as dirty or ugly, she may miss the marvels and beauty of growing a baby in her uterus and pushing the baby out through her birth canal; instead she may get caught up in the blood and mess of birth and regard it as a crisis event.

Susan was a first-time mother who carefully selected her birth attendant and birth place. She told us, "I feel that just as the sexual act is a consummation of love, birth is the consummation of pregnancy." She went on to conclude, "The right environment for birth is like the right environment for sex."

None of these relaxing techniques will work if you are bound up in fear (see "Rx for Healing Fears," page 135). The imaginative powers of your mind are endless. Let them work for you during birth.

A POTPOURRI OF RELAXATION AND COMFORT TIPS

Here are some favorite ways to relax that mothers we know brought to their births:

- **Visualizing favorite foods.** One child-birth educator reminded her prenatal mothers: "*Stressed* spelled backward becomes *desserts.*"

- **Favorite scents**. Some mothers bring their favorite smells, such as peppermint or spice, to give off a pleasant aroma during labor.

- **Favorite rollers.** Tennis balls and paint rollers make nice back massagers.

- **Birth balls.** We have a twenty-eight-inch-diameter rubber ball we use for physiotherapy for one of our children. Pregnant mothers visiting our home love to sit on it. This type of ball is also helpful for labor. Sitting and rolling on a physio ball can relax the pelvic muscles. Be sure you master this exercise during pregnancy, lest you roll off at the height of a contraction. This round, rubber labor aid is available in physiotherapy catalogs. Ask for a ball with a diameter between twenty-four and twenty-eight inches. Inflate to desired comfort.

- **Bean bag chair.** As with birth balls, you are not likely to find this squishy little nest in your local maternity ward. You might need to bring your own. A soft cloth

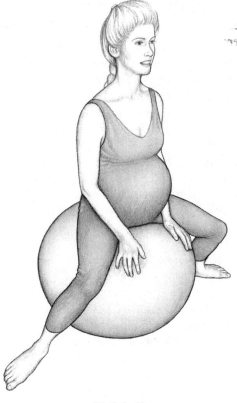

Birth ball

cover feels best, if you don't mind a few stains, or if the bean bag is vinyl, cover it with a blanket. Sink into this supportive nest and sprawl your limbs over the sides. Use oval or rectangular bags, large enough to allow you to lie on your side. Bean bag stores are happy to add or subtract the little foam beads inside to suit your comfort.

- **Foam wedges.** Tapered foam wedges, inexpensively bought at upholstery shops, can be placed behind your lower back while sitting or beneath your abdomen while side-lying to give support and relieve discomfort.

- **Birth notes.** During pregnancy collect encouraging quips that relax and empower. Write them on 3 × 5 cards and bring your treasured collection to birth. These bits of wisdom may be memorable lines from birth books you've read, verses from poems or Scriptures, or humorous limericks. An affectionate verse we enjoy is:

  I wish I were a teddy bear.
  No one cares how fat they are.
  And the older they get, the more
       valuable they are.

  Listening to a gentle voice reading their favorite scriptural verses gives some women borrowed strength. And hearing your loved one reading a deeply meaningful lyric from a love song can not only melt you in the present, but will provide a moment of tenderness in your birth memory that you will keep forever.

- **Hot and cold packs**. Heat and cold ease labor pain by changing blood flow and pain perception in local tissues. Apply these readily available aids to tense back, abdominal, and perineal tissues. Try a warm shower jet well aimed at those aching lower back muscles; or a hot-water bottle or warm water–filled rubber surgical gloves nestled against your lower abdomen. Moist heat, such as a warm towel soaked in hot water, wrung out, and wrapped in a waterproof pad can relax tense abdominal or thigh muscles. Most birthing units have a blanket warmer where you can get a steady supply of warm items to place against hurting areas. While most mothers prefer warm comforts, some get better relief from cold packs, such as ice water in a rubber glove or in a hot-water bottle or a pack of fro-

zen, chopped veggies. Cover ice packs with cloth; no bare ice to bare skin, please. A cool cloth applied to a hot forehead by a caring hand may be the best method for the moment. Sucking on a cold, wet washcloth can be just what you need for a dry mouth during the hot and heavy phases when even nibbling on ice chips is too much of a bother.

- **Acupressure.** Acupressure is like acupuncture, but it's done with the fingers. Also known as *shiatsu* (from the Japanese *shi* for finger and *atsu* for pressure), this pain-relieving method is based on stimulating pain-controlling points around the body. Practitioners of this technique can teach a couple during pregnancy which points control which areas of the body. We do not have personal experience with this skill, but we know women who have employed acupressure specialists to help ease their labor pain. There are easily accessible books that teach these skills.

- **TENS**. Transcutaneous electrical nerve stimulation (TENS) is a pain-easing technique that is used in pain centers mainly for postoperative pain. TENS is being used to ease labor pain, and it is most helpful with continuous pain like that of back labor rather than with the rhythmic pain of contractions, which allows for rest in between. A TENS unit, about the size of a deck of cards, is held in the mother's hand. Wires from the unit are attached by tape to areas of the mother's skin, usually around the lower back. When mother senses a contraction or back pain coming on, she operates the electrical-current generator to send tingling sensations into the skin and muscle. The mother can adjust the level of electrical stimulation as desired. Practitioners of both acupressure and TENS believe that pressure and electrical current interfere with the conducting of the pain signals and stimulate local endorphin release. These mechanisms decrease either the local sensation or the awareness of pain.

WATER FOR BIRTH

Tops on the Sears family's easier labor list is the simplest, most available, and least expensive tool for a more comfortable labor — water. Our only regret is that it took us seven babies to discover it. Water ranks as the most effective yet undervalued labor assistant.

While new in America, water is a familiar tool in labor and birth in other countries. Water-birthing was used in Russia in the 1960s, and during the seventies and eighties French obstetrician Michel Odent studied the benefits of laboring in water in hundreds of women using "water pools" (oversized tubs). He shared his discoveries with the rest of the world in his book, *Birth Reborn*. Once the French, widely respected for their sophistication, tested the waters for this new approach, it gained worldwide respectability, if not acceptance. Until the 1990s, few American hospitals were willing to get their feet wet, preferring to stick with more traditional approaches to birthing. But because the studies showing the value of laboring in water are so convincing, we predict that for hospitals who wish to stay in the baby business, labor pools will soon be as standard as birthing beds.

Why Water Works

Water relieves pain during labor because of the law of buoyancy, known as Archimedes'

principle, which says that an object in water will displace a volume of water equal to its own weight and be acted upon by an upward force. Simply put, water gives a pregnant mother a lift. When a laboring mother gets into a deep pool of water she feels almost weightless as the water supports her muscles and bones. This spares energy for the hardworking uterus. As thigh, back, and abdominal muscles relax, the birth passage muscles also relax. When Martha opted to use water in her seventh labor, she was experiencing sharp pain down low in front. She had tried all the standard maneuvers but simply could not relax enough. Once in the water, it took several contractions before she found the position that best allowed her muscles to relax. Then the internal relaxation that had been eluding her finally came, and the pain literally melted away. But it wasn't instant relief; she had to experiment and be in the water long enough to let the buoyancy work.

The deeper mother is immersed in the pool, the greater the weight-reducing effects and the more the counterpressure on her tissues. Mothers enduring back labor are especially grateful for the almost instant relief that the counterpressure on a hurting back brings. As the back muscles relax, so can the internal tissues, allowing baby more leeway to make his maneuvers, especially when his head is in a posterior position.

Water labor fits in nicely with our philosophy that what's good for the mother is good for the baby. Water is relaxing. A relaxed mother houses a healthier baby. In contrast, stress and anxiety cause the release of stress hormones, which may not be in the best interest of mother or baby. To protect the vital organs, such as the brain, heart, and kidneys, stress hormones steal blood from nonvital sites (and the body under stress considers the uterine muscle a nonvital organ). If blood flow to the uterus is short-changed, baby can become oxygen-deprived. So it is likely that a baby receives increased oxygen when mother takes a nice warm bath.

Water is releasing. Contractions and water are a perfect match: Mothers feel that contractions come in waves. They speak of an ebb and flow. Enclosed in the privacy and security of her own "womb," mother escapes from foreign interventions and is free to improvise without inhibitions. Water frees her body to float into the most comfortable position as she finds one that eases contraction discomfort. Water frees her mind to tap into her deepest labor instincts, letting go of external tensions and internal memories that may have a hold on her. Next time you get into a swimming pool see if these feelings don't ring true. There is a surrender of mind and body in water that may not be possible on land.

Water tricks the pain-sensing system. Immersion in water acts like a continuous total-body massage, stimulating temperature- and touch-sensitive receptor nerves in the skin. These stimuli bombard the nervous system with pleasant sensations, virtually gridlocking the gate to painful stimuli. It would take thousands of fingertips to reach the same number of receptor sites in the skin that can be stimulated by a nice warm soak.

What Water Research Shows

Not only does our personal experience make us champion the cause of water laboring, but research also shows that laboring in water is safe and beneficial. From 1985 through 1993 approximately eighteen hundred women labored in Jacuzzi-type pools at the Family Birthing Center in Upland, California. The center's director and obstetrician, Dr. Michael Rosenthal, told us that women who used water almost always experienced shorter, easier labors, and experienced a cesarean-section rate one-third that of traditional hospital births. Water labor was particularly useful for mothers desiring a vaginal birth after cesarean. One birthing center specializing in water labor reported an 87.5 percent VBAC success rate. A study comparing eighty-eight women who spent one-half to two hours of their labor in a warm bath versus a "no bath" control group showed the following results: cervical dilation was 2½ centimeters per hour in the water mothers compared with 1¼ centimeters per hour in the control group; the descent of the water mothers' babies was twice as fast; and the mothers in water experienced less pain. More gain for less pain — that's a good deal.

Mothers labeled "high risk" because of high blood pressure showed a dramatic reduction in blood pressure within minutes of immersion in the pool. Concerning the use of water in labor and birth Dr. Rosenthal comments, "The use of water for labor and birth is a sane, intelligent, practical and safe procedure. It's humane; it restores control of birthing back to women; and it eliminates the need for many medical interventions that are clearly counterproductive when compared to the amazingly simple 'intervention' of allowing a woman to sit in warm water."

Using Water for Labor

While you should feel free to create your own movements when laboring in water, here are a few suggestions we personally have found helpful.

- Try bath-water temperature (usually body temperature or slightly less). The bath should be at least two feet deep to cover the mother's abdomen when she kneels or squats. To encourage freestyle movements, the pool should be at least 5½ feet wide.

- The best time to take the plunge is when active labor begins, usually between 5 and 8 centimeters' dilation. Getting into the pool too early may cause labor to stall (this could be used to an advantage in a long, latent phase where the mother is exhausted yet has trouble resting and sleeping, especially if she has no access to sedatives). Many women find water labor particularly comforting during transition when freestyle movements assist baby to find the path of least resistance. Most women find that when their contractions come on like tidal waves, they're glad to be in the pool. If your contractions on land become so overwhelming that you feel you are about to sink, you may find that being in water will keep you afloat.

- Back labor is a sure signal to get wet and improvise to your back's content. The counterpressure of the water will ease the pressure of contractions. Rather than staying in pain, stay in the water.

- If a previously active labor stalls while you are comfortably floating in the pool, it's best to get out and walk, kneel, or squat on land to get your labor going again after you've rested. Once contractions resume with increasing intensity, it's okay to reenter your "womb."

- Besides easing the pain of unmanageable contractions, water can sometimes jump-start a stalled labor. So if your labor is going nowhere, go to the pool. One mother told us that water helped her con-

tractions restart because she had the water at nipple level. The splashing of the water against her nipples stimulated contraction-producing hormones.

- Unless you're advised to the contrary, it's safe to use water labor even after your membranes have ruptured. That's when you're most likely to need water anyway. While theoretically there is risk of infection, centers with significant experience in water labor report no increased infection rate in women using water after their membranes rupture, as long as the woman is in active labor and as long as proper infection control standards are followed. (These standards are explained in "Resources for Water During Labor and Birth," page 157.)

- It is rarely necessary to leave the water for fetal monitoring. Underwater handheld monitors are available for intermittent fetal monitoring, or the nurse can use the fetoscope on the bulge protruding just above the surface. Also, the nurse can put a plastic bag over the usual Doptone monitor.

- Don't expect water to wipe all sensations away. It decreases pain, but it may not completely drown it out. How you move in the water is often just as important as the water itself. Let being in the pool bring out the mermaid in you.

- If your hospital or birth center does not offer a labor pool, try taking a shower. A well-directed warm water jet is a boon to back labor. If you're laboring at home, a shower or bath will be a welcome friend. Sometimes it's not only the feel of water that relaxes but also the soothing sounds of the shower running or the tub filling. Use these sounds to imagine ocean waves,

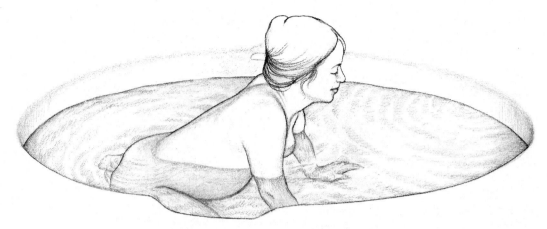

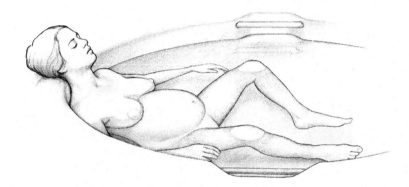

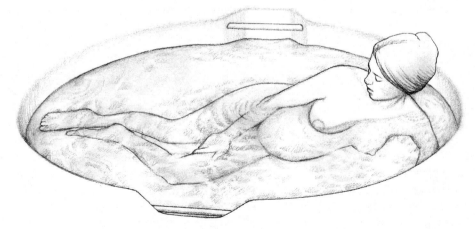

Labor pool

a babbling brook, or a rushing stream accompanying the waves of your concentration.

- Rent a pool. If your birth place doesn't offer a labor pool (birthing centers often have their own, as do midwives) and you wish to use one, you can rent a portable pool (see list of resources, page 157). Make sure you alert your physician and birth place of your intentions before you rent the labor pool. If you face resistance, show your doctor the list of references to water labor on page 262. Maybe the birth place will get the clue that they are lacking a valuable tool in their establishment.

- When to get in and out of the water is a matter of choice. Be sure to enter and exit the pool between contractions. For most women, when they feel the urge to push, it's time to get dry.

Using Water for Birthing

Our water suggestions in this book are mainly for the use of water in labor, not water-birthing. But if water works so well and your water labor is so manageable, why not just stay submerged to birth your baby? Water births are perfectly safe when done properly, but culturally we are not used to them. For the western mind-set, water-birthing conjures up a back-to-nature, counterculture image. Physicians and hospitals are just getting used to water labor. Perhaps someday water births will gain medical respectability. Meanwhile, most of the objections to water-birthing lie in people's minds more than in reality. In fact, birth centers with the experience of nearly a thousand water births report excellent outcomes for mother and baby, often better than for traditional births in beds.

Many water births are unplanned. They just happen because the mother is so comfortable that she feels "Why rock the boat? I'll just have my baby right here." It is perfectly safe to do so as long as baby is brought above water right after birth. The school of water-birthing that practices slow emergence can be dangerous. In the slow-emergence method, baby is left under water for a while to "ease the transition to life outside the womb." Proponents believe that as long as the cord is pulsating, baby is getting enough oxygen. Opponents counter that since the placenta begins to separate from the uterus within seconds after birth, less oxygen is available to the baby, and they argue that cord pulsations are an unreliable measure of satisfactory oxygen delivery. We definitely discourage slow-emergence birth. Perhaps we can humble ourselves enough to take a tip from creatures of the sea. Whales and dolphins shuttle their newborns to the surface immediately after birth. Certainly, these mammals have a lot more experience with water-birthing than we humans do.

Water labor is not a passing fad. We believe it is here to stay, mainly because it makes sense. Nor is it new and radical. In the overall span of human history what's new and radical is birthing on the back with an epidural. It's only a matter of time until water labor becomes part of mainstream obstetrics. If your hospital is worried about liability, explain to them that there is no other obstetrical intervention that is so simple yet carries such a low risk and at a lower cost. Weigh the costs and risks of five dollars' worth of water versus a $1,500 epidural. This simple and inexpensive labor-saving tool belongs wherever birth is taking place.

Resources for Water During Labor and Birth

- *Waterbirth. The precise guide to using water during pregnancy, birth and infancy.* Janet Balaskas and Yehudi Gordon, M.D. (London: Unwin Hyman Limited, 1990).
- *Global Maternal/Child Health Association,* P.O. Box 366, West Linn, OR 97068 (800) 641-BABY. This organization rents and sells birth tubs, and refers couples to waterbirth practitioners and birth centers.
- *Family Birth Center,* 1125 East Arrow Highway, Upland, CA 91786 (909) 946-7001.

Don't expect to soak comfortably in a warm tub throughout hours of painless labor and then hop out and quickly birth your baby. Water is only one tool in your whole labor-management kit. The most successful labor-easing program combines intermittent warm water immersion with upright activity, such as walking, kneeling, and squatting. A bit of mermaid plus a bit of human activity is a winning combination.

TOUCHES FOR BIRTH

Birth partners take note! One of the simplest ways to help a mother relax during labor is right at your fingertips. Massage is one of nature's oldest proven remedies for mind tension and muscle tension, and it's a handy helper for birth. Studies show that laboring mothers who were given frequent doses of caring and appropriate touches during labor were less anxious and handled their contractions better. Here is how mother and birth partner can develop the right touch.

Why Touch Works

Besides pain receptors, touch receptors reside in the skin. When you stimulate these receptors, you speed "feel good" messages to the brain. These messages reach the brain faster than their rivals, the pain signals. Touch messages can fill up the brain with good feelings so that there is less room for painful feelings. The pain messages don't go away if there isn't a place for them. They just keep circling around until the touch messages pull out and make room for them. This is why prolonged touch may be necessary.

Vary the site and intensity of touching. The same stroke eventually bores the brain and gradually loses its competitive edge — a phenomenon called *habituation*. Another reason for changing touches is that different strokes produce different messages. The most sensitive and easily touchable areas are the hairless body parts: fingertips, lips, palms, and soles. Stimulating these surfaces produces the fastest nerve impulses, and there are more places for these in the brain. Perhaps this explains why laboring women often massage their lips with lip balm. Many a woman has made it through labor having her feet rubbed. And don't forget the pleasurable feeling of a well-timed kiss on the lips.

Along with these superficial touch receptors are other sensors, lying deeper in the skin. These pressure-sensitive receptors bombard the brain with even more competing messages. This is why pressing or kneading often makes a deeper impression than a light rub. The more types of touch you try, the more stimuli occupy the brain and literally keep the pain out of your mind.

Practicing Touch

Labor support is definitely a hands-on job. During your prenatal practice sessions learn the right touch. For couples who are out of touch with the benefits of massage, pregnancy is a good time to make this a part of your relaxation repertoire. Instead of waiting until labor to discover where to rub, practice different strokes on different parts of the body so that both of you can work out a touch partnership that is most likely to produce good feelings at birth. Prenatal practice is also helpful in training your partner's muscles so they don't become tired so quickly during the real event.

Learning the right touch. Mothers, show and tell your birth partners where and how you like to be touched. Rehearse together until you both understand what touches feel best. But remember, the rub a mother likes during pregnancy may not be the touch she wants during labor. Every mother has certain spots she wants rubbed at various stages of labor, and every birth partner has his own personal touch. Birth partners, learn to identify, by sight and by touch, where your mate shows tension, and work on these spots. Get a feel for your job. Stay tuned for frequent "rub where it hurts" signals that demand a quick response and just the right touch.

As a rule, male birth partners do not touch their laboring mate as often or as long as do female assistants. Labor-support women whom we have watched frequently massage for hours on end, because they know a massage can make an incredible difference in the comfort of labor. Encourage your male partner to make a conscious effort to go beyond what he naturally may think would be adequate "touch time" and to keep a hands-on approach. If this is uncomfortable for your partner or he feels too pressured, consider adding a labor-support professional to your team. She can fill in the gaps and allow him the freedom of doing what he does best — loving you and encouraging you in a manner that is most comfortable to him.

Rubbing the wrong way. Birth partners, don't take rejection of your advances personally. Laboring mothers are supersensitive to every stimulus, especially touch. And this is one time in their lives when women are not known or expected to be polite. An unanticipated "Stop that!" may set you back a few strokes, but that is because you may have unknowingly touched off an irritating response rather than a pleasant one. It's not a rejection of your touch altogether. One mother was disturbed when her husband moved her bangs in the opposite way she combed them. Some women reject "tickle" touches, and feathery fingertip strokes, but prefer a down-to-business firm pressure. Many childbirth classes advocate using "tools," such as tennis balls or paint rollers. Expect some areas to be off-limits (in some women the abdominal bulge); touching these spots irritates rather than relaxes. Also, expect the "hot spots" to change at different points through labor. The touches that were desirable at 3 centimeters may need modifying or changing totally at 7 centimeters to be interpreted as pleasant or helpful. There's a right time and a right place for all birth touches.

Little touches mean a lot. As you and your partner work out a massage technique, you may find subtle strokes that either trigger pleasure or touch off resentment. Stroking down in the direction of the hair, for example, is usually pleasant, while rubbing upward against the hair shaft goes against the grain, a feeling many mothers find irritating. Try demonstrating to your partner the type, rhythm, and pressure you enjoy most as you massage him. He'll learn quickly and appreciate your touch. When teaching someone how to massage to your liking, be sure to instruct them in an affirming way: "A little bit lower and softer please. . . . Yeah, that's great!"

Types of Touch

During your childbirth class your instructor will demonstrate various types of massage for labor. Massage is best with skin-to-skin contact, using a nonpetroleum vegetable oil, such as one recommended by massage instructors. Experiment with different strokes using different degrees of pressure such as the following:

- Light caressing, stroking with fingertips and palms, is welcome on the face and scalp.

- Deep pressure is usually preferred for large tense muscles, such as shoulders, thighs, and calves.

- Kneading (squeezing and releasing with the whole hand) may be particularly helpful for large muscle groups, such as shoulders, buttocks, thighs, calves, and feet.

- Counterpressure (continually pressing with the heel of your hand), applied to the lower back area, is a welcome relief for back labor (see "Rx for 'Back Labor,'" page 216).

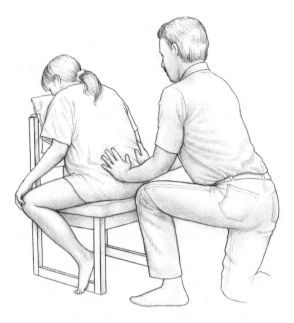

Use counterpressure to relieve back pain

Touch Relaxation

The tension-releasing technique of touch relaxation draws on an age-old physiologic principle of conditioned response. You condition a person to expect a pleasurable event to follow a familiar stimulus. To benefit from this technique, during your final few weeks of pregnancy, you and your birth partner can practice these exercises: you tense a muscle, he lays a hand on the spot, and the two of you work out what kind of touch will relax the area. With repetition you and your partner will establish touch cues and responses. For example, you tense your shoulder blades, your partner perceives where you are tense, and he puts the right touch on the area; by a conditioned response, you relax your shoulders and look forward to your partner's continuing the massage.

Mother's Action	Partner's Touch	Mother's Response
• Frowns and grimaces, a sign of tense facial muscles	• Applies pressure on both temples, releases when frown relaxes; or strokes forehead side to side as if smoothing out the wrinkles	• Relaxes facial muscles
• Arches her back and tenses her back muscles	• Kneels behind mother, kneading her tense back muscles	• Relaxes back muscles

Touch relaxation conditions you to relax and release at the first reminder of muscle tension. You allow the tension to flow out of yourself into your partner's hands. This special touch prompts you to expect pleasure to follow muscle tension, not pain. When you first sense a contraction coming, your mind and body will be conditioned to release rather than tense.

BREATHING FOR BIRTH

Breathing is so automatic you do it in your sleep. So why learn how to breathe for birth? Every strenuous exercise causes the body to alter its breathing patterns for best performance. Since birthing is one of the most strenuous exercises humanly possible, it stands to reason that the better you breathe, the better you birth.

You will naturally experience your body's need to change the rate, depth, and rhythm of its respirations throughout this event. Rather than rehearsing a prepatterned way to breathe during different phases of labor, allow your body to respond naturally to the stress of labor and work with its cues. It is also beneficial to know how to guide your breathing to avoid the pitfalls of panic, tension, and hyperventilation.

A Breath of Fresh Air

Back when breathing patterns were the hallmark of prepared-childbirth classes, much of what was taught was indeed a lot of hot air. Mothers and their partners rehearsed formulated breathing patterns called *patterned breathing* for the various phases of labor. But what was learned in class often failed at birth. Lamaze graduates entered the labor room armed with these breathing techniques, and, like inspired robots, clicked into a canned breathing pattern within a millisecond of every uterine twitch. The intent of the complicated breathing patterns was to give a woman something to do so she wouldn't notice how much labor hurt, and give the partner something to do to feel like an active participant in the labor. Typically, however, what happened was that the woman would abandon "the breathing" in frustration once in the grip of an overwhelming contraction. We remember a mother who went to pieces during transition, confessing, "I forget how I'm supposed to breathe!"

Today's childbirth instructors have simplified breathing techniques so they are easier to understand and carry out. They have created a more flexible approach to encourage women to practice and adapt whatever breathing pattern works for whatever stage of labor they're in. If you sense our bias against giving too much importance to breathing techniques for birth, it is intentional. Also, breathing styles are a lifelong pattern. Sedentary women tend to be chest breathers while athletic women tend to be abdominal breathers. To try to "correct" established breathing patterns and change them for birth would in itself make a woman nervous. Specific breathing techniques should be just one of many tools in your whole bag of birth tricks and, we believe, one of the least important. A professional labor assistant who works in our practice shared her experience of breathing techniques with us:

As a labor and delivery nurse for ten years, I have observed and been involved in a thousand-plus births, and out of those I have seen only four couples use patterned-breathing techniques successfully throughout labor. Most women become so frustrated with the concentration it takes to continue and change breathing patterns, that they find "the breathing" confuses and stresses rather than relaxes them. They find breathing isn't sufficient to distract them from the intensity of the late active phase and transition contractions. They then either switch intuitively to an internal focus and to consistent deeper, slower breathing to relax them and tune into working with their body, or turn to medical pain-relief measures, such as epidural anesthesia.

Breathing Through Your Birth

Proper breathing through your birth does not guarantee "breezing" through your

birth. But many women will attest to the fact that keeping breathing slow and even is a valuable tool for relaxation. It delivers the most oxygen to you and your baby with the least amount of effort. Breathing too fast and too deep (see "Avoiding Hyperventilation," page 163) or not breathing at all (see "Don't Hold Your Breath," page 162) is unhealthy for you and the baby. But you can use natural breathing patterns to your advantage. As your contractions begin to demand your attention, assume a comfortable position; totally relax all muscles and allow your head to lean back if supported, or fall forward as if imitating sleep. Your breathing should be at a comfortable, slow rate with normal depth. If you notice that you are feeling out of breath, funny, or lightheaded, you are unphysiologically altering your normal breathing pattern. As you get a few good contractions under your belt you'll settle into breathing that is relaxing and comfortable for you.

As the intensity of contractions increase, you may desire to add an element of concentration and comfort to your breathing. When a contraction begins, take in a deep breath, then gently blow out as if you were inhaling peace and exhaling tension. Your exhale now becomes your body's cue to release tension; as you blow out, you go limp all over, especially in your abdomen and pelvis. This is not the cheek blow used for birthday candles, but a long, steady release of air involving both abdominal and chest muscles. Continue to breathe normally, but inhale through your nose (to keep your mouth from getting dry), and exhale through your mouth with a gentle, long, relaxed blow. This breathing will not take you out of yourself and away from your task, but will assist you in purposely relaxing

Don't Hold Your Breath

Blow out the scene of blue-in-the-face breathing for birth. During the pushing stage you usually will feel urges to push with each contraction. You will need to take in a deep breath and bear down. But there's no need to hold your breath longer than the bearing-down reflex lasts — usually only around five seconds. Prolonged breath-holding and pushing (ten to fifteen seconds or more) until your eye vessels pop is unnecessary and unhealthy for you and baby. You both need all the oxygen you can get during the final sprint. Research has shown that this type of breathing (called the *valsalva maneuver*) causes the following unphysiologic changes in the body: increased pressure in the chest, which slows down the return of blood to the heart and lowers blood pressure; less blood, containing less oxygen, to the uterus; and fetal heart-rate changes, suggesting that baby is not getting enough oxygen.

Better than prolonged tight-lipped breath-holding is breathing the baby out by short periods of bearing down as the urges come. As the contraction begins, wait until you feel an urge to push. When it comes, breathe in deeply and bear down for about five seconds, then release that air and repeat the sequence as the urges come. This allows your diaphragm and abdominal muscles to help in pushing the baby out — and ensures that they will have the fuel to do so. Always keep your mouth open and your jaw relaxed. You can allow air to be released while you are actively bearing down if that feels better. Also, breathing out helps the pelvic floor muscles relax rather than tighten, as happens with breath-holding and straining. Also, breath released out rather than held behind tight lips conveys a releasing attitude from the top part of the body to the bottom, a sort of open mouth–open birth canal message.

If you are one of the few women who do not experience the urge to push, you should follow this same sequence and give short bursts of pushing as the contraction nears its peak. You may find that doing so will bring out a natural urge to push after a few times faking it. In studies in which women were encouraged to do whatever came naturally, they pushed around three to five times during a contraction and in short, frequent bursts lasting around six seconds. Most of the time the women would naturally exhale rather than hold their breath, and if they did hold their breath, the breath-holding seldom lasted longer than six seconds. Research on different methods of breathing while pushing showed the best oxygen delivery to mother and baby occurred when the bearing down lasted between four and six seconds. Following instincts makes sense.

Avoiding Hyperventilation

Breathing too fast and/or too heavily, called *hyperventilation,* is a classic example of too much of a good thing. The natural inclination is to overbreathe when stressed. Instead of keeping the proper balance of oxygen and carbon dioxide in the blood, hyperventilation blows off too much carbon dioxide and causes lightheadedness, dizziness, and tingling sensations in fingers, toes, and face. Here's how to keep your breathing in balance during labor.

- Recognize that you are stressed, but do not choose flight or fight, both of which are inappropriate for labor. Get your mind off the stress and back to acceptance and surrender.

- Avoid the fast panting style of breathing. It tires you out, tenses your upper body, and shortchanges your oxygen intake — and may progress to hyperventilation.

- Use natural breathing patterns (see page 161) with a comfortable depth and slow rate. If hyperventilation occurs, first slow down your breathing. Frequent reminders about hyperventilation and constant support during subsequent contractions will help you avoid it. Also, if you're struggling with slowing your breathing, you can rebreathe

your own air by tightly cupping your hands around your nose and mouth or by wearing a surgical mask over your nose and mouth. This will restore the proper balance of the oxygen and carbon dioxide in your blood.

- During fast breathing periodically take a blowing-off-steam breath — one deep breath followed by a long drawn-out blow.

- If you're the quick-panic type and your fast breathing is escalating, have your partner (who presumably is not also hyperventilating) conduct the breathing and try to follow his counts at around twenty per minute; then institute other relaxing measures (e.g., massage, water, and changing positions) to take your mind off your fast breathing.

every part of your body. Between contractions you return to sleep-imitation breathing — not focusing on your respirations, but conserving energy and making the most of the lulls your body allows you.

For most women the scenario described above is adequate to get them through the entire labor, especially if a supportive partner is able to remind and model a slow, relaxed rate of breathing for her when contractions threaten to be overwhelming. A loving reminder during the tough times, either in front of her face or near her ear, saying, "Follow me, sweetheart, listen to my breathing and stay with me — you can do it," can keep her on track. Sometimes the intensity of each inhalation and exhalation increases, yet it's best deliberately to keep

the rate unchanged to provide a feeling of being anchored securely.

For other laboring women, as the intensity of the contraction increases, they will automatically speed up their breathing rate as a natural response of their body to cope with the stress. Dr. Bradley, the obstetrician who originated The Bradley Method® of childbirth education, learned his approach to breathing by observing animals giving birth. Animals, such as horses, don't pant during stress because these animals sweat to relieve heat. Dogs and cats, however, because they don't sweat, pant when giving birth. We discourage panting during labor because it is not physiologic for humans, and it will lead to hyperventilation. Partners must make sure this increased respiratory

How Physiologic Breathing Helps

Breathing is emotionally tied to your ability to relax and your power to accomplish. You breathe a sigh of relief after completing a formidable task. Before climbing a tree, even a child looks up and takes a deep breath of determination. There is something psychologically and physiologically good about how we express our feelings through our breathing. Slow, deep, rhythmic breathing communicates peace and safety to mind and body. Fast, spasmodic breathing communicates fear, anxiety, and danger. If a woman breathes like this during a contraction she's telling you she's very tense and fearful — definitely not relaxing. Physiologic breathing delivers enough oxygen to the mother to fuel her efforts and to the baby to ensure a healthy passage. Emotionally, the role of physiologic breathing is to help relax the mother.

rate does not bring about a tense body. If the breathing becomes too fast, communicating panic, the partner can help by breathing along, pacing the rhythm back down to a steady, slower rate so the feelings of calm and safety can return. They must also be alert to the mother's need to slow her breathing back to a normal resting rate between contractions to avoid hyperventilation, panic, and loss of resting periods between contractions. The partner may speak gently to her as the peak of the contraction passes, "Okay now, Jennifer, start slowing down, it's easing off. That's right, let this one go and rest." A cue to help her do this is called a "releasing breath." As a contraction ends, encourage her to take one last deep breath and slowly blow it out as if to blow away any tension that has built up, in preparation to rest and forget about that contraction.

Many childbirth classes spend a fair amount of time dealing with specific breathing techniques in the event that the mother encounters a premature urge to push. As we discuss on page 221, some birth attendants and nurses believe that a woman should not push (even when she has an overwhelming urge to push) until her cervix is completely dilated. This is a controversial issue. Many times little "grunting" or "cheating" pushes will finish dilating the cervix safely and relieve much discomfort for a laboring woman. In the rare case that you do get an urge to push before you are 6 centimeters dilated, or your cervix is swelling with the pushing pressure (diagnosed by your birth attendant during a vaginal exam) and must have some relief before it will continue dilating, your breathing can assist you. Continued slow breathing in through the nose and out through the open mouth helps prevent pushing, and decreases the risk of hyperventilation. But don't expect it to be easy or comfortable — it takes concentrated effort.

If your birth attendant advises you not to push (such as during final crowning), try this breathing technique to interfere with the urge to push: do quick blowing breaths at the peak of each contraction. This is not a puffed-out cheek blow, but a relaxed blow with somewhat pursed lips, similar to keeping a feather aloft in the air. By blowing out the air, you ensure that air pressure in the lungs will not add to your urge to push. Return to slow breathing to recover, as the contraction and need to push dissipate. This breathing should be necessary for only two or three contractions. In these difficult moments, remember that your baby is about to be born. It will soon be over and well worth it.

While it is not necessary to memorize specific patterned-breathing techniques to prepare for labor, it is helpful to become familiar through daily practice with the sensation of breathing in through your nose and out through your mouth, and with blowing out slowly in conjunction with relaxing and getting into a comfortable position. Relaxing doesn't come naturally for many people, so commit to daily practice. And remember, the three goals of your breathing through birth in order of priority are: to deliver adequate oxygen to mother and baby; to relax; and to give rhythm to the waves you ride.

10

Easing Birth Pains — How the Doctor Can Help

PAIN RELIEF DURING LABOR and birth requires a partnership between you and your doctor. As a prepared and informed mother you work with your body and mind to achieve needed comfort, and the birth attendants offer their own suggestions and remedies (natural and medical) to complement what you're doing. But before you automatically ask the doctor to open his medical bag, give your own body a chance. You may be surprised at what powerful pain relievers you bring to birth. Signing up for an epidural before giving your body a chance to deal with labor would be devaluing your own abilities. On the other hand, to enter birth with a headstrong resolution against taking any medication no matter the circumstances may be equally unwise. While a no-medication mind-set can work as a powerful motivator for most mothers, it can deprive some of a safe and satisfying birth experience. Learn all about your options before labor and think about what you might want to do in various situations. This will allow you to be flexible in making on-the-spot decisions about medical pain relief should the need or desire arise.

THE TRADE-OFF

As long as women have had babies, birth attendants and mothers have searched for the ideal pain reliever — one that works for mother and is safe for both mother and baby. Whenever an analgesic is injected into your body there is a trade-off. In order to get the benefits of pain relief you must also accept the risks. No drug has ever been proven to be perfectly safe for mother and baby during childbirth. Before asking for or agreeing to any medical method of pain relief during labor ask yourself these questions:

- Do you fully understand the benefits and risks of the medication to you and your baby?
- Have you first tried all of the natural pain-relieving methods? Are they working well enough to make the pain manageable?
- Is the fear of more pain or the pain itself the major issue? Fear is best self-controlled (see page 135); overwhelming pain can be medically controlled.
- How well are you managing? Are you able to keep on top of your contractions while

your labor is progressing normally? Or is pain overwhelming you? Are you becoming exhausted? If the natural ways of coping are not helping, and you find that you are fighting your labor, it may be in your best interest and your baby's, to request some medical pain relief to help you go on.

- Are you at your absolute limit of handling any more contractions; or do you just need a little medical assistance in relaxing so that you can again refocus and go on? This distinction may help you choose between a mild narcotic for relaxation and epidural anesthesia designed to eradicate most feeling in your lower body.

- What stage of labor are you in? If you are sure you "want to die" and want medical relief at 2 centimeters, the choice of medical relief may be much different than when you are in transition — close to pushing. If you are laboring and progressing rapidly, see if you can get through just the next contraction — take it one at a time.

Don't be afraid to ask your obstetrician or anesthesiologist to explain the risks and benefits of the medications advised. Any doctor worth his or her diploma expects to be drilled respectfully about drugs going into your body and your baby's body. The fear of pain in childbirth may prevent a woman from asking about the side effects of drugs. The doctor wants to ease pain so much that he or she may subconsciously suppress the fact that no labor drug has ever been proven safe. This is the human element — both mother and doctor want to believe that the medicine will work and that it is safe. But the doctor cannot guarantee either one. What the doctor could do is learn more about nonmedical pain relief, which carries risks to no one.

It helps to enter birth with realistic expectations about what you and your doctor can do. Your doctor's goal is the same as yours: maximum comfort for you with minimum risk. If your goal is totally pain-free childbirth, you are likely to be disappointed. This is rarely achievable because giving a mother enough analgesia during childbirth to eradicate the pain totally is unacceptably risky. And as with all obstetrical interventions, once you open the door to one unnatural guest, others are likely to enter. The best that you and your doctor can shoot for is to arrive at a labor-management strategy that allows your pain to be manageable — less pain, rather than pain*less.*

If you decide ahead of time that you are going to have an epidural, then you will not be motivated to take relaxation training seriously and you won't be able to apply those needed skills in labor. Multiple studies have shown that women who take prepared-childbirth classes experience less pain during labor and, even if they do need or request pain-relieving medication, they require lower doses. An epidural only covers over pain; it doesn't deal with the tension in your system. So you would still have the negative effects of tension inhibiting your labor. Don't ignore relaxation — you need it with or without medication.

NARCOTIC PAIN RELIEVERS

Narcotics have been used to ease the pain of childbirth for more than a hundred years. Best known of these is Demerol, but there are other popular narcotics, such as Fentanyl (a synthetic relative of Demerol) and narcotics that are combined with an antagonist to lessen the undesirable side effects: Stadol, Numorphan, and Nubain. Every drug has risks and benefits, and because two persons, mother and baby, are involved, it's doubly important for parents to understand what these drugs do.

Effects on Baby

There are no benefits of narcotics to the baby, only risks. When mother takes a narcotic so does baby. Within thirty seconds after the drug is given intravenously to the mother it enters baby's circulatory system at around 70 percent of the concentration in mother's blood. While it is hard to know exactly how the drug is affecting the baby in the womb, common sense tells us the effects must be similar to those experienced by the mother. Electronic fetal-monitoring tracings of babies whose mothers have received narcotics during labor have shown heart-rate patterns that are different from normal. Research has also shown that narcotics produce changes in the fetal electroencephalograms and can decrease fetal respiratory movements. The significance of these changes is unknown. Narcotics may have a greater effect on the baby than on the mother for two reasons: the baby's central nervous system may be more susceptible to the effects of the narcotic since the blood-brain barrier, which is there to prevent outside substances from entering the brain, is more permeable; also, the baby's immature liver and kidneys are less able to break down and excrete the drugs. The baby is thus not only less able to handle the narcotic, but also less able to get rid of it. While in the womb, the baby uses the placenta as an additional excretory system to get rid of substances such as drugs. But once

baby is born, this extra help is cut off, and the drug remains in baby's system longer. (This is why doctors prefer to give narcotics earlier in labor, so that the placenta is able to help get rid of the drug prior to birth.) The peak effect of a narcotic on the nervous and respiratory systems is around two hours after administration, but the effects may last four to eight hours. Babies born to mothers receiving Demerol during labor show varying degrees of respiratory depression, feeding difficulties, and behavioral disorganization. These undesirable effects last varying lengths of time, depending on the dosage and the time between administration and delivery. Narcotics given during labor have been detected in babies' bloodstreams eight weeks after birth. While some studies reassuringly conclude analgesics and anesthetics do not harm the baby (studies show that Nubain does not cause respiratory depression in the infant), some researchers believe the contrary. The fact is, no one knows for sure!

Effects on Mother

Narcotics are noted for their unpredictability. Different people react differently. While some mothers receiving narcotics get a lot of pain relief during contractions, most describe the feeling as "only taking the edge off." Narcotics reduce pain perception, but never eliminate pain completely. In general, narcotics do not obliterate the pain, they simply make it more tolerable. Some mothers describe it as more of an escape from their labor rather than pain relief. For some, this euphoria is pleasant, while others dislike the fuzzy feeling that puts them out of touch with their labor. Also, if the effects of the medication compromise your ability to walk, your labor progress could be slowed.

For some mothers, a well-timed dose of analgesia when they are "losing it" can break the cycle of overwhelming pain and exhaustion, and actually help them regain the ability to work with their labor. Other women don't experience this trade-off. They feel that the amount of pain relief was not worth losing the rhythm and the sensation of their labor. One mother's helper may be another's hindrance.

The good news is that narcotics, unlike epidural anesthetics, seldom slow the progress of labor unless given too early. But if they are given during the early stages of labor, narcotics (as with all analgesic agents) may decrease uterine activity, slow cervical dilatation, and slow the progress of labor. Some women react to narcotics with nausea, vomiting, and dizziness, and others we have interviewed do not like the "spaced-out" sensation, feeling that it keeps them from thinking clearly in making decisions about their labor, or even from responding well when a contraction is upon them. Also, medical personnel have observed that narcotics during labor can interfere with mother-infant bonding. A spaced-out mother and a spaced-out baby don't make good first impressions on each other.

Using Narcotics Wisely During Labor

Take a balanced approach toward narcotics in childbirth. In most cases it is best for mother and baby not to use narcotic analgesia during labor. But there may be circumstances (e.g., the position of the baby) when the difficulties of labor overwhelm natural coping mechanisms and it would be unhealthy not to seek outside help. Consider these ways to lessen the amount of narcotic analgesia you need and the effects on your baby:

- Try all the natural pain-relieving suggestions listed in chapter 9: relaxation techniques, water, massage, and, most important, changing positions during stages of labor.

- If you are investigating narcotic pain relief, labor and delivery nurses will tell you that the drug Nubain is effective in "taking the edge off," and it causes the least amount of the spaced-out feeling, nausea, and vomiting. You should know, however, that the second dose doesn't seem to be as effective as the first in many women, so timing is important. You won't need a second dose if the first dose gets you back on track and labor progresses quickly enough to get you into pushing. Most relaxed mothers find the pushing stage to be manageable without medical pain relief.

- If you feel you need narcotic help, the intravenous route may be preferable because the relief is quicker and wears off sooner. Following an intravenous injection you usually feel some relief within five to ten minutes, and it will last around an hour. Intramuscular injections may require half an hour to an hour to take full effect, but the relief may last three to four hours.

- If you have an intravenous, request a heparin- or saline lock, which allows you mobility during labor (see page 217 for use of this device).

- There is seldom a reason to use narcotic analgesia before you are in active labor, and, in fact, this may stall your labor. But it is sometimes advisable to use a sedative in a long drawn-out prelabor to help mother sleep. Otherwise a mother may enter active labor already exhausted.

• To minimize the effects of the narcotic on your newborn after delivery, try to avoid an injection within one to three hours of birth, so you can take advantage of the placenta to help clear the drug from baby's system prior to delivery. While the exact moment of birth is anyone's guess, your birth attendant can usually give you a time after which a narcotic would not be safe. Once you have the urge to push it's best to say no, otherwise the baby may be born at the time when the effect of the narcotic peaks, and he may need resuscitation or an injection of the narcotic antagonist Narcan to reverse the effects. Varying amounts of a drug may persist in a baby's body for weeks after birth and result in temporary feeding difficulties and disorganized behavior.

EPIDURAL ANESTHESIA

While some mothers want to hug their anesthesiologist after being given an epidural, others have mixed feelings. Many laboring women praise their epidural as a "gift from heaven," but others feel that the experience put them in the role of a passive patient (a "beached whale," as one mother put it), unable to participate actively in the birth. Hailed as the Rolls-Royce of obstetrical analgesia, this magic medicine may allow women to give birth without pain, but not without a price — to mind, body, and bank account. Some anesthesiologists believe that severe pain not relieved by relaxation and comfort measures should be considered a complication of labor, and is therefore in need of treatment. The best benefit of the epidural may be the option of knowing there is a way out, that overwhelming labor pain is no longer necessary.

How Epidurals Are Given

If you choose to let someone poke a needle into your back and place tubing next to your spinal cord, you really should know what's going to happen. To understand your doctor's explanation of the anesthetic options there is a bit of anesthesia language that you should know. *Analgesia* refers to reduction of pain without the loss of movement. *Anesthesia* refers to a complete blockade of sensation and movement. Most epidurals contain both an anesthetic agent and a narcotic analgesic. The doctor can

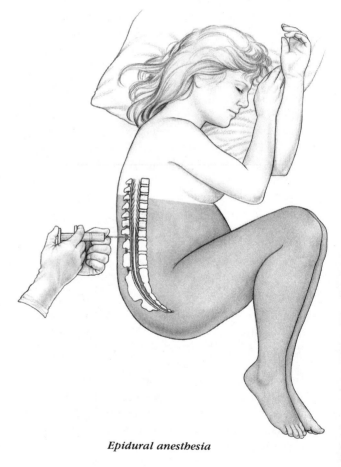

Epidural anesthesia

vary the dose of each according to how little pain and how much movement the
mother needs or desires. Except when the
epidural agent is a narcotic only (in this
case it would be called *epidural analgesia*),
the doctor will use the term "epidural anesthesia." The term *epidural* means the anesthetic will be placed in a space above or
around (*epi* in Greek) the *dura* — the
sheath around the spinal cord. The nerves
that carry the labor-pain signals to the nervous system all pass through the epidural
space. When medication is injected into the
epidural space, these pain signals are
reduced or blocked. The word *spinal* refers
to the space within the dura containing the
spinal cord, spinal nerves, and cerebrospinal
fluid. An anesthetic "going spinal" means the
medicine has entered that space and will
travel up the spinal canal.

To prevent the drop in blood pressure
that often accompanies an epidural you will
be given a liter of intravenous fluids. As you
sit or lie with your back rounded, the doctor or nurse will scrub your lower back with
an antiseptic solution. It will feel cold. You
will feel a bee sting–like feeling as the doctor injects a tiny bit of local anesthetic to
numb the area. When the area is numb, the
doctor painlessly inserts a larger needle
between the spinal bones at the level of
your waist. When the needle enters the epidural space the doctor injects a test dose to
be sure the needle is in the right place and
to determine that you are not allergic to the
medication. Once the needle is properly
positioned the doctor threads a flexible plastic catheter through the needle into the epidural space, and then removes the needle
leaving the catheter in place. You may feel
only a slight burning pressure or a transient
shooting sensation like an electric shock
down one leg. Within five minutes of the

doctor's injecting the medication you may
begin to feel numb from your navel down,
or you may notice that your legs are feeling
warm and/or tingly. After ten to twenty minutes, the lower half of your body feels completely or partially numb depending on the
type of anesthetic used.

If you are receiving a continuous epidural, the tubing is connected to a special
pump that is programmed to infuse a certain
amount of medication continuously, and this
is periodically adjusted to meet your level of
comfort. If you opt for an intermittent epidural, a top-off dose is given as soon as the
previous dose wears off and you begin to
feel the contractions again. The anesthesiologist cannot always control the exact level
of loss of sensation. Most mothers will experience numbness from the navel down, others will experience some loss of sensation as
high as the nipples, and still others may
notice patchy areas on their skin where they
can still feel sensations. The doctor or nurse
will rub all over your skin to detect your
level of sensation.

Once the epidural anesthetic is injected,
safety measures are taken. Your blood pressure will be monitored every two to five
minutes until your vital signs are stable, then
every fifteen minutes thereafter. You will be
positioned on your left side, with the head
of the bed up at a 30-degree angle. You will
be turned from side to side approximately
every hour to keep the pain relief even on
both sides of your body. The sensation to
empty your bladder will be impaired, requiring a urinary catheter to be inserted. Electronic fetal monitoring must be done to
ensure that the baby is also handling the epidural well. While the epidural is functioning,
the doctor or nurse will do periodic sensitivity checks to be sure that the level of
numbness is not too high and causing

"Walking" Epidurals

The newest epidural anesthesiologists have in their bag of pain relievers is one that relieves pain yet allows some movement. This marvel is achieved by mixing a morphinelike narcotic (an analgesic) with an anesthetic, thereby reducing the dosage of anesthetic needed for pain relief. As a result, the pain pathways are blocked but the motor nerves are partially spared. Dubbed the "walking" epidural (though women are seldom able to walk during an epidural), this technique makes it possible for mothers to feel the urge to push and retain the ability to do so while still experiencing varying degrees of pain relief. You and your doctor negotiate a balance: how much pain relief you need versus how much movement you need. Adding narcotics to the magic potion means that the onset of pain relief is more rapid (five to ten minutes versus ten to twenty minutes without the narcotic), lasts longer, and is better than the anesthetic agent alone. With this new combination mothers supported by their birth partner can stand, squat, kneel, and push. When only a narcotic analgesia is given, some mothers can even stand and walk with support. However, epidurals using only narcotics are seldom effective in eliminating the pain associated with labor. And with anesthetic agents (those that numb sensations and take away the ability to move), mother must remain horizontal until her body has adjusted to the epidural, because of the danger of falling blood pressure if she is upright. With the added narcotic analgesia there seems to be no more effects on baby than with the anesthetic agent alone. With these new combinations you get the best of both worlds: pain relief and more active participation in birth.

---

breathing difficulties and that the level of pain relief is sufficient for your desired comfort. After the epidural catheter is removed, the numbing effects wear off within a couple hours.

To some women whose memories of previous births are marred by excruciating pain, the availability of epidural can encourage them to have another baby. As one mother told us, "After my first birth I swore I would never go through that again. With my second birth I had an epidural. It was marvelous. Now I can't wait to have another baby." But before you rush to call in the anesthesiologist, remember there are risks and benefits to consider. Here are the questions mothers ask most frequently about epidurals.

QUESTIONS YOU MAY HAVE ABOUT EPIDURALS

I want to know about what goes into my body. What questions should I ask my doctors?

Try to consult three sources: your obstetrician, mothers who have had epidurals, and your anesthesiologist. Ask your obstetrician about when he or she thinks they should be used and what types of epidurals are available. Find out if you have any special conditions that would make an epidural either advisable or unadvisable. Ask mothers who have had epidurals about their feelings (physical and emotional) or lack of them — when the epidural went into effect. What would they do differently next time? Be sure to interview mothers who had epidurals at your chosen hospital, since the level of anesthesia skills varies among anesthesiologists. Interview your anesthesiologist, if that's possible, before labor day. Do the anesthesiologists have special training or expertise in obstetrical anesthesia? Quiz him or her on the risks and benefits. Explore your options for the type and timing of the medications. Obstetrical anesthesia is changing so rapidly that information you read in books and magazines may be out of date. When we were researching this subject and talking to anesthesiologists about the side effects of a particular drug or procedure, we would frequently hear, "Oh, we don't use that anymore!" Don't forget to ask how much the procedure costs. The fee for epidurals varies from $500 to $1500.

Are there different types of epidurals? How would I know which to choose?

There are many types of epidurals. *Continuous epidural* means that the pain-relieving medications are continuously infused around your spinal cord. In an *intermittent epidural* the anesthetic is injected periodically into the tubing either on a regular schedule or "as needed." Each type has advantages. Continuous epidurals offer constant pain relief without the roller-coaster effects sometimes experienced with intermittent top-ups; less blood pressure instability; and a lower overall dose of medication is needed. Some anesthesiologists believe

that patient mobility and the quality of pain relief are better with continuous epidurals; others feel intermittent top-ups allow mothers to regulate more easily the balance between the level of pain they can tolerate and the degree of movement they desire. Discuss with your anesthesiologist the pros and cons of continuous and intermittent epidurals. The new gold standard of epidural anesthesia is the combined use of an anesthetic agent and a pain-relieving narcotic, which allows the mother more freedom to move. (See "'Walking' Epidurals," page 172, for an explanation of this new type of epidural.)

You may not want or need the epidural after you are through the most difficult part of labor. Discuss with your obstetrician or anesthesiologist the advisability of allowing the epidural to wear off to see if you can manage the pushing stage without medical pain relief. While some mothers desire the pain-relieving effects of the epidural throughout their entire labor, others want to let it wear off in the pushing stage so that they can find their own most comfortable position (usually upright) and better use their body movements to participate in the baby's birth. If you choose an epidural, be sure to discuss the types of analgesic agents with your anesthesiologist so that together, in partnership, you can work out a plan tailored to your individual needs. It is best to ask for the type of anesthesia that will give you the most pain relief with the least restriction of movement.

Could an epidural harm our baby?

The truth is no one knows for certain. Anesthesiologists and obstetricians regard epidurals as totally safe for baby, and there is much research to back up their claim. Studies have shown that newborns of mothers who had epidurals showed no adverse effects in Apgar scores, neurologic effects, or changes in blood chemistry. But some of the drug that enters mother's bloodstream also crosses the placenta into baby within minutes. There is evidence of changes in fetal heart-rate patterns as shown by electronic fetal monitoring following an epidural, but the significance of these changes is unknown. Doctors must be a little worried about the effect epidurals have on the baby, since it is usually hospital policy that a mother having an epidural must also have electronic fetal monitoring. Some observers report that newborns whose mothers had epidurals are more likely to show feeding difficulties and more disorganized behavior in the weeks after birth, but these correlations are hard to prove. Recent studies show that when newborns are placed on their mother's abdomen immediately after birth, the babies whose mothers were not medicated during labor made crawling movements toward their breasts more than the babies of medicated mothers. Though studies suggest that epidural agents don't harm the baby very much, there is no research proving that these anesthetics and narcotics don't harm baby at all. The current tools for measuring effects of drugs on babies are imprecise. It is fair to say that there has never been a drug proven conclusively to be safe for a baby in the womb.

Because it works and is apparently safe for mother and baby, epidural anesthesia for childbirth became very popular very fast. Its acceptance mushroomed long before its safety was proven. There are questions about its use that are not yet answered. For example, doctors have long observed that some mothers, for an unknown reason, develop a fever following an epidural, but this finding has been dismissed as an easily treatable nuisance. New research, however, has shown that when mother gets overheated, so does the baby inside; in fact, the baby may be much warmer than standard thermometers detect. Estimating that as many as 5 percent of babies develop high fevers following an epidural birth, these researchers raise an important question: "Could high fever harm a newborn's brain?"

Epidural-induced fever also poses problems in the medical care of the newborn. To the pediatrician, fever in a newborn is a serious red flag that must be thoroughly investigated. Is the fever "simply" due to the drug or is there an infection present? A doctor is often obligated to order a battery of uncomfortable and expensive tests to track down the cause of the fever and often needs to treat the baby just in case there is an underlying serious infection.

Like many other drugs and procedures, epidural analgesia is "generally regarded as safe" (GRAS) by the FDA. The key word here is *generally,* a hedge that means we really aren't absolutely sure. So we're left with our internal safety monitor — common sense. There are obstetrical situations in which an epidural helps the mother have a healthier labor and thus indirectly helps the baby. But there are instances when an ill-timed epidural interferes with the normal progress of labor and therefore may not be received kindly by the baby. Before you take a leap of faith and sign the consent forms, obtain information from reliable sources about the safety of any drug or procedure for you and your baby, and learn exactly what it will do for you.

Is having an epidural safe for me?

It depends on whom you ask. Remember, almost everyone has a bias in favor of epidurals. Doctors want them to be safe because this is the best pain-reliever they have ever had to offer for childbirth. Hospitals want epidurals to be safe because it further justifies the mothers' being in the hospital rather than in a birth center or at home. And mothers want comfortable births. The cards are stacked in favor of epidurals, and that may cloud objectivity.

It is true that the majority of mothers breeze through an epidural delivery with no immediate complications and have long-term memories of a satisfying birth experience. But as soon as that magic medicine enters your body, your birth experience changes. Rather than being an active participant in your birth, you become an observer, a patient on the receiving end of the technology that is directing your birth. Since the lower half of your body is weak, you are now dependent upon others to move you. As long as the drug is doing its job, you may get less attention from your caretakers. The medical staff will turn you, check the monitor, the intravenous line, the correct dosage, and the position of the epidural catheter, do your perineal hygiene and empty your bladder, but they sometimes forget that there is a whole person at the end of the tubing. You can be a less passive patient if you ask for an epidural that allows you some feeling and some movement (see "'Walking' Epidurals," page 172).

Epidurals are strong medicines that are not without side effects. Ideally the drug would stay where it's put and affect only the pain-carrying spinal nerves. But that area of the body is richly supplied with blood vessels, and some of the medications may enter mother's bloodstream, setting off the following possible complications:

Shivering. This commonly occurs even in women without epidurals. Epidurals con-taining dilute concentrations of narcotics may actually reduce shivering. Besides being unpleasant and contributing to feelings of being out of control, shaking uses up energy, possibly diverting oxygen from your uterus and your baby. Some women are significantly bothered by the shaking, and even with assurance to the contrary, they are convinced "something is wrong."

Falling blood pressure. The drugs used to give epidural anesthesia may cause your blood pressure to drop, compromising blood flow to your uterus and baby. To prevent this complication the doctor will "hydrate" you by giving a lot of fluid intravenously.

Confined to bed. If you are given an epidural anesthesia that does not allow you much movement (best to request your anesthesiologist to administer the newer type, which allows you to move), you spend more time lying on your back. Besides the fact that the back-lying position diminishes uterine activity and the progress of labor, this position is potentially dangerous for baby since the weighty uterus may compress the blood vessels along your spine and compromise blood flow to your uterus and baby. Obstetrical nurses are aware of this complication and will position you on your left side, but here again you must rely on help from someone.

Long-term backaches. With or without an epidural, some mothers experience backaches for months after childbirth. However, this problem is more common in women receiving epidural analgesia. A recent study showed that 10 percent of women delivering naturally experienced backache lasting longer than six weeks; nearly 20 percent of women who received epidurals experienced long-term backaches. Presumably this is the result of strain on the back muscles while anesthetized. Normally when you are lying in a way that hurts your back, your muscles cry pain and you naturally adjust your position to one of comfort. But anesthetized muscles don't signal a need to move. Consequently you can lie in a muscle-straining position but not feel the effects until after the anesthesia wears off. Problems can be minimized if your caregivers support your hips and normal lumbar curve with pillows and rolls of sheets during labor.

Itching. Generalized itching is one of the most common side effects when narcotics are used in epidural anesthesia. This is more a nuisance than a serious medical problem and a trade-off some mothers gladly accept.

Spinal headaches. On rare occasions (more common with difficult epidural insertions) the epidural needle may accidentally enter the spinal canal, producing a "spinal tap," more commonly called by anesthesiologists "a dural puncture" or "wet tap." When this occurs, spinal fluid may leak through the needle hole in the dura (the thick covering containing the spinal cord and spinal fluid), producing a mild to severe headache that may last from hours to days. These headaches can be effectively treated, but sometimes the treatment also has side effects. Uncomplicated epidurals do not produce headaches.

Nerve injuries. Injuries to spinal nerves from epidural analgesia and anesthesia have been estimated to occur in one in every ten thousand epidurals. These injuries usually produce an area of numbness or weakness in one leg. The good news is that virtually all of these symptoms subside over several weeks to months and are seldom permanent. However, they can be disturbing to a new mother.

Other possible side effects. Seizures and difficulty urinating, necessitating bladder catheterization, which increases the risk of a urinary tract infection, are also possible side effects. On rare occasions the anesthetic enters the spinal column and travels high enough to depress the muscles used for breathing.

Technical problems. Even in experienced hands, problems can arise in placing an epidural. Anesthesiologists use surface landmarks on your back to locate the proper spot in which to insert the epidural. If you have excessive swelling over your back or are overweight, the epidural may be difficult and sometimes slightly more painful to insert. The epidural needle may bump up against the bones of your spine, increasing the likelihood of backache following delivery. There is also a greater chance that the epidural won't take completely. These problems occasionally mean replacing the epidural. On rare occasions, the catheter has broken off and become lodged in the spinal canal, requiring surgical removal.

The epidural doesn't take. In at least 1 percent of mothers there are windows of unanesthetized areas, where breakthrough pain may appear. These problems are usually corrected by adjusting the epidural catheter and/or administration of the medication or by changing the mother's position. In rare instances, because of the woman's anatomy or scar tissue from previous epidurals or trauma, the anesthesiologist is unable to obtain a satisfactory epidural. Spotty epidurals are also more common in women who are obese or have excessive swelling due to toxemia.

How might an epidural affect my labor?

Unless begun too early (before you are 5 centimeters dilated), epidurals seldom have any effect on the duration of the first stage of labor. Most studies, however, do show that an epidural can prolong the second stage of labor. Whether and to what extent this happens varies among women and also depends on the type and dosage of medication. A prolonged second stage of labor seems to occur more often in first-time mothers. In some women who are having dysfunctional labor patterns, an epidural may actually accelerate labor, probably by relieving the fear, pain, pelvic tension, and consequent exhaustion. In general, be pre-

---

The Pros and Cons of Epidurals

Advantages

- Pain relief is adjustable from complete to partial.
- Relieves pain while still allowing movement (varies with dosage and type of epidural).
- Mother is awake, even for a cesarean section.
- May enhance labor progress if mother is exhausted.
- May enable a gratifying birth experience if natural coping mechanisms fail.
- Just knowing it's available reduces the fear of birth.
- Presumed to be safe for mother and baby.

Disadvantages

- Restricts movement and active participation in birth.
- May lessen a mother's feeling of accomplishment.
- May lessen a mother's trust in the powers of her own body.
- May prolong the second stage of labor by depressing the urge to push.
- Safety for baby not conclusively proven.
- Expensive ($500–$1,500 in 1993).
- Increases the likelihood of forceps or vacuum-suction delivery.
- Increases the likelihood of needing pitocin augmentation.
- Possibly increases chances of needing a cesarean.
- Can cause fetal heart-rate pattern changes of unknown significance.
- Technical problems may occur, such as difficulty inserting needle into the right space around the spinal cord.
- Headaches may occur if the epidural goes spinal.
- Increased intervention needed: intravenous, EFM with internal monitoring, urinary catheter, blood-pressure monitoring, etc. (which also increases the cost of the delivery).
- May cause low blood pressure, shivering, nausea and vomiting, generalized itching, long-term backache, difficulty urinating, respiratory depression.
- May cause newborns to show irregular feeding patterns and more disorganized behaviors.

pared for a longer labor if you opt for an epidural.

Expect to need some intravenous pitocin administration to boost your epidural-dampened labor along. In unmedicated births there is a natural surge in oxytocin (called *Ferguson's Reflex*) during the second stage of labor, helping to push baby out once you are fully dilated. In fact, oxytocin has been measured to be higher during the second stage of labor in mothers not having an epidural. In managed labors, epidurals and pitocin go together. One slows labor, the other speeds it up. Pitocin-induced contractions are so strong that mother needs an epidural to ease the pain. Epidural-muffled contractions need pitocin to make them stronger. A champion of unmedicated birth might ask in this case if two wrongs can make it right.

Some mothers feel that epidurals take away not only the pain of birth but also the pleasure. In unmedicated labors, mothers get natural relief from their own natural narcotic pain relievers and the feel-good hormones, endorphins. Mothers having epidural anesthesia have been shown to have lower endorphin levels. On the positive side, however, epidural anesthesia can also lower the levels of circulating catecholamines. High levels of these hormones can produce dysfunctional uterine contractions and decreased blood flow to the placenta in mothers who are experiencing severe pain. When the catecholamine levels drop after the epidural anesthesia, the uterine contractions may become regular. Emotionally, mothers having epidural anesthesia report very different birth experiences from mothers who had a nonmedicated birth. Mothers choosing epidurals often observe the workings of their bodies much like a bystander. In a nonmedicated birth, the mother tends to experience the lowest lows at the most

difficult point of labor, and the highest highs as she births her baby. She experiences tremendous relief, accomplishment, and the joy of her reward's arrival. It is important to reflect on your birth value system and decide which type of experience you most desire to give you "birth satisfaction."

Finally, with an epidural expect your body signals to be a bit out of sync. If the epidural obliterates both your normal sensation and your ability to push (the higher dose anesthetic agents do, the lower dose combined with narcotics often don't), you will need outside coaching to tell you when to push, and these external signals may not be as well timed as your natural cues. Sometimes mother and doctor decide to let the anesthetic wear off during the final stage before delivery so the mother can feel her urge to push.

Am I more likely to have a forceps delivery if I have an epidural?

Yes. Studies have shown that a mother is twice as likely to have either forceps or vacuum extraction if she has an epidural. The less efficient uterine contractions may keep baby from rotating naturally, and the diminished urge to push may keep baby from coming down. But the need for instrument assistance to get baby down and out is less with the newer epidurals (those with a lower-dose anesthetic combined with narcotic) because mother retains some ability to move her muscles and can participate better in pushing her baby out.

Does having an epidural increase my chances of having a cesarean birth?

It is difficult to glean from the studies and from interviewing anesthesiologists a definite answer to this question because there are so many variables connected with cesar-

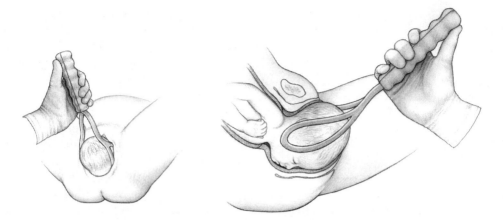

Using forceps to assist delivery

ean birth. Studies claiming that epidurals increase a woman's chance of needing a cesarean section are retrospective and poorly controlled. Some studies actually show a decrease in cesarean-section rate in hospitals with an increasing use of epidurals during labor. Most authorities discount the worry that epidurals increase the mother's chance of needing a cesarean, but in our experience, any departure from labor the natural way opens the door for further interventions that can lead to a cesarean.

One possibility for an increase in cesareans following an epidural, especially in women who choose to have epidurals early in labor (before 5 centimeters), is an increased chance that the descent of the baby's head will be arrested by baby's awkward positioning in the pelvis. When a mother has no anesthesia and has normal muscle tone in her pelvis, she is able to walk and vary positions, allowing the baby to twist and turn and find the way of least resistance down through the pelvis. When an epidural takes effect, her pelvic musculature may relax dramatically and her movement may be restricted. If baby is posterior and the head is not flexed or is awkwardly turned even slightly, the reduced tone and movement in the pelvis may not encourage the baby's head to correct its position. In turn, the contractions will just bang baby's head against the pelvis and arrest progress, causing "failure to progress."

Some anesthesiologists we have interviewed feel that any increase in the number of cesareans might be related more to the mother's mind-set than to the epidural itself. A woman who decides to have an epidural before going into labor may bring ideas and attitudes to birth that set her up as a likely candidate for a surgical birth. Epidurals do sometimes cause worrisome changes on the electronic fetal monitor that may trigger "obstetrician distress" and send the mother off to the operating room. By putting yourself in the dependent, nonparticipating role in birth, you open yourself up to the domino effect: The epidural slows down labor; pitocin is given to get contractions going again; the pitocin-induced contractions are harder and longer and produce fetal-distress patterns on the electronic fetal monitor; and the obstetrician decides on surgery. On the other hand, an epidural may prevent some cesareans. We have seen mothers whose tension prevents their progress or whose labors are stalled from sheer exhaustion; but following an epidural they are able to rest and regain their strength and continue on to a vaginal birth.

What is the best time during birth to get an epidural?

An epidural given too early may stall labor, too late and you are already over the worst. Obstetricians do not usually advise an epidural in women under 4 to 5 centimeters' dilatation. Be certain that your labor is already well established before considering this form of pain relief. Since the end of the first stage of labor (transition, from 8 to 10 centimeters' dilatation) is usually the most difficult, you might consider an epidural when you are around 6 to 8 centimeters dilated — before the worst pain would hit. If you are a second-time mom or a first-time progressing very quickly around 8 centimeters, you may want to forgo the epidural at this point since you are probably only a short time away from pushing — when the epidural would not be helpful to your progress or have time to take effect. Many mothers don't realize that the sensations of pushing are very different from those of first-stage labor and are often not perceived as painful, so that an epidural would not be needed for pain relief. Also, remember the decision-to-effect time (the time between deciding on an epidural and its being in place and relieving pain) can be at least thirty minutes.

Are there situations in which I should consider an epidural?

The decision about using any intervention boils down to whatever is in the best interest of mother and baby. To illustrate when an epidural is a wise move, here is the story of how a couple in our practice handled this decision. Pregnant with their first baby, Jan and Tony wanted to birth their baby "right." They did all their homework and chose their birth attendant, childbirth class, place of delivery, and labor-support person with the care befitting one of life's most important events. They informed themselves about all the options available to them and prepared a customized birth plan that took all possible contingencies into account. Midway through labor this super-prepared couple realized the natural way wasn't working. Jan walked, knelt, soaked, and squatted. Tony rubbed, supported, and defended. And the labor-support person and obstetrician performed their roles perfectly. But Jan felt that she had used all her resources to cope with the pain and was now becoming exhausted. Because the couple had learned about all the alternatives that would help labor progress, Jan could make an informed decision about whatever help was available so that she could achieve her goal of a gratifying birth experience. She opted for an epidural, which allowed her to rest and recharge her strength. "Sure, there was a twinge of 'I-couldn't-do-it-naturally' remorse, but I knew when to say when and I feel good about my decision." Jan went on to push out a nine-pound baby. This couple viewed epidural anesthesia as one more tool available to them in their quest for a satisfying birth.

And we have witnessed this scenario: A mother is so exhausted her labor stalls. For the reason of "failure to progress" the doctor advises a cesarean and the mother is so worn out she will agree to anything that will get the baby out. In preparation for the cesarean she has an epidural. But while the surgical staff is making preparation for the operation, to the surprise of everyone, including herself, she pushes out her baby. This mother had nothing to lose by having an epidural as she would need one for the operation anyway. This is an example of how the epidural can be a trade-off in choosing one intervention to avoid another.

There are also medical situations that would indicate an epidural as the best choice, including very high blood pressure as a result of toxemia of pregnancy. The stress of labor may push the mother's already high blood pressure into a danger zone resulting in a cesarean section. By accepting an epidural not only would her stress level be decreased but the epidural may decrease her blood pressure enough to buy some time to deliver vaginally safely.

III

EXPERIENCING BIRTH

THE BIRTH OF A BABY is loaded with emotion and meaning at least equal to the load of physical sensations it brings. Most people watching a birth in person or on film will feel a catch in their throat the moment that precious head emerges. Many weep with joy and reverence at that moment. In this part we will take you through real birth stories, help you find your best positions for labor and delivery, and give you clues to both recognizing what's happening in your body at each stage of labor and knowing what you can do to help your labor progress more efficiently and comfortably.

Best Birthing Positions

JUST AS THERE'S NO SINGLE position that suits everyone for making love, there's also no one right position for all laboring mothers. Obstetricians prefer mothers to birth in the lithotomy position (lying on back with feet in stirrups) because it is easier to deal with complications should they occur. Birth reformers rightly counter that complications are more likely to occur in the lithotomy position.

The right positions for your birth are the ones that help your labor progress most comfortably and efficiently and help baby find his or her way down the path of least resistance. Often, the most comfortable positions for you are likely to be the best positions for baby, too.

WHY BIRTHING POSITIONS MAKE A DIFFERENCE

Learning why positioning makes a difference, rehearsing various moves and birthing postures prenatally, and giving birth in a supportive environment where you are free to improvise are the best ways for you to choose a position that will work for you.

How Back-Birthing Began

The horizontal mind-set for birthing prevailed for one hundred years. Doctors learned this method in obstetrical residencies. Even though some counterestablishment books and childbirth classes preached walking during labor and vertical births, most women stayed in bed, because this was the only position they knew about and they were reluctant to ruffle the established way of birthing. Until birthing women regain their "birthright" of upright birthing positions and change the mind-set of their caretakers, birth for many is likely to remain a less than satisfying experience. For more on the history of birthing positions, see chapter 2, "Birth — Then and Now."

Why Upright Is Best

Let's answer this question by first showing why back-lying is both unsafe for baby and uncomfortable for mother. The answer lies in a principle we studied in grade-school science — the law of gravity. When a laboring mother lies on her back, gravity pulls the bulge toward her back. This abnormal position does two abnormal things. It gives

Five Reasons Not to Birth on Your Back

- It will hurt mother.
- It can harm baby.
- Labor slows.
- Episiotomy or tears are more likely.
- It makes no sense.

the mother a backache; and, by compressing the major blood vessels that run along the spine, it also reduces blood flow to the uterus. These unhealthy events snowball: the mother's blood pressure may decrease; the baby may get less blood and less oxygen; uterine contractions become less efficient; progress of labor slows; and mother has to push the baby out uphill. And with legs up in stirrups she needs to have her perineum cut. In sum, mom and baby hurt.

Now see what happens when mother sits up or stands or even leans against her partner: gravity pulls the baby down since the mother's body position is now in harmony with the forces of nature instead of working against them; the baby's head pushing better against the cervix helps it dilate more quickly; the baby is in a better angle to approach the pelvis and negotiate the easiest path through the birth canal. When the pressure is off a mother's back, and she has gravity as her birth partner, she hurts less, her uterine contractions are more efficient, and she makes better progress. There's a Native American saying: "If you lie down the baby will never come out."

Being upright for birth not only gives baby an easier angle for delivery, but it also widens the passage. When you're up and out of bed your pelvic joints, loosened by the

hormones of pregnancy, are free to move and accommodate the little passenger with the large head and broad shoulders. While sitting or lying down, these bones aren't as free to move, and your pelvic outlet narrows. In addition, vertical birthing allows more natural stretching of the birth-canal tissues and is kinder to the perineum, making episiotomy unnecessary and tears less likely.

What Position Does Research Support?

Over the past two decades research has made a strong case for the upright position in birth. Experts (veteran mothers and obstetrical researchers) conclude that women who move about during labor and are upright for birth experience less pain and need less analgesia; have shorter labors; have smaller and fewer vaginal tears and get fewer episiotomies; have babies who show less fetal distress on electronic fetal-monitor tracings and have better blood and oxygen supplies.

Beware the "Patient" Image

Veteran birth attendants report an interesting observation about women who spend most of their labor in bed. When the doctor visits a laboring woman and sees her walking around her room, strolling the halls, or laboring in the arms of her birth partner, the doctor perceives that all is going well, mother is managing nicely, and no intervention is needed. But if the obstetrician observes the mother struggling a bit in bed, she is a target for intervention. Being in bed makes a woman seem dependent, sick, and in need of intervention. The doctor feels obliged to do something. While sometimes the mother does need pain relief, at other times her behavior merely triggers the domino effect of multiple unnecessary interventions. Delivering in positions other than lying on the back is standard birthing procedure to most midwives but still foreign to most obstetricians. The birth scene of a mother in the squatting position, supported by her partner from behind and her obstetrician kneeling to receive baby from below has not yet made the obstetrical textbooks, but this kneeling position is not beneath the medical profession. The best birthing position is the one that works for you. Choose the birthing environment that encourages you to improvise positions and a birth attendant who will accommodate your wishes.

FINDING YOUR BEST BIRTHING POSITION

There is no single position that suits every mother at all times during birth. You must be free to create your own. Here are some labor-tested positions that veteran mothers birth by.

Squatting

The best birthing position used by mothers the world over is squatting.

Why Squat

This position is labor-friendly to both mother and baby for the following reasons:

- speeds progress of labor
- widens pelvic openings
- relaxes perineal muscles so there is less tearing
- relieves back pain

- improves oxygen supply to baby
- facilitates delivery of the placenta

Now squat and feel what happens in your pelvis. Your upper leg bones, the femora, act like levers to open your pelvic bones and widen your pelvic outlet. Research shows that changing positions from lying down to squatting can enlarge the pelvic outlet 20–30 percent. That's good news for any tight-fitting baby coming through. While you're squatting, your uterus is in the best angle for delivery and it utilizes your labor friend — gravity. When you're delivering in the back-lying position, the baby must work his or her way through a narrow, curvy tunnel. Change this scene to squatting and baby now has a better route through a straighter, wider passage.

When to Squat

Squatting is usually the best position for speeding labor. It makes contractions more intense because it positions baby's head to put pressure against the cervix. If contractions during squatting are overwhelming but your labor is progressing well, try a more comfortable position. Squatting is seldom necessary during the first stage of labor while your cervix is dilating. It's better to avoid tiring your legs and save your energy for pushing in the second stage. Ideally, begin to squat when your birth attendant announces that your cervix is fully dilated and the second stage of labor has begun or is near. Certainly, the urge to push is your signal to squat. For best efficiency, squat during contractions: as soon as the contraction begins, squat and push; then sit back or bend forward on your knees to rest between contractions. When using the squatting position your second stage of labor is likely to be shorter but may also be more intense.

How to Squat

Most western women are not used to doing a lot of squatting, so the more you practice this position during pregnancy, the easier your birth squatting will be. Place your feet at least shoulder-width apart and descend gradually; don't bounce. Move your knees at least as far apart as your feet and plant your feet flat on the floor. If you have trouble keeping your feet flat, wear a shoe or slipper with a low heel. Keeping the weight on the outside of your feet reminds you to keep your knees far apart. Another reminder to open your knees is to clasp your hands together and rest your elbows on the inside of your knees.

Squatting can be tiring. Try these variations on the squatting theme:

The supported squat. In this position your partner sits or squats behind you, toboggan-style, with his back against the wall or bed or supported by a chair. Or he can sit or squat in front of you, holding your hands for balance.

The standing supported squat. This squatting position takes best advantage of gravity and provides the best angle for delivery. As you relax down into the squat, you take the weight off your feet and melt into the arms and against the body of your partner. And in this position the body tells the mind to relax. The key to a satisfying birth is surrendering your mind and body to the forces of labor. The dangling or hanging squat reminds you to let your body go, releasing your abdominal muscles completely, looking like you are eleven months pregnant. When you let your body go, your mind is also likely to get the surrender message, and you'll find the sensations become

Holding Tips for Birth Partners

For supported squatting to work best, practice this routine before the final performance. Otherwise you may not trust yourself to hold your mate comfortably, and she may not trust you, causing her to waste energy and tense her pelvic muscles. When standing behind the mother, place your feet shoulder-width apart. You'll get the best traction with bare feet. Hold her under her arms and allow her weight to ease back onto your thighs. Keep your back straight but bend your knees slightly. Rest her buttocks on your knees. Place your arms far enough through her armpits in front of her so that she can grab on to your hands or forearms if she wishes. If you need back support, try leaning back against the wall while standing or sit behind your mate toboggan-style. Continue supporting her after the contraction is over, until she leans forward into the kneeling position or back into a sitting or semireclining position. Rest between contractions.

more like pressure and less like pain. Let it all hang out with each contraction. If you tense and brace your abdominal muscles, it will hurt.

Try the "squat for three" position if you have two willing and able birth partners to support you.

While human beings make the best squat props, here are alternatives: lean against the wall, sit-squat on a toilet seat, or hold on to a chair, the edge of a table, or the squat bar on the birthing bed if available (wrap a

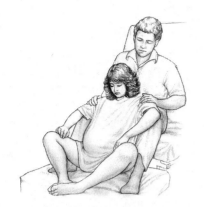

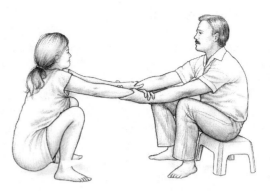

Squatting in birthing bed using partner for support

Supported squat

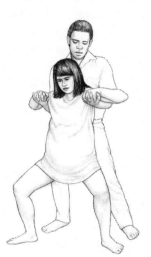

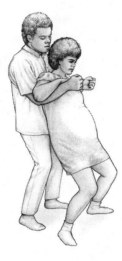

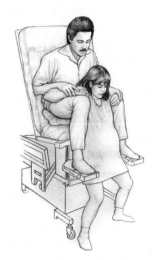

Supported squat

Supported squat (leaning against partner)

Supported squat using birthing bed

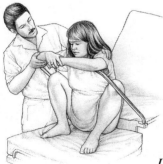

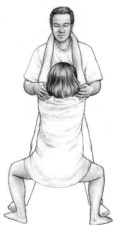

Using squat bar

Dangling supported squat

towel around it as a cushion). It's better not to bounce while squatting as this strains your muscles and joints. Some women ease their pain and speed their labors by swaying side to side during a squat. Don't strain to prop yourself. Use people, pillows, furniture, walls, whatever prop takes the weight off your feet, pressure off your uterus, and ultimately lets you surrender your whole self into birth.

Birth attendants are more comfortable with side-birthing and semisitting rather than squatting because they can better see what's going on. But birth attendants are able to assess adequately both the baby and mom in a variety of positions. You seldom have to "get back in bed" to do fetal monitoring, vaginal exams, vital signs, and so on.

Kneeling

A natural extension of the squatting position when the going gets tough, kneeling on the floor on a pillow, leaning against a chair, or getting on all fours can provide a welcome relief from the intense contractions in the upright squatting position. The all-fours position is especially helpful if you're having back pain, trying to turn a posterior positioned baby, or if your labor is accelerating to an unmanageable intensity and you want to slow it down a bit. If you are trying to speed things along, rather than getting on hands and knees, keep your abdomen more vertical and your knees well apart to widen your pelvis. And don't forget pillows under your knees and for your head to lean against. While kneeling, many women feel a natural urge to sway their hips from side to side. This can help a posterior baby rotate to anterior. You can improvise other variations of the kneeling position and you'll probably have the urge to do so. If you're using a birthing bed, kneel on the drop-down section and lean against the bed.

Kneel-Squat Position

Another variant is to kneel on one knee while squatting with the other leg. Alternate knees and try rocking or swaying between contractions.

Knee-Chest Position

A valuable variant to kneeling in labor is to assume the knee-chest position or even to curl up into the fetal position with your bot-

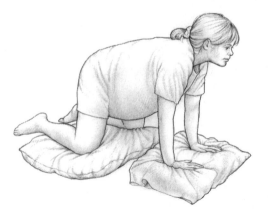

Kneeling on all fours

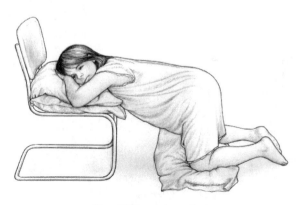

Kneeling against chair

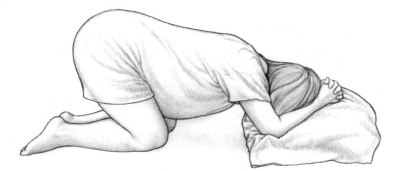

Knee-chest position

tom higher than your head. This position moves baby's head away from the cervix. This pose may soften the intensity of the contractions if they become intolerable, counteract the urge to push if that is medically necessary (for example, if your cervix still has an unripened "lip"), or slow a generally overwhelming labor.

Standing and Leaning

During the first stage of labor you may be most comfortable walking a lot and stopping during contractions. Rather than just standing there unsupported, take some weight off your body by leaning against the wall or a piece of furniture, by putting one foot on a chair, or by embracing your partner. We have beautiful memories of embracing during contractions. Your birth partner provides more than a valuable pole to lean against. He has caring arms and a reassuring voice. Besides, men love to feel needed.

Bill notes: I remember Martha hanging on to me during a contraction. I felt her heavy breathing and her hardening abdomen. In a way I felt I was experiencing labor with her but I had the painless part.

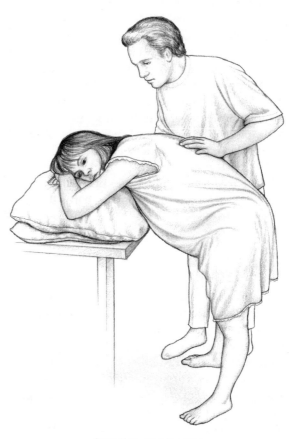

Standing and leaning

Ode to the Toilet Seat

Have you ever wondered why veteran laboring mothers spend a lot of time on the toilet seat? This natural labor throne is readily available at just the right height. Moreover, mother's pelvic and leg muscles are already used to being on it. Finally, it may be the only place in the whole world a laboring mother can find solitude. Perching on the pot is not only a comfortable retreat; it also makes good obstetrical sense. Mothers often return to this familiar place to "jump-start" their labor. As mothers who share their intimate birth secrets relate, contractions on the commode are often stronger. The abdominal straining and pelvic muscle movements used in defecation are similar to those used in second-stage labor. Sitting on this familiar throne seems to remind these muscles to perform. And this familiar sitting prompts the bladder to empty making more room for baby. Being in the semisquatting posture — knees far apart with pelvic muscles relaxed — is a proven recipe for a better birth. To ease a strong contraction while sitting, place a pillow on top of a bedside table in front of the toilet. Rest your head and chest on the table while keeping your knees apart during the contractions.

Obstetrician Michael Rosenthal refers to the toilet as a "self-cleaning porcelain birthing chair." Needless to say, obstetrical staff fear that a toilet seat used in labor may become a toilet seat used in birth. The procedure for pushing on the toilet is that once the baby's head crowns, the mother simply stands up for the birth, and the baby is safely received into the hands of the birth attendant. We know of an experienced mother who deliberately asked for a last-minute potty break just to shake up a hospital staff who were constipated in their rigid ways of labor.

Sitting

If you find your contractions overwhelming in the squatting position, you may find them more manageable while sitting. Sit astride a low stool, toilet seat, chair or birthing bed angled as a seat. Best is a sit-squat position on a low stool. Studies comparing mothers sitting during labor with those lying on their backs showed the upright mothers had shorter second-stage labors, their pelvises widened (but not as much as while squatting), they had less blood loss during delivery, and the measured oxygen supply to the baby was higher.

Side-Lying Position

While gravity aids birth, you can't stay upright for twelve to twenty-four hours of labor. Many women find relief between contractions, even during them, by lying on their side. Theoretically, it's better to lie on your left side to prevent the uterus from compressing the major blood vessels that run along the right side of your backbone.

Though the side-lying position doesn't take advantage of gravity as your ally, it still keeps your uterus off your back and may afford a few winks of much needed rest — and a way to slow down a labor that is going

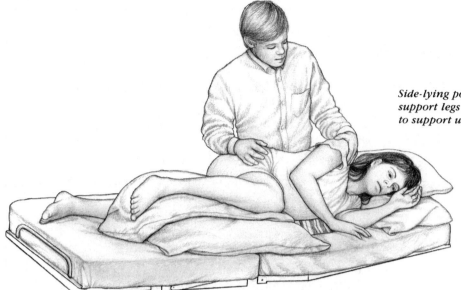

Side-lying position using pillows to support legs and head and a wedge to support uterus

too quickly. Create your own pillow nest: a pillow or two under your head, one supporting your top knee, one behind your back, and another under the bulge. (See figure on this page.) During a strong contraction you can either remain lying on your side (if you need to slow birth down) or quickly roll into a kneel or up to a squat and then return to your side-lying nest afterwards. If you prefer to push or even deliver on your side, a birth attendant or your partner can hold one leg up, which widens the pelvis.

If and when possible, design your labor movements and create your own birth nest based on what works best for you — and require the birth attendants to respect these. Rehearse these popular birthing positions during your childbirth classes and your prenatal exercises. During labor, use whatever position works, when it works, and feel free to change as labor continues. The freedom to move about during labor and vertical birthing are proven keys to a more satisfying birth.

Minding Your Progress

A labor checklist to ease pain and aid progress:

P POSITION ——————→ Change position frequently if, for medical reasons, you must stay in bed.

R RELAX AND RELEASE —→ Use massage, mental imagery, breathing, music, etc., to relax your mind and muscles.

O OUTPUT ——————→ Urinate every hour; a full bladder creates painful spasms.

G GRAVITY ——————→ Let gravity help you. Be upright: sit, kneel, squat, stand, walk.

R REST ————————→ Between contractions, rest and let go of any tension from the previous contraction; don't fearfully anticipate the next one.

E ENERGY ——————→ Check your energy level. Snack when hungry; drink to avoid dehydration.

S SUBMERGE —————→ If the going gets rough, get into a labor pool. Otherwise use a tub or shower.

S SUPPORT ——————→ Throughout labor enjoy continuous support from your partner and professional labor assistant.

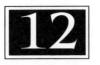

Labor and Delivery

AS THE BIG DAY NEARS it's normal to feel a bit of stage fright as the reality that you are going to have a baby hits home. While no two births are the same, there are some general patterns that most mothers experience, and by understanding these stages you'll be able to understand what's happening to you.

PRELABOR SIGNS

By the end of pregnancy, most women are getting tired of feeling bulky and uncomfortable. As your due date comes (or passes) you may become impatient, anxious for something to happen. Here are signs that announce birth day is near.

Dropping. You may notice a shift of the bulge into your lower abdomen as baby descends deeper into your pelvis. This is called *dropping* or *lightening.* This descent may occur as early as two to four weeks before delivery in first-time moms, or as labor begins in multiparas. The shift in baby's position takes the pressure off your diaphragm and you can breathe more easily. Dropping relieves pressure on the stomach,

easing heartburn. But now the pressure is on your pelvic organs and baby makes her presence felt in that direction, especially on your bladder.

Low backache. This is not the usual tired ache familiar through much of pregnancy. It's different. These sensations are not only the result of pressure from your pelvic passenger but also the increased stretching of the sacroiliac joints as baby gets heavier and drops. Many women now find it hard to get comfortable in any position, and sleeping becomes more difficult.

Frequent urination and bowel movements. As baby presses on your bladder expect frequent urges to urinate. The birth hormones acting on your intestines cause a sort of preparatory cleansing; some women experience abdominal cramps and diarrhea. If you find yourself running to the bathroom more than sleeping at night, try this: As you get into bed, assume the hands and knees position. Do forty pelvic rocks, which will work your baby up and out of the pelvis slightly to reduce some of the pressure on your bladder. Then, do not stand up or allow your body to be upright but immediately lie down on your side for sleep. This trick may get you an extra hour or two of sleep before another bathroom trip is necessary.

Cramps and swelling. Menstrual-like cramps are a reminder baby has dropped into the pelvis. Also, baby's head pressing against the nerves and blood vessels in your pelvis may cause cramps in your thighs and swelling of your ankles. Frequent position changes ease the cramps, and putting your feet up eases swelling. If you experience frequent thigh cramps, stretch the muscle that is cramping. Rather than picking up your foot and hopping around, stretch the cramping leg out with the foot flat on a cool floor surface. If you must sit a lot, place one foot on a footstool and alternate feet. Get up and stretch now and then and move around.

Bursts of energy. In contrast to feeling the usual fatigue and inertia in the final weeks, you may one day get the urge to tidy, sanitize, or redecorate the whole house, as if the most important person in the world will soon be your guest. This nesting instinct is normal, and the activity breaks the boredom of those endless last weeks. Don't overdo it. Conserve your energy for the final event. A spent mom is not ready to begin labor.

Increased vaginal discharge. You may notice increased vaginal discharge of eggwhite consistency, perhaps with a slight pink tinge. This discharge is not as noticeable as the "bloody show" described later.

These signs simply tell you that something's about to happen, but not necessarily when. Some women experience these signs a few weeks, others a few days, before B-day. Some mothers don't notice any specific changes at

---

Different Times for Second-Timers

With the first vaginal delivery it may take a half hour or more once you see or feel your baby's head at the perineum until full delivery of the head. Then one push for the shoulders and quickly baby's body comes out with little resistance. After the second or third baby, one or two pushes is all that is needed from crowning to delivery of the whole baby. And birth attendants have to hang on tight to keep the slippery infant from eluding their grasp if mother is not lying on a soft surface.

---

all. And the timing and intensity vary with each pregnancy. None will give a definite answer to the question, "When will my baby be born?" Besides these prelabor signs, here are some more definite indications that labor is imminent.

Prelabor contractions. Braxton-Hicks contractions (see page 199 for explanation) change as labor day approaches. They may go from being simply uncomfortable to downright painful, particularly in your lower abdomen. They may also become more frequent. In fact, in your eagerness for labor to begin, Braxton-Hicks contractions may send you to the phone to tell your birth attendant, "This is it!" (Before you make the call check page 199 for the difference between prelabor and labor.) Many women experience these contractions like a tightening belt inside the abdomen that contracts, releases, and tightens again. These off-and-on contractions may go on for days or weeks before delivery, and they eventually turn into the "big one." Use these practice contractions to get in some relaxation practice, and see if your relaxation skills help make the contractions less uncomfortable. You may find you need to become more skilled in relaxation.

Bloody show. As baby's head descends, the lower uterus accommodates by changing from cone- to cup-shaped. The prelabor uterine contractions cause the outlet of the uterus, the cervix, to relax and thin out — a process called *effacement.* Here's what's

---

When to Call Your Doctor

When to make that long-awaited "I am in labor" call depends on your individual obstetrical situation, but in one of your ninth-month prenatal visits be sure to ask your birth attendant, "When should I call you?" There may be specific concerns about your pregnancy that merit an early call. If this is your fourth baby and your past labors were short, call early. Obviously, if any of the emergency signals occur call your doctor immediately (see page 203). But if this is your first baby and your first contraction and nothing seems abnormal or worrisome, you can let your doctor sleep until morning, even if you can't. When in doubt, call; you've paid for the privilege. No need to feel apologetic for false alarms.

It's important to be diligent and share the responsibility for your health care. Call your physician to inform him or her of "what's happening." Be prepared, if all is well and there are no warning signs or problems (see page 203) to say, "My water broke at 11:00 P.M. The water is clear and my baby is moving normally. I am tired and would rather rest at home until contractions begin and intensify. How about if I call you during the night if things dramatically progress and I'll watch for anything worrisome? [Your physician

may review with you what to watch for.] Otherwise, I will call you at 8:00 A.M. and we can make a new game plan if you feel it is necessary." If you take some responsibility and verbalize a preference toward your care, your doctor is much more likely to comply with your request and make medical decisions according to your best interest and not what is legally safer.

Before calling, make an at-home contractions chart (see page 209), as your birth attendant needs this information to advise you when to go to the hospital or birth center. When to leave home is an important decision. Leaving home too early deprives you of the comfort and relaxation of your nest and is likely to prolong labor. Leaving too late means a mad dash with heroic driving, which is not in your birth plan. Unless otherwise instructed by the birth attendant, first-time mothers should go to the hospital or birth center when contractions are becoming increasingly strong and occurring around five minutes apart (see "When to Go to the Hospital," page 214). For multiparas it's wise to leave home a bit earlier. Upon arrival at your chosen place of birth the nurse or birth attendant will check your progress and then call your doctor.

happening. Imagine pushing a softball or grapefruit through the neck of a turtleneck sweater. Notice that the fabric shortens (or effaces) as the ball presses against it. As the cervical canal thins out, the mucous plug that had corked the cervix comes loose, and the mother notices a discharge of mucus mixed with blood (see figure on page 227). This "bloody show" is a sign that baby's on her way down and will soon be coming out. The color of the show can vary from light pink to brownish red; the blood comes from tiny blood vessels that break as the cervix effaces. The amount of blood may be only a spot or as much as a teaspoonful. The amount of mucus may be copious and the texture may vary from thin and stringy to a thick, gooey blob.

To many women the passage of the mucous plug is an obvious one-time event, for others it may slowly be discharged as it breaks up and is passed with your normal vaginal mucus. Sometimes it comes out on the doctor's glove during a routine vaginal exam and you may never notice it. Generally, after passing the mucous plug, most women will be in labor within the next three days. But, it's still possible to hang on for as much as two weeks.

Leaking water. The most promising sign that your baby is about to be born is your bag of water breaking. But the bag of water breaks prior to labor only in around one in ten mothers. More often the membranes don't break until you're well into labor, or until the birth attendant breaks them. (For what to do when your water breaks, see page 206.) If you are already in labor when your membranes break, expect your contractions to take a giant leap in intensity. When the water cushion is gone, baby's head acts like a hard wedge directly stretch-

ing open your cervix. Now baby's presence is going to really be felt.

Intact membranes are for the protection of baby and mom. With the membranes intact through the slow early phase of labor, infection is kept away. Also, the fluid bag decreases the pressure on your baby's head through the early hours of uterine contractions, and helps to distribute the pressure of the head onto the cervix more evenly during dilatation. Studies show that spontaneous rupture of membranes (ROM) between 2 to 4 centimeters' dilatation has the most effect on stimulating and speeding the labor process. Sometimes the mother is sleeping, unaware of labor when the water gushes and then the contractions "start" with alarming intensity. Other times the water starts leaking or gushes and contractions don't start for hours or even at all.

Martha notes: For first-time births those first contractions can be scary. You've never experienced feelings like this before and labor seldom goes the way you rehearsed in class. The first sign of labor with my first baby was my water breaking at 3:00 A.M. after a trip to the bathroom. After about ten minutes contractions came on like gangbusters. They didn't start out mild and gradual like the books said. I didn't have the benefit of a slow buildup or of the cushion of water. Rather I went quickly from no contractions to full, active labor. Probably, though, contractions had been occurring for a while as I slept. Because I had no previous experience, I thought these contractions were the mild ones and thought how on earth would I handle them when they got stronger — but they never got stronger. I have since learned to tell the women in my childbirth classes that, unless a problem is occurring, once your

Labor Versus Prelabor* Contractions — How to Tell

Labor Contractions

- Follow a pattern, become progressively more regular, stronger, longer, and more frequent.

- May feel like strong menstrual cramps; may have low backache with discomfort radiating around to the lower front. Deep internal pressure feelings increase and may radiate into the thighs.

- Intensified by walking.

- Don't stop when you're lying down or changing activity.

- Internal exam by birth attendant reveals cervix is softening, thinning, or effacing, and dilating progressively.

- Usually has "show" — pinkish mucus.

Prelabor Contractions

- Irregular, don't become stronger, longer, or more frequent.

- May not be uncomfortable or may be mildly uncomfortable in the lower front and groin. Uterus "balls up" and feels very hard to touch.

- Not changed or they go away by walking.

- Stop somewhat when you're lying down or changing positions. Decrease or disappear while you're taking a hot bath or shower.

- Some effacement and slight dilatation may occur before labor begins but there is no significant change from one exam to the other.

- Usually no show or there's a brownish mucus.

If you are in doubt about whether you are experiencing labor or prelabor, time your contractions for an hour. As a general guide, if you have had six or more contractions during the hour and they are lasting at least thirty seconds (see "Sample At-Home Contractions Chart," page 209) and are increasing in intensity, chances are good you are in labor.

Many women will, however, have a number of episodes (usually in the evening) when they will have two to four hours of regular contractions (five to ten minutes apart) that are even a bit uncomfortable (pulling in the groin area), but that eventually peter out. Don't be discouraged by these "this is it" starts that turn out to be prelabor. The more work you do in preparing your cervix prior to labor, the less work you will have to do in labor.

If you are concerned about your progress, or are anxious about yourself or your baby, contact your birth attendant for him or her to assess your situation and reassure you that all is well.

* *We prefer the terms "labor" and "prelabor" instead of "true" and "false" labor. There is no such thing as a "false" labor contraction. Prelabor (also called Braxton-Hicks) contractions may go on for weeks and they do save work: toning the uterus, adjusting baby's position, effacing the cervix, helping to get the delivery system in order for the time when labor begins.*

Labor Language

Every profession has its jargon, and obstetrics is no exception. To help you understand what your birth team is saying about you and your baby, here are the terms you're likely to hear.

Descent. Baby dropping down into the pelvis.

Dilatation. Refers to the opening of the cervix that either follows effacement (see below) or occurs along with it. Your birth attendant measures the degree of opening in terms of centimeters. At the beginning of labor most first-time mothers may be 1 or 2 centimeters dilated. "Ten centimeters dilated" means your cervix is completely open. Obstetrically speaking, you are in labor if your cervix is dilating.

Effacement. The thinning of the cervix from a thick-walled cone to a wide cup containing baby's presenting part (see below). Your birth attendant measures the degree of effacement during the exam. "You're 0 percent effaced" means the cervix has not yet started thinning; "You're 50 percent effaced" means it is halfway; and "You're 100 percent effaced" means your cervix is totally thinned out.

Engagement. The presenting part is at Station 0 (see below). "Your baby's head is engaged" means that it is settled into the pelvis.

Floating. Baby's presenting part is above the pelvic inlet, or at −4 Station (see below), and could be pushed back up easily.

Gravida. The total number of pregnancies. Both this term and *parity* (see below) will be listed on your chart. G 1/P 0 means this is your first pregnancy. G 111/P 0 means a currently pregnant mother had two miscarriages. Often the term "primiparous" or "primip" is used for a first-time mother, and "multiparous" or "multip" for a woman who has had a baby before.

Lie. The position of your baby in your uterus — either *longitudinal* (vertical to the pelvis, which is normal and most common) or *transverse* (horizontal across the pelvis, which is uncommon, and a potential reason for a cesarean section).

Parity. The number of births a woman has had.

Position.   Refers to the locations of baby's head in the pelvis. If the back of baby's head faces forward toward your pubic bone, baby is said to be "anterior." If the back of baby's head faces toward your tailbone, baby is said to be "posterior." Anterior is the ideal position because it allows the smallest diameter of the head to pass through the birth canal. Either a posterior head will either have to rotate to anterior, which makes labor last longer and causes more back pain, or baby will be born posterior (i.e., face up as the head emerges), causing more back pressure in pushing.

Presenting part.   The part of the baby resting over the cervix. In 96 percent of labors, baby is head down, also called a "cephalic" or "vertex" presentation. In 3–4 percent of cases, baby is breech (feet or buttocks first). Rarely, baby will be jackknifed or flexed so far forward that the shoulder presents first, or baby's head will be tipped backward, causing a face presentation.

Ripe.   Refers to the softening of the tissues of the cervix near term. "The cervix is ripe" means that you are near labor because the cervix will be able to start effacing and dilating.

Stages of delivery.   Divided into three: the first stage is the dilatation of the cervix. It begins when your contractions are regular and ends when your cervix is completely dilated. The second stage is the passage of the baby through the birth canal and begins when the cervix is completely open and ends when your baby is delivered. This stage is the actual birth. The third stage is the delivery of the placenta.

Station.   How far down baby's presenting part is in the pelvis. Station 0 is the middle of the pelvis, where the birth attendant feels the projections of the pelvic bone, called "spines." Each centimeter above (minus) or below (plus) is a station. Station 0 means the widest part of baby's head has entered the pelvic inlet. "Your baby is at +4" means his head is all the way through the pelvis and you can now see his head.

contractions get so strong that you almost can't handle them any longer, that's the strongest they are likely to get. Somehow your body will know when it's reached its limit. To mothers who may be jealous of my fast labors, I say, "Give me the slow buildup textbook labor anytime!"

IF YOUR LABOR DRAGS

In "classic labor," the woman notices the progressive nature of the frequency and intensity of her contractions. On vaginal exam, her cervix shows a response to these contractions. But there are some early labors that drag. Often referred to as *prodromal labor,* this is actually a day-long prelude to active labor. It is almost like another phase of labor for some women, especially first-timers. Prodromal labor may be considered as a very drawn-out early or "latent" phase (although there is nothing latent about the mother's experience) that slowly effaces the cervix over two or three days. In first-time mothers this effacing work is often done over a period of a couple of weeks, so labor can officially start with the cervix nearly fully effaced. Prodromal labor is not only difficult to interpret, but also difficult to endure — physically and emotionally. In this type of early labor the uterine contractions characteristically drag on with little or no acceleration in their frequency or intensity and very little or no cervical dilation. An example of prodromal labor would be a woman having contractions every eight to ten minutes for three full days during which her cervix effaces 75 percent but dilates only 2 centimeters. The contractions are not usually overwhelmingly painful during this time, but they are strong enough to keep the woman awake and in need of some com-

fort measures. The greatest difficulty with this kind of labor is the exhaustion and discouragement that a woman feels. These feelings snowball into making mild contractions seem strong and the prospect of dealing with the "real labor" yet to come seem overwhelming.

The couple may find it difficult to make wise choices when the labor is not progressing the way the childbirth classes and books say it should. They may become angry and alarmed at how much it hurts and how long it is taking to make even a small amount of progress, and they can easily begin to suspect the woman's body of malfunctioning. They realize that by the guidelines given to them of when to go to the hospital, it is not time yet. But once contractions have been present for a while, they lose confidence at home and figure somebody better do something to make this birth happen. This sets them up for snowballing interventions that will deliver the mother rather than assist her in giving birth. The following ideas may help you make the right birthing decisions in this type of labor:

Get some sleep. If you have difficulty getting to sleep or staying asleep because of the contractions, try self-help or ask for medical help. Take a warm water soak in a full tub. Sometimes this alone will slow the contractions enough for you to doze for a while. When you wake up the contractions will be less intense, or you will awaken to more intense contractions, rested and ready to cope. While you are resting in the tub, explore any possible psychological barriers, such as specific fears (see "Fear — Labor's Foe," page 134) that may subconsciously be keeping you from accepting your labor. You may not be ready yet to surrender to the demands of labor and may be fighting or resisting the contractions. For those who do not object to alcoholic beverages, some birth attendants recommend the relaxing properties of wine. Many times the combination of a bath and a glass of wine will induce a restful sleep. We do not condone alcohol use throughout your pregnancy as it can affect your baby's development. Wine, however, under these circumstances is medicinal. Ask your doctor's opinion on this remedy.

If you are still unable to sleep during prodromal labor, ask your doctor for an oral sedative to help relax you and induce sleep. To keep a closer eye on you, some doctors may put you in the hospital and give you an injection of a drug such as morphine to induce sleep. This will relax you and cause you to sleep through the contractions for a few hours. Then you will awaken to find that you are 3 to 4 centimeters dilated and rested enough to face active labor. It is generally better to rest at home through a dragging labor rather than in the hospital. Being in the hospital for this can backfire because of the frequent interruptions in your sleep the staff must make to assess you and the baby. There is also the possibility that you may not progress at all; then you'll face all the induction interventions since you're already admitted.

Once you have gotten some rest, are feeling a second wind, and the contractions are continuing, try prodding your labor along by walking, staying in a vertical position, or stimulating your nipples (see page 99). Also, if your membranes are intact, your birth attendant may suggest an enema or a dose of castor oil to stimulate your bowels and produce prostaglandins, a natural labor stimulator. The drawback to castor oil and enemas for inducing labor is that you may have intestinal cramping for a while. If, however, your contractions stop, it would be better to allow yourself to sleep rather than anxiously working to get labor going again. Sleep is a lingering labor's best friend. Don't leave home without it.

Don't run out of fuel. Drink whenever you are thirsty and eat whenever you are hungry. Nibbling and sipping during a lingering labor keep you from getting dehydrated and keep your blood sugar adequate, which will help prevent exhaustion (see "Eating and Drinking During Labor," page 213).

Be aware of signs that something may be going wrong. If you are doing well with the prodromal period at home and desire to remain there until labor picks up, be aware of any warning signs that may need medical attention, such as the following:

1. You have decreased fetal movement. Most babies kick around six to ten times in an hour when they are awake. If your "kick count" of movements is less than that, drink some juice, change your activity, and tune in to the baby. If it takes more than one hour to get ten movements again, call your physician and go to your doctor's office or to the hospital for further evaluation. (See "Fetal Movement Counting," page 97.)
2. Your uterus stays hard even between peaks of the contractions and the contractions never seem to go away.
3. You have excessive vaginal bleeding (fresh blood in greater amount than a menstrual period).
4. You notice a green or discolored fluid coming from your vagina.
5. An internal alarm signals you that there may be a problem or you see

signs your doctor has instructed you to be watching for. If you feel the need to call your doctor and he or she wants to evaluate you, or you just need to see your doctor for reassurance that everything is okay, try to be examined in your doctor's office rather than in the hospital. When you are exhausted it is easy to get sucked in to staying in the hospital and beginning interventions to "get this thing over with" once you're there. If your doctor establishes that you and your baby are tolerating this trying time well, your greatest need is to get some rest and not be pushed into hard labor, which you are too exhausted to tolerate.

Be patient. A watched pot never boils. You may be tired of sitting around watching your uterus. If your mate is acting impatient, send him shopping or to work. If you are scared to be home alone, have a friend labor-sit for a while. Remember, if you put yourself into the hands of the hospital system before you are in active labor, you could be signing up for one long continuous list of interventions. (For an example of a labor that drags see "I Should Have Slept!," page 237.)

IF YOUR LABOR STALLS

You've been laboring for hours and your birth attendant does an internal exam and announces "Nothing's happening!" Before you get into a counterproductive cycle of discouragement and anxiety causing diminished uterine contractions, consider the following.

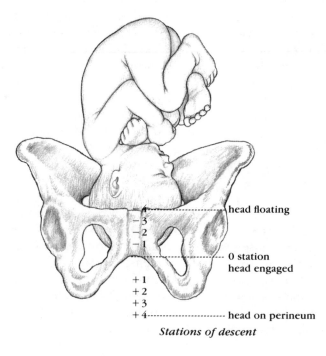

head floating

0 station
head engaged

+ 1
+ 2
+ 3
+ 4 ---------------- head on perineum

Stations of descent

What's Progress?

Your birth attendant measures how far along you are by the two *D's* — *dilatation* and *descent:* how many centimeters your cervix is dilated and how many centimeters your baby has come down. Obstetricians have a rule of thumb that calls for a one-centimeter-per-hour dilatation and one-centimeter-per-hour descent (1.5 for "multips") after active labor has begun. But these are rules of thumb of obstetricians, and they do not necessarily reflect the ideas of your uterus. Some uteruses have a pace of their own. These average "times" simply help birth attendants monitor labor and alert them to the possibility that your contractions may need assistance. Varying from the average does not necessarily mean your labor is abnormal or your baby is in trouble.

Many times there is other necessary work to be done before the cervix is able to dilate and baby is able to descend. For instance, in a first-time mother the cervix may need to efface almost completely before it will open to even 3 or 4 centimeters. So if you've put many hours into effacing but not dilating, you still have made good progress. The same holds true for descent: if you've spent the last two or three hours of labor getting the baby to turn from posterior to anterior so he can descend, but have no other progress by the standard measures, you have still made a very positive change and should go on encouraged in your labor. As long as your cervix is dilating some, and your baby is coming down a little, and it has been determined through monitoring that both members of the laboring pair are healthy — that's progress!

Don't watch the clock. You may not really be stalled, but just slowed down. The uterus has its own pace. It is not in a hurry, nor should its caretakers be. Banish all clock watchers from the birth room. You don't need discouraging messages like "still at" or "seems stuck." Remember, lulls in labor are normal and they allow you to rest and recharge.

Review your progress notes. Do those things that help labor progress (especially relaxation techniques and position changes) and not those things that slow your labor (e.g., spending a lot of time on your back hurting and worrying).

Put your hormones to work. Once you get to the second stage of labor your body's reflexes automatically trigger a surge of contraction-enhancing hormones. But before you get that far, you may have to get them going yourself. Try techniques that encourage your body to release oxytocin, such as nipple stimulation. Kissing and cuddling with your partner may also help labors that are slow starting. Where membranes are still intact, veteran birthers have used sexual intercourse to get the birth hormones going. (Sperm contains prostaglandins, which help to ripen the cervix.) If you're a bit uptight physically and emotionally, your body is probably producing stress hormones, which interfere with the hormones responsible for a properly functioning labor. Get into a deep tub with warm water (around 97° F). The water will relax you, decreasing the nonproductive hormones; and getting the water level right at your nipples will stimulate the release of contraction-producing hormones.

Are you out of fuel? Are you dehydrated or calorie-deprived? Drink to quench thirst and eat lightly to satisfaction during early labor to keep your energy reserves up for the big work ahead (see "Eating and Drinking During Labor," page 213). A couple of tablespoons of honey works well if you are further along when, because of the possibility of vomiting and aspirating, eating may not be allowed.

Get more efficient. To conserve energy, enjoy R & R & R (rest and relaxation and recumbency) between contractions, but let gravity and movement work for you during the contractions. Get up and get moving. Alternating on-your-side rest with upright movement usually keeps contractions coming. During the pauses in the action, the uterus should rest and so should everyone else. Keep the crowd quiet. Keep your bladder empty. Go to the bathroom at least once every hour.

Turn on medical help. If you have tried all your home remedies and your cervix is no wider or your baby no lower, your doctor or midwife may advise some medical assistance. The possibilities are prostaglandin gel applied to your cervix to entice it to soften and dilate, intravenous pitocin to stimulate contractions, or analgesia to break the pain-exhaustion cycle. A well-timed dose of pain reliever (into your muscle, vein, or by epidural) may help you regain some energy and make some progress. Sometimes sleep is what you and your uterus need, and medication can allow you to take a nap.

Turn off medical help. If your labor was previously progressing but stopped shortly after an epidural was begun, consult with your doctor about turning it off and allowing the anesthesia to wear off. You can always turn it back on again if needed. If you are a victim of the bedridden patient scene (continuous epidural, intravenous,

and continuous electronic fetal monitoring), ask to be released from these confines. If your doctor wants an I.V. in place and continuous monitoring, request a heparin lock for your I.V. and telemetry monitoring, and be on your way. Take a walk. Take a shower, or soak in the tub. If you feel your birth nest is overpopulated, request some privacy. Keep the help that helps and banish those who hinder. Make a "Do Not Disturb" sign like the ones in hotel rooms and place it on your hospital room door while you are sleeping.

WHAT TO DO WHEN YOUR WATER BREAKS

Throughout pregnancy your baby nestles snugly in his custom-made swimming pool. The water is called *amniotic fluid,* and the "bag" containing the fluid is called the *amniotic membrane.* In most mothers the membrane remains intact during early labor, which helps cushion the baby's head as it pushes against the cervix. In most labors the membranes rupture on their own, at the time that's right for that particular labor. There is no pain when membranes rupture since there are no nerves. In about 10 percent of mothers at term the membranes rupture before labor begins, and 80 percent of the time this signals that labor will begin within twenty-four hours. Sometimes the membranes rupture prematurely before term; this requires vigilant obstetrical surveillance to prevent baby from getting an infection. The membranes can develop a slow leak any time during pregnancy, but they usually seal themselves without problems. This swimming pool refills itself every three hours, so the lost fluid is replenished quickly.

The final breaking of the bag of waters may occur as a slow trickle, possibly during a cough, causing you to wonder whether this is the "real thing" or if you have just wet your pants. A trickle indicates that the membranes likely broke high up in the sac. If the break occurs low, near the cervix, you feel an internal "pop" followed by a gush of fluid. After the initial gush or trickle expect more water to come out for a while, especially with contractions. Usually you will have no trouble telling the origin of the liquid coming out of you: Amniotic fluid is normally clear and is either odorless or has a weak musty odor. Urine is yellow and a sniff test will confirm the diagnosis. And if you've been doing your Kegel exercises you will be able to stop the trickle of urine. Sometimes it's difficult to tell amniotic fluid from vaginal secretions, and your doctor may use a litmus test to identify the fluid. Vaginal secretions are acidic; amniotic fluid is alkaline. Vaginal secretions usually cause your panties to be only moist, but leaking amniotic fluid, even in little trickles, will make the crotch of your panties wet.

When Your Membranes Rupture

If your membranes rupture by themselves, you should do the following:

- Note the time, amount (gush or trickle), and color (clear, bloody, green) of the fluid.

- Notify your birth attendant. The advice you receive will depend upon whether or not your pregnancy is at term, the color of the fluid (green fluid due to meconium may indicate stress on the baby and should be evaluated promptly), and how much baby has already descended, which will be known from your regular weekly checkups. If baby has not yet dropped, your birth attendant may advise you to go immediately to the hospital or birth center or will come check you if you're having a home birth. The concern here is that the umbilical cord could precede baby's head down the birth passage and be squeezed, a serious emergency condition called *prolapsed cord.* If, however, baby's head has already dropped your practitioner may advise you to stay home until regular contractions increase and you really are in active labor.

- Do not put anything into your vagina after your water breaks. The amniotic membranes are no longer sealing out the germs. Avoid tampons, intercourse, and unnecessary vaginal exams.

- Shower instead of soaking and soaping in a tub. Obstetricians usually discourage immersion in a tub after the membranes have ruptured because of a theoretical risk of infection. Authorities experienced in the use of water labor have not found an increase in infections with immersion after rupture of the membranes if there are frequent active contractions, which keep everything moving forward and out. But it is probably prudent to reserve the tub for when you are actively laboring.

Artificial Rupture of Membranes (AROM)

Mothers, hold on to your bag of waters. It is there for a reason. Before you let anyone tamper with your membranes understand the benefits and risks of this procedure. Your doctor may advise AROM (also called *amniotomy*) to induce an overdue labor, to jump-start a stalled labor (although not all obstetricians agree that this does any good, considering the risks), or to insert internal fetal-monitor tubing and electrodes. But there are risks to this premature break. The bag of waters protects the baby from infection and makes labor more comfortable for the mother. The amniotic sac allows the forces of contractions to be more evenly distributed during stretching of the lower uterus and cervix — better than a hard head pushing against these tissues. Besides increasing the risk of infection, AROM, if performed when baby's head is not yet engaged, may result in prolapse of the umbilical cord (see page 48) and serious fetal distress. If your birth attendant recommends AROM, discuss the risks and benefits, and participate in the decision.

WHAT TO DO WHEN YOU'RE OVERDUE

Your due date arrives, but your baby doesn't. You wonder if this pregnancy will ever end. Your doctor starts to wonder if baby is all right. Meanwhile, you snarl every time an impatient friend remarks, "What, are you still pregnant?"

Much of the tension surrounding due dates and pregnancies that go beyond them comes from a misunderstanding of what the term means. This produces needless worry when the day arrives and nothing happens. The actual medical term is *estimated due date* (EDD), and that's all it is — an estimation. You can calculate your EDD by identifying the first day of your last menstrual period, counting back three months and adding seven days. However, only around 5 percent of babies are born on their actual due date. Biological systems don't follow precise mathematical timetables. The length of menstrual cycles varies, as does the length of time babies stay in the womb. How quickly your uterus grows, the time when your doctor first hears baby's heartbeat, and the time when you feel the first kick, all help to confirm the due date or raise questions about it, but the timing of these signs varies from mother to mother. Even ultrasound exams are not infallible when it comes to predicting when baby will be born. It's better to think in terms of a due month or time of the month rather than to focus on a specific day. Instead of September twenty-first, think of your baby's arrival date as late September.

Why the Worry?

You look at the circled day on your calendar. You look at the bulge in front of you and wonder how much bigger it can get. Your doctor starts to schedule tests to see if baby is okay. What's going on? Statistically, babies who stay in the womb beyond forty-two weeks' gestation have an increased risk of not surviving or of having a more difficult delivery. One concern about staying too long in the womb is that the placenta will cease to function well, and the baby will outgrow the placenta, shrivel up, and be born too small. This happens in only about 10 percent of babies who go beyond forty-two weeks. A greater concern is that the overdue baby will get too big, leading to a more difficult delivery or a labor that fails to progress.

What to Do?

You have three choices. First, you can just have patience and wait for the baby to be born in his or her time. Second, your doctor could intervene and induce your labor. Third, your doctor can closely monitor the health of your overdue baby and intervene only if necessary. Recent studies cast doubt on the overdue-baby worry and suggest that less aggressive approaches may be the best. Let's examine each of these approaches.

Simply wait. Have patience and trust that nothing will go wrong. Statistics are on your side. After delivery the majority of babies who were thought to be postterm appear to be right on time after all with no signs of problems. Only about 4 percent of babies are truly postterm, and the majority of these are variants of normal and go on to a good outcome regardless of management. But because of the slightly increased risk of problems, simply waiting forever may not be the safest choice. The question is what kind of medical management to choose. You have the following two options.

Take no chances. Your doctor can artificially induce your labor in various ways.

Prostaglandin gel can be applied to your cervix to ripen it and stimulate labor. Or, your doctor may elect to rupture your membranes artificially (if baby has descended low enough to make this a safe procedure) and induce your labor with pitocin. But because you may not really be overdue and in most instances your baby is perfectly safe staying inside for a while longer, this aggressive intervention may not be the best choice. Induction can lead to a less than satisfying birth experience with more complications than would have occurred if nature had been allowed to take its course.

Wait and watch. This is the most prudent course for most women who are overdue. Watching means your doctor will monitor your baby's well-being by a series of tests, usually a daily kick count (see "Fetal Movement Counting," page 97), a nonstress test (see page 98) three times a week, and an ultrasound twice a week to determine amniotic fluid volume. If baby is all right,

Sample At-Home Contractions Chart

Time of Onset	How Long?	Minutes: Start to Start of Contractions	Comments
1:02 A.M.	60 seconds	5 minutes	Continued to walk — emptied bladder
1:06 A.M.	65 seconds	4 minutes	Backache, restless, drank 2 oz.
1:10 A.M.	50 seconds	4 minutes	Contraction stronger
1:13 A.M.	35 seconds	3 minutes	Bloody mucus
1:17 A.M.	80 seconds	4 minutes	Trouble relaxing, called Dr. S.
1:22 A.M.	60 seconds	5 minutes	Went into tub

you can safely wait for nature to act in due time. If these tests suggest baby's well-being may be in jeopardy, your doctor may suggest artificially inducing labor. Depending on your particular obstetrical situation and the results of these surveillance tests, your doctor may also advise ways for you to stimulate your own labor (see page 99). A recent study comparing artificial induction with the watch-and-wait approach showed no difference in the outcome of the babies.

Whatever you do when you're overdue, remember your role in labor. Your doctor assesses the well-being of your baby and reassures you that baby is all right. You do your part by relaxing during those seemingly endless final weeks. By worrying about your baby and convincing yourself of the riskiness of going beyond the circle on your calendar, you may further delay the onset of labor. Remember, fewer than 1 percent of babies reach forty-three weeks' gestation, the point at which complications significantly increase. It's important to monitor the postterm baby responsibly, but not to overdo either the anxiety or the interventions.

LABOR BEGINS

Some mothers ease into labor gradually and cannot pinpoint exactly when it begins. In others, the first contraction is overwhelming and there is no doubt baby is on the way. Even though the experience of labor is extremely individual, here are the general patterns that are true for most women.

The First Stage of Labor

Once contractions occur at regular intervals and don't let up, you'll know that your real work has begun. You will hear your birth attendants talking about how "far along" you are. (This will be on everybody's mind, especially yours.) Here is the labor language that tells how your labor is progressing. Labor has three stages and the first stage has three phases: *latent* (also called *early labor*), *active,* and *hard* (also called *transition*). Some women are able to recognize these as distinct phases; for others they seem to blend together. And the length of these phases is variable. Most women, especially first-time mothers, begin labor with slow contractions that gradually become more intense and closer together; other labors come on hard and fast. The average (and that's all it is) length of labor for first-timers is thirteen hours; for multips it's eight hours. Most of the difference between the two is time spent in the early phase of the first stage. (Don't take any of these numbers we give you as gospel, since they were derived from large studies of laboring mothers in the fifties — a time when most moms were stationary during their labors and hospital birth attendants had little knowledge about how to help labor progress.)

Early Labor

For most women this is the puttering-around phase. If this is your first baby expect this early labor to last eight hours (or many more). You can safely spend this time at home. It is also called the latent phase because for many women the phase goes unnoticed or unrecognized as labor. During this phase your cervix effaces (thins out) and begins to dilate, reaching 3 to 4 centimeters. Contractions gradually become closer until they're about five minutes apart. As they become more frequent, they also last longer, from thirty to forty-five seconds, and they become increasingly intense.

The Magnificent Muscle

Picture your womb as an upside-down pear encircled by hundreds of rubber bands representing muscles. These fan out primarily over the top large part of your uterus, the fundus. The lowest, narrowest part of the uterus, the cervix, does not contain much muscle but is thick and fibrous. During prelabor, the pregnancy hormones ripen or soften the firm cervix, and during labor the muscles of the upper part of the uterus pull it up over baby like a turtleneck sweater stretching over a softball. These large muscles are also pushing baby downward. So during labor your uterus is really doing two things — pushing and pulling (much like when you put on a pair of pants with elastic ankle bands: you push your leg down into the lower part of the pants and at the same time pull the band up over your ankles). During labor and delivery these actions change the uterus from pear-shaped to tubular. For the uterus to do its work the upper and lower segments must work in harmony. The upper contracts and hardens while the lower softens and relaxes and opens. This magnificent muscle group acts like no other group in your body. After flexing (shortening), other muscles usually relax and return to their original length. Uterine muscles function differently. The muscles remain at their progressively shorter length at the end of each contraction. That's why your uterus gets smaller during and after birth.

Other Important Labor Muscles

During the first stage of labor your uterine muscles do all the work. No deliberate pushing on your part is necessary. After the upper part of the uterus has done its main job — pushing baby down and pulling the fully dilated cervix up — the uterus continues to contract to push baby out. But it needs the help of your abdominal muscles. Rest these muscles during the first stage of labor so they will be ready and willing helpers when needed later. Unlike the muscles in your uterus, which are involuntary (they contract automatically), your abdominal muscles are voluntary (you control them). And when they are relaxed, contractions are much less uncomfortable.

Many of the signs discussed under prelabor may actually occur during the early phase: the bloody show, the bag of waters breaking, loose bowel movements, backache, and restlessness. During this early labor try to stay comfortable and conserve energy for the work to come. If labor begins at night try to go back to sleep or at least rest. Go on doing the things you would normally do. Take a shower, have an easily digestible dinner (see "Eating and Drinking During Labor," page 213), or enjoy a walk. Walking during early labor keeps you upright and allows gravity to help baby settle down into your pelvis. Use or practice your relaxation techniques. Take it easy between contractions. Get done what you have to, but don't overdo it. Finish packing your bag (see "Packing for Birth," page 232) and call your birth attendant and labor-support person(s). Expect mixed feelings: excitement that birth is near, apprehension

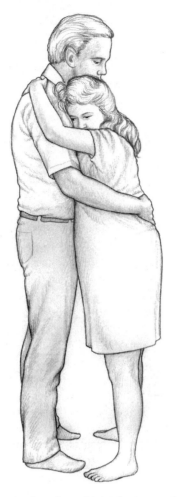

Embracing partner for support during contractions

about what's ahead. At this stage many women feel euphoric and chatty. There's no need yet to concentrate on labor or retreat into quieter places.

The early phase is usually the longest part of labor and the easiest. You are not too uncomfortable, and in a relaxed way you can do your normal activities for the time of day. Toward the end of the early phase, even while your contractions are still relatively manageable, you may feel the need to

retreat, become introspective, and tune out what is going on around you. A laboring mother's emotions, if she heeds them, are usually ahead of her uterus. This is the signal that the active phase of labor may follow shortly and intense contractions may soon be upon you. This turning-inward feeling is the best and most reliable signal that it's soon time to go to the hospital, or at least to notify the hospital, birth center, or your midwife. Some mothers go to the hospital too early if they go strictly by the "numbers" the book, class, or doctor gives them. The timing of the labor process can vary greatly; you may have contractions every two to three minutes, but if they are short and very mild, it is not necessarily established labor or active labor. Your emotional status is sometimes a better evaluator of the situation at hand.

Besides resting up physically and emotionally for the big work ahead, walk a lot during early labor. If you find that most of the discomfort is in your back at this time, it is probably due to the posterior position of the baby — with the back of her head and spine against your backbone. To alleviate pain, spend your resting moments on all fours or standing and leaning forward on your partner or a sturdy piece of furniture. This will encourage a posterior baby to turn before it gets deeper into your pelvis — avoiding the harder work later in labor.

With a posterior baby, labor is usually slower because the baby's head does not fit as well into the pelvis and so the descent is not as efficient. An inefficient labor pattern can result because the head is not fitting well into the cervix. There is also often a need for medical pain management, such as an epidural, followed by pitocin augmentation because of slow progress; instrument assistance; or cesarean section if the baby

---

Eating and Drinking During Labor

Once upon a time women were discouraged from eating during labor, not for any nutritional reason, but in case the mother needed an emergency general anesthetic. If vomiting occurred under general anesthetic, food in the stomach could be aspirated into the lungs — a potentially fatal situation. Today, except in a true emergency, most women needing a cesarean birth opt for epidural rather than general anesthetic. (If you have a special situation that makes a general anesthetic a high probability, calories and fluids will be given to you intravenously.)

Doing work requires calories and fluids, and the hard work of baby birthing is no exception. Eating and drinking during labor are not only safe, but necessary. Try these labor-friendly food suggestions:

- Grazing (small, frequent nibbling) throughout labor is easier on the squeezed intestines than gorging on large meals. Labor slows the digestion process.

- Stick to proven favorites that you consumed during pregnancy and know you can easily digest. For most women, proven labor-friendly snacks include crackers, gelatins, and light soups.

- The best energy-providing and stomach-friendly foods are carbohydrates: fruits and juices for quick energy, grains and pasta for a steady supply of time-released energy. Honey provides a quick burst of energy at a low point, especially if you don't feel like eating.

- Avoid gassy foods, fatty and fried foods, and carbonated beverages.

- Don't become dehydrated — it throws your body's physiology off, depletes your energy, and slows labor. As you progress in labor, your body diverts some blood and energy from your digestive system to the system working the hardest — your uterus. Therefore, if you overload, even on liquids, your stomach is likely to expel its contents. Take sips after every other contraction, a thirst-quenching job your partner can assist you with. Here is a time-tested recipe for "laborade":
1/3 cup lemon juice
1/3 cup mild honey
1/4–1/2 tsp. salt
1/4 tsp. baking soda
1–2 calcium tablets, crushed
Add water to make one quart. Another 8 ounces of water may be added for a milder flavor, or you can flavor with your favorite juice.

---

becomes wedged in the pelvis. Most posterior babies do turn themselves by the end of the first stage of labor; about 5 percent need manual or forceps rotation, and occasionally a posterior baby emerges face up.

Active Phase of Labor

The real work begins with active labor as your body gets down to the business of dilating your cervix. The active phase is also called the *acceleration phase* because your

contractions become stronger, longer, and more frequent, with your cervix dilating to 8 centimeters. The contractions during the previous stage are usually no big deal, but just when you are deciding "it's not so bad after all," you find yourself dealing with a whole new ball game. Now, the overwhelming intensity of the contractions may catch you by surprise, and you can't soften them simply by busying yourself. They demand your total attention and you need to click

When to Go to the Hospital

If this is your first contraction and your first baby you may want to rush to the hospital at the first cramp, but such urgency may not be in the best interest of you or your baby. During one of your ninth-month checkups be sure to ask your caregiver the "when?" question. You may have a special obstetrical reason for going to the hospital early.

For most mothers the best odds for a safe and satisfying birth come with laboring at home as long as possible. Presenting yourself at the hospital too early may give you a case of performance anxiety. Soon after check-in the clock starts ticking and the pressure to progress begins. Early arrival opens the door for questionable interventions that may shake your confidence and slow your progress. Also, you're no longer queen in your castle, but a "patient" in someone else's domain. The house rules are not yours. It is common for labor to slow down or even stop when a woman in early labor moves to the hospital. So realize you still have the option of returning home if you arrive at the hospital and find that you are only 2 centimeters dilated.

For most first-time mothers it's time to make the trip when contractions:

- number at least 12–15 in one hour
- occur consistently less than five minutes apart
- last at least one minute
- are strong enough to stop you in your tracks, demand your attention, and require you to muster up comfort-producing techniques to manage them

A good rule of thumb to go by so you don't get to the hospital too early is *4–1–1:* contractions *four* minutes apart, lasting *one minute* and consistently for *one hour* or more.

These symptoms are signals to get to the hospital in a hurry:

- sudden gush of a lot of blood (more than a menstrual period)
- sudden excruciating pain in the uterus that feels different from a contraction
- persistently feeling faint
- an inner voice telling you something is going wrong

on the pain-easing techniques you have been rehearsing. If your contractions stop you in mid-sentence and you can't talk through them, chances are you are well into active labor. At some point in the active phase you will go to the hospital, birth center, or summon your midwife.

Upon arrival your birth attendant or obstetrical nurse will check baby's progress downward and your degree of dilatation. Soon after the onset of this active phase of labor, most women are around halfway dilated — 5 centimeters. At this point you may be overjoyed at the progress you have made and reassured by the rather manageable labor so far; or, you may be discouraged and disappointed, if it has taken you twelve hours or more of discomfort to get this far. Here is where your feelings may become as intense as your contractions. How can you survive another twelve hours? Take heart: the rest of your labor, while more intense, is likely to be more productive and therefore faster. Contractions come every three to five

A Practice Run

For a safe, uneventful journey to the hospital, take a dry run before delivery day. Find out before the last-minute rush where to park, which hospital entrance to use (night and day entrances may be different), and the easiest way to the labor ward. To make this ride a safe and comfortable one, pillow your nest in the back seat but make sure you can still fasten your seat belt over your hips below the uterus. In case your water breaks en route, cover your "car-bed" with plastic — either a sheet, a shower curtain, or a garbage bag. Choose the least bumpy and most direct route and be sure to take your favorite music. If you live a long distance from your birth place, rather than waiting until you are in active, intense labor, and risk an out-of–seat belt car ride while you try to manage your contractions, leave your home earlier in labor and check in to a hotel or go to a friend's house that is near your birth place. Then take the short ride to your birth place when you are ready. Don't forget to preregister. When those contractions take over, neither you nor your birth partner will be in the mood to fill out forms.

minutes and their duration lengthens to forty-five to sixty seconds.

In this active phase the time to full cervical dilatation is usually three to four hours. But, remember, don't spend much time comparing yourself with "average times" during any stage of labor. Many labors have lulls and plateaus where you stop dilating for a while, and no one should worry about that. Each uterus has its own clock and it doesn't reveal its timings until after each stage of labor has passed.

Transition

Between the first and second stage of labor lies a phase of birthing that most mothers would like to skip. In fact, one way to recognize transition is when the laboring woman declares "I don't want to do this anymore." For most women this is the most difficult time of their whole labor. But when it's finished you are, as it were, over the hump.

A Not-So-Grand Entry

When you arrive at the hospital it is best to sneak nonchalantly past the information desk, and, assisted by your partner, amble toward the labor ward. Making a grand appearance in the hospital lobby or emergency room is likely to get you the royal invalid treatment — a bumpy ride in a narrow wheelchair. If this chariot ride is standard operating procedure, time your dash between contractions or demand a pit stop to move around during your contractions. Purposely going slowly from your car to your room is a great, relaxing way to kill time. Don't be embarrassed to lean against the wall or your partner for support. Just smile and assure well-meaning "rescuers" that you are doing fine and prefer to move along at your own pace.

Rx for "Back Labor"

The most common contributor to back pain during labor is a posterior position of the baby. Women often ask, "How will I know if my baby is posterior?" This position is often detected by the skilled hands of a birth attendant palpating the mother's abdomen or feeling the top of baby's head during a vaginal exam once labor is progressing and the bag of water is gone. Most often, however, the mother gives a clue that baby is posterior by saying "All my pain is in the back" or "The contractions are so strong in my back that I hardly feel anything in the front." If you find yourself making similar statements in labor, try the following suggestions to ease your back pain:

- Keep off your back. Lying down, particularly on your back, will only intensify the pain by pressing baby's skull into your backbone, and will immobilize your coccyx, which needs to be able to flex.

- Spend much of your labor time on all fours, on your knees, or in the knee-chest position. Besides relieving some of the pressure on your back, these positions allow gravity to help baby turn as the heaviest part of baby's body (the back of the head and torso) is drawn toward the floor.

- Do pelvic rocking. While you are in the hands-and-knees or knee-chest position, rock or swivel your pelvis in a circle to encourage baby to turn.

- Keep moving! Walking encourages your pelvic bones to move more freely, which helps baby twist and turn and find the path of least resistance through your pelvic passage. Think twice before asking for epidural anesthesia relief in back labor. Being confined in a horizontal position without the freedom to move lessens the chances that baby will move into a better position and increases the likelihood of a forceps or cesarean delivery.

- Take the plunge. Immerse yourself in a tub of water. (See the benefits of water labor, page 152.) The deeper the water, the more you are free to rotate — as is baby.

- Other back labor aids (see page 151): counterpressure and back massage, hot or cold compresses, TENS, and a well-aimed shower jet.

What's happening in your body. You are getting ready for the second stage of labor when you will push your baby out. Your cervix is dilating the final few centimeters and baby is beginning to descend into the vagina. The reason transition can be so intense and confusing is that the birth muscles are transitioning from one job (dilating cervix) to another (pushing baby down and out). This double-duty for the muscles sends double messages to your body — pull cervix over baby, push baby through cervix. Both are very strong forces going on at once and you can become disoriented.

What you may feel. Transition is often the phase of maximum pressure on the muscles surrounding the cervix and, because of the intense sensations, you have a harder time keeping your muscles relaxed. Therefore, this can be the time of maximum pain. Your contractions during the active phase may have felt like gradually increasing waves that you could ride and stay afloat. Now your contractions feel like tidal waves and you may wonder if you can ride out this storm. The contractions may come on every two minutes and usually last a minute to a minute and a half. Before you have a chance to

Do You Need an I.V.?

Most women don't, but some women do. The reason for giving intravenous fluids during labor is to make sure mother receives adequate fluids since dehydration interferes with the mother's overall physiology and can hinder progress. If your stomach is too queasy to hold down fluids or you are too anxious to eat or drink, an I.V. can add the necessary fuel for your labor. But even in this case, ice chips and popsicles or frequent sips of liquids is a preferable method for getting fluids into mother. The presence of a catheter in your hand implies that you are sick, restricts your mobility, and instills fear. There is some experimental evidence that giving mother too much I.V. sugar may stimulate insulin release and induce low blood sugar in the newborn. Some obstetricians feel more comfortable having an I.V. in place in case of emergencies, such as falling blood pressure and excess bleeding, or if labor-inducing medicines are needed. Mothers counter that if they are low-risk and these things are unlikely to happen, why do they need an I.V.? Consider these alternatives. If you have a medical reason for an I.V. or there is a high probability of problems during labor, a precautionary I.V. would be wise. If your labor is progressing normally, you are low-risk, and you are able to eat lightly and drink to satisfaction, an I.V. is unnecessary. If the I.V. is necessary or your obstetrician insists, request a saline or heparin lock setup. (The needle is placed in your hand or arm but not connected to tubing or a pole. It is periodically flushed with saline to keep it open in case it is needed.) Note that if you choose or need to have an epidural anesthesia, an I.V. is nonnegotiable for safety reasons. If you feel that the I.V. is a sore spot inhibiting your labor, make your views known. The medical team wishes you to have a safe birth, and, as much as possible, a satisfying birth. You may be able to negotiate these desires.

recover from one, the next one begins. They may have more than one peak of intensity with little letup in between. By the time you muster up your coping techniques and take charge, the contractions seem to be overtaking you. Feelings of doubt and of being overwhelmed are normal. You may ask, "Is everything okay?" or insist, "I can't go on."

As baby rounds the curve from womb to vagina expect backache and bowel pressure. You may experience diaphragm tensing causing hiccups and belching. Some women in transition feel nauseated (and may vomit), feel a catch in their throat (an early form of the pushing urge), have hot and cold flashes, feel flushed, or shake all over, especially in the legs. Being irritable, unpleasable, and hypercritical goes with the territory. While some women let go with all their emotions (and it's healthy to feel free to do so), others become quiet and introspective, retreating into their self-therapy of mind over matter. You can be at both your best and your worst during transition.

Expect to learn a lot about yourself and your relationship with your partner during birth. One mother described these feelings that occurred during her transition:

Sounds Laboring Women Make

Many women find power, and therefore comfort, in letting go with a yell, a prolonged moan, or a grunt when the going gets tough. Called "sounding," these often involuntary gut sounds stimulate pain release and seem to muster up surges of inner energy. Go ahead and make noise or be quiet — whatever works for you. You don't have to be embarrassed about or apologize for the noises you make during birthing. Do prepare your partner for a noisy experience. Otherwise your labor sounds may be interpreted as a sign that you are "losing it" and your partner may want to do something to fix the problem and keep you quiet. Keep your mouth and throat relaxed as you vocalize, since a tense mouth is likely to carry over to tense birthing muscles. As free as you should feel to express yourself in labor, there are types of vocalizations that can make labor more difficult for you. If you find that the pitch of your moan is rising to a scream, you will probably find your body tensing and fighting the labor process, and you can frighten yourself (and the women in the next room as well). Keep your sounds long and low to assist in relaxation and letting go.

To illustrate the energy that emoting puts into labor, recall the famous "grunt" that tennis star Monica Seles uses to put more power into her serve. At the 1992 Wimbledon match authorities forbade her to add noise to her slams, arguing that such outbursts were unbecoming to the event. Without the aid of her grunt, Seles lost the match.

I was rather embarrassed after the delivery was over knowing how verbal I had been during transition. I had pictured myself as able to be peaceful and quiet even through the toughest part of labor. So I was shocked and disappointed that I had verbally expressed my feelings and cried out with the intensity of the pressure. Later, my husband changed my whole perspective when he made this comment: "Sherri, you are an expressive and vocal person. What would make you think that at the point of maximum stress in your life you would be anything but who you are?" That somehow eased my mind and gave me dignity to know I had coped through difficult moments in an individual and effective way for me.

The good news is that transition is the shortest phase of labor, sometimes lasting through only ten or twenty contractions, seldom longer than an hour. These seemingly overwhelming contractions are signs that you are making progress. Transition is the highest hurdle you will have to go over and it's literally downhill from then on. By the time you feel you've reached the absolute end of your tolerance, you've reached the end of transition.

What birth partners may feel. A woman's sudden mood changes, often out of character, may come as a shock to her partner if he is unprepared for the trials of transition. It's the time during labor when many men mistake normal birth discomforts for something going wrong, and they panic. A normally loving touch may be perceived as irritating, "Quit playing with my hair!" Charges such as, "You did this to me," or "You aren't doing anything right," can shake even the most committed partnership. Women in transition usually aren't rational, and they aren't expected to be. The mother may throw off her inhibitions with her covers. Men, don't take transition personally. It's normal to feel frightened if your laboring mate is coming unglued. It's normal to feel helpless because you can't "fix it" for her. Transition means change — a change like she's never experienced before and probably will never experience again. Even if she snaps at you to "get out," stay with her, reassure her, praise her, and try to keep her on track. This is your chance to be at your best, to be the hero of the moment. Transition trials soon will pass, but the memories of your support will last a lifetime.

What you can do. Transition is a time when even the president of the Drug-Free Childbirth Society may wish for relief. It's normal and okay to ask for medication at this point, but before rolling up your sleeve for the needle, consider this: taking analgesics during transition is not good timing for the baby, since the peak effect may occur around delivery time and depress baby's breathing. From your point of view, by the time the shot takes effect, transition is likely to be over and the medication may then compromise your ability to participate fully in the pushing stage. Remember that the feeling that you can't go on any longer is a sign that you will soon be ready to push. This timing issue is true for an epidural as well. By the time it is placed and takes effect, you would probably be ready to push,

and that's the time when the benefit of the epidural can turn into a detriment. In most cases it is desirable that the epidural be wearing off (or at least decreased) to allow the mother to push effectively. Remember, during transition it is common to feel you are near the end of your labor rope and are most vulnerable to any suggestion that could put you out of your misery.

THE SECOND STAGE OF LABOR

Entering the second stage of labor is like heading for the finish line in a marathon race. You may feel elated that birth is near, but worried about whether you will have enough energy left to get there. Just as you feel like dropping out of the race, some extra force pulls you up. You are relieved that the most difficult or painful part of labor is over and excited that there will soon be a baby for you to hold. You are now fully dilated and you and baby are ready to negotiate the final stretch, the journey through your birth canal.

Second-Stage Stats

Contractions may last sixty to ninety seconds and occur every two to four minutes or space out slightly to every three to four minutes once pushing begins. With long labors the intensity of the uterine contractions may decrease. The average length of the second stage is one to one-and-a-half hours in "primips" (first-timers), and much shorter in "multips"; but there is wide variability in these times. Some second-stage labors may last as long as three or four hours. Epidural anesthesia may prolong the second stage at least in first vaginal births. This is primarily the result of the decrease

Real Quotes from Women in Labor

Early/Active

"Like really strong menstrual cramps."

"Like having awful gas pains."*

"Pulling and stretching right above my pubic bone."

"My lower back hurt so bad I couldn't even feel anything in the front."*

"I was doubled over during a contraction from severe pain in my lower abdomen, then between them I felt fine. It was weird."*

"Mild cramping — not really pain."

"A wave starting at the top of my uterus going to the bottom."

"Uncomfortable, but tolerable pain."

"I'd be walking along comfortably, and then the pain would stop me in my tracks and take my breath away."*

"Severe cramps from hip bone to hip bone."*

Transition

"Tremendous pressure very deep in my pelvis."

"I had to focus intently on deep breathing to keep my head on straight in order to deal with the overwhelming power of the contractions."

"Like someone was pulling apart my legs, ripping me up in the middle."*

"I was sure my back was breaking."*

"I had only two transition contractions, but they were incredibly overpowering. I was so glad I could then push and *do* something with the pain."

"Not much different from the other strong contractions, but more pressure as the baby was coming down."

"I felt I didn't have a break. The pressure and pain stayed even between contractions."*

"Nonstop pain — no starts and stops."*

"Nobody told me it was going to hurt this bad."*

"It was awful — but I did it!"

Pushing

"Wonderful compared to transition."

"Like a Mack truck inside trying to get out."*

"Excruciating pain all in my rectum."*

"Wanting to have the most intense bowel movement of my life."

"Irresistible, overpowering."

"I thought I was going to burst, but I didn't."

"The most earthy feeling I've ever experienced."

*   *These feelings are not "normal" and they signal the woman to make a change, such as in position, or to apply relaxation or comfort measures.*

or absence of the urge to push, which affects the quality of the pushing effort.

To give you a much needed rest between full dilation and the onset of pushing, there can be a lull in the action dubbed "the time of peace." This ten- to twenty-minute reprieve is like a pit stop in the race allowing you to refuel and recharge before the final lap. Use this time-out period to rest up for the final sprint. After a short rest, mothers often experience a renewed motivation, a surge of energy, a sort of second wind to begin the final dash.

Your cervix is fully dilated and effaced so

the sensation that accompanies dilation is gone, too. Also, when you are actively "working" with your contractions by pushing (instead of just "taking it" as you had to do in the previous parts of your labor), you can "push away" much of the remaining discomfort. Here's how the labor nurse attending the birth of our first grandchild motivated our daughter-in-law to become an effective pusher. She told her to "get mad at the pain and push through it." This gave Cheryl a way to visualize herself actually pushing and it helped her see how pushing would be an ally to beat the pain. By "pushing through" the pain to get the baby down, the mother finds out that pushing effectively feels much better than if she tries to avoid pushing.

During the first stage of labor your uterine contractions did most of the work getting baby down into position for birth. Your main role was to adjust your mind and body to accept the labor contractions, abandon yourself to the wisdom of your body, and allow it to operate more efficiently. In the second stage, while uterine contractions still assist delivery, it's up to the rest of your muscles to finish the job. It's as if the uterus says to the body, "I've got the baby down for you, now you help get the baby out."

Oh, That Urge to Push!

Around the time your cervix is fully dilated you may feel an overwhelming urge to push or bear down. It is an involuntary action — you find that you pushed in response to a contraction rather than thinking about it first. Mothers describe this feeling as "irresistible," "overpowering," "like having a hard bowel movement, but much more intense." To some it "feels wonderful compared to transition" or "The most earthy feeling I've ever experienced." When and to what degree women in labor feel this bearing-down impulse varies, and some women don't have an urge to push at all. For some women, the urge to push occurs before full dilatation. Early pushing sometimes is not helpful, and can actually do harm, if your cervix is unyielding to the pressure. Your birth attendant will advise you to hold back by having you breathe as if blowing out a candle or getting into the knee-chest position to relieve the tremendous pressure on the cervix. The pressure of the baby's head against this resistant tissue may traumatize the cervix, causing it to swell, impeding further dilatation. But, if a trial of pushing isn't hurting you, it probably isn't hurting your cervix, and most attendants will let you follow the urge to bear down. And it is comforting to note that an urge to push at less than 6 centimeters is extremely rare. If this premature urge should occur, and despite your best efforts your cervix begins to swell and not dilate, this is one instance where an epidural can be a positive intervention. The epidural will remove the urge to push, allowing your pelvic musculature to relax, decrease the force on the cervix, let the swelling diminish, and resume dilating.

Here's what triggers your urge to push. When baby's head stretches the cervix and pelvic floor muscles, microscopic receptors in these tissues trigger the urge to bear down and also signal your system to release more oxytocin, the hormone that brings on uterine contractions. These natural reflexes telling you to push and telling your uterus to contract are meant to work together, so the timing is important. Why push? Contracting the abdominal muscles and bearing down puts pressure on the uterus to increase the force pushing baby down and out.

Here are some pushing pointers Martha

Pushing for Birth

Short, Frequent, Instinctive Pushing	Prolonged, Strained, Commanded Pushing
• spares mother's energy	• tires mother
• preserves facial blood vessels	• breaks skin and eye blood vessels
• enhances uterine contractions	• may work against contractions
• gently stretches perineal tissues	• strains or tears perineal tissues
• stabilizes mother's blood chemistry	• upsets mother's blood chemistry
• ensures oxygen available to baby	• disrupts baby's oxygen supply
• decreases likelihood of episiotomy	• encourages use of episiotomy

has used in her own labors and a few that experienced veterans have shared with us.

When to push. Bear down when you have to, not when someone tells you to. The best effect comes when you and your uterus work together. Manufactured pushes waste energy; instinctual pushes are more efficient because you and your uterus work in sync, pushing at the same time. Wait until you have the overwhelming urge to push before you bear down. You may have two or three pushing urges per contraction or you may feel it as one long continuous urge. The urge may come on at the beginning of a contraction or after the contraction has intensified a bit. Listen to what your body is telling you. Don't put up with an overbearing cheering squad yelling, "Push! Push!" "Bear down harder!" "Hold your breath!" "You can do it — try harder!" These well-meaning but counterproductive taskmasters only tire mothers and tear perineums. Called *directed pushing,* this bad birth scene is a carryover from the days when mothers were so medicated and immobile that they couldn't feel when to push or couldn't push properly even if they could feel it.

Somewhat directed pushing may be necessary in births in which mother doesn't feel the urge to push either because that's just her sensation pattern or because an epidural is masking this normal reflex. In this case, the nurse or a labor-support person will tell you when to push, saying something like this: "As soon as your contraction begins" (you will feel it, the electronic fetal monitor will show it, or a hand on your abdomen will sense it) "take a deep breath, tighten your abdominal muscles, relax your pelvic muscles, and bear down for five to six seconds either holding your breath or gradually blowing it out. Repeat these pushes three or four times during the contraction and rest when your uterus does." If directed pushing makes you feel out of sync with your contractions, request that the epidural be allowed to wear off and get into a more upright position if that is helpful.

For a mother who is experiencing a precipitous second stage (meaning the baby is coming so fast you don't need to add your own pushing), the best position to use is side-lying with someone holding your upper leg. Then you either pant or blow to keep from pushing so birth can be as gradual as possible under the circumstances. A hand on your perineum for support feels good. This happens more often with mothers who have already had one or more babies with a short pushing stage. You will know this applies to you if your perineum starts burning with your first pushes. The burning sensation is your cue not to push.

How to push. Bear down just as much as you have to in order to get the job done. It is neither necessary nor healthy to strain with all your might "until your eyes pop out" or you are "blue in the face" (called *purple pushing*). Push with as much pressure as you comfortably can. Short (five to six seconds) and frequent pushes (three to four per contraction) are less exhausting for mothers, and deliver more oxygen to baby than prolonged pushing. After five to six seconds of bearing down, let the air completely out of your lungs and refill with enough new air to push through the next five or six seconds. This sounds like a short time, but it really isn't when you are working this hard. If the birth attendant feels that a longer push would help at a particular moment, he or she will ask you to stick with the push a bit longer. But in general you orchestrate your own efforts. To avoid strained pushing, keep your chin up off your chest while pushing, but not to the extent that it causes you to strain your neck and arch your back, which is a less-productive painful push.

Long, strained, and untimely pushing is hard not only on mother; it's also hard on baby. Prolonged bearing down with prolonged breath-holding leads not only to maternal exhaustion but also deprives the baby inside of oxygen. Because research validates what mothers' instincts tell them, childbirth educators and birth attendants no longer advise directed pushing and now encourage a more natural approach to bearing down.

Position yourself for pushing. As we have repeatedly stressed, the more upright you are, the more efficient your pushing is. While most mothers push in a semisitting position, consider the benefits of squatting. When squatting you are in the perfect position to push efficiently. If you are in the usual semisitting position, the favorite of birth attendants because it gives them a good view, change to a squat if you need to. Sitting on your coccyx bone is often a painful and nonproductive pushing position. What is more important — for your birth attendant to have a good view, or for you to have a good birth? When you are in a semisitting position, the coccyx (which is designed to flex outward during birth) is immobilized with your weight on it, closing the outlet somewhat; but more upright positions allow it to move out of the way. At least stay well up off your back, or you'll be pushing baby uphill. When you wish or need to speed up your progress, squatting or sitting on a toilet seat may stimulate your urge to push and take advantage of gravity to get baby down. If the contractions and discomfort are coming on faster than you can handle, the side-lying position will slow them down a bit. And don't forget to ask your anesthesiologist to turn down the epidural if you don't feel the urge to push and baby is not coming out.

Take your time. You may sense that the medical staff wants to speed up your second stage of labor. The reason for their concern is the long-held belief that a shorter second stage is better for babies. Obstetricians worry that too long a squeeze in the birth canal may harm baby and, since baby may get less oxygen during contractions, they reason that the fewer the contractions, the safer the journey. But new research is putting the worries about a long second stage to rest. Properly managed and properly monitored, long second-stage labors do not bother babies. Don't be alarmed if the electronic fetal monitor bleeps slow down during your contractions, as long as they bounce back to normal after the contraction is over. This is a normal and harmless slowing of baby's heart rate during contractions.

Don't worry; trust your body. Some mothers hold back pushing either because it hurts or because the rectal pressure worries or frightens them. In either case, the solution is to relax your pelvic floor muscles. The application of warm compresses to your perineum can help you relax. And don't let inhibitions about stooling interfere with your work. There may not be any stool in your lower bowel now if you were able to have the self-administered enema early in labor, or if you had the prelabor diarrhea, which tends to clean out the lower bowel. But even if some stool is pushed out, you won't be aware of it, and your birth attendant will quickly wipe it away to keep things clean and pleasant for the new arrival. Even though you've never experienced these birth sensations before, it's important to trust that your body is designed beautifully for birth and that it knows just what to do. The elasticity of your perineum is an awesome feature of the design. After the birth, you'll marvel at how it happened. As the moment of birth approaches, visualize the graceful unfolding of tulip petals as a way to comprehend this miracle moment.

This is your body bringing forth your baby, and it is awesome.

Protect your perineum. As baby's head descends further down into the birth canal you will want to give more attention to protecting your perineal tissues from tearing. The first few urges to push may take you by surprise, prompting you automatically to tense instead of relax your pelvic floor muscles, which will create pain. After you have gotten used to these urges, you'll want to keep your pelvic floor muscles relaxed as you feel the pushing urge beginning. (Here's where practicing relaxing your Kegel muscles really pays off. See page 62.) Think of opening up, blooming, releasing, letting out. Birth partners can help by smoothing away frowns, tight lips, and clenched jaws, praising the mother, encouraging her that soon the baby will be here, and perhaps offering light, appropriate humor to relax the star for her "opening" performance. This would be the time for perineal massage (see "Perineal Massage," page 93). Also, be kind to your perineum by staying off your back and out of stirrups. Side-lying and upright positions (as opposed to semisitting with legs pulled up) decrease pressure on your perineum and allow for maximum relaxation, stretching, and accommodation of the baby to your birth canal. In these positions you are less likely to tear or get an episiotomy.

Crowning

The first glance of a puckered scalp delights all the birth watchers. Your baby still has a corner to round and a bone to bend under. During the final inch or so of descent the top of baby's head may peek out during a contraction only to retreat back in, like taking two steps forward and one step back.

This courtesy may be baby's way of slowly stretching the tissues, protecting the perineum that births her. Once baby's head bends under your pubic bone, it won't be able to slip back anymore. There will be more and more bulging of the perineum. You may want to reach down and touch your baby's head, a normal and healthy reflex that is just the touch you may need to orient those last few pushes and to encourage you that your birthing journey is soon coming to a happy ending. When your birth attendant announces, "Baby's crowning," this means that your perineum is fully stretched, fitting like a crown around baby's head. You will feel a stinging, burning sensation that can be frightening if you don't understand what it is. (Grab the corners of your mouth and pull. Notice the stretching and burning sensation. Magnify this for birth.) Now your birth attendant will advise you not to push, to protect your cervix and your perineum. Better to ease baby out gently. Once your perineum is fully stretched the pressure naturally numbs the nerves in your skin and the burning sensation will stop.

Once your baby's head fully crowns, the next contraction may bring the head out. Let baby negotiate the final exit. Your attendant will continue to remind you not to push. The stinging sensation is also your body's signal to stop pushing. Listen carefully to this signal and the final instructions from your birth attendant. Before complete crowning your obstetrician or midwife will massage and gently stretch your perineal tissues (a maneuver called "ironing") and support the perineum during birth to minimize tearing and avoid an episiotomy. You may feel the exact moment your baby's head emerges. This is the moment to relish your

---

A Father's Touch

A custom that some birth attendants encourage and many parents love is for father to help "catch" his baby. The birth attendant instructs you how and where to put your hands on baby's head as both of you ease your son or daughter out. For three of our eight babies I was first-string quarterback, being the first to hold our babies. That first touch our babies may not remember but I shall never forget.

---

accomplishment and imagine that within a few seconds you will be holding the reward for your labor. Then baby's head turns as the shoulders maneuver under the pubic bone. After the shoulders are out, one at a time, the rest of baby's body slithers out into the hands of your birth attendant.

Martha notes: I love to participate in bringing my baby onto my abdomen by putting my hands around baby's chest as soon as her arms are free. That is an indescribable moment as I feel baby's body slipping out and I already have my hands around that precious little bundle.

After the mucus is cleared from baby's nose and throat and the cord is cut, baby is draped tummy-to-tummy for you to hold and comfort.

THE THIRD STAGE OF LABOR

This stage of labor — delivery of the placenta — is brief and usually easy compared

Labor at a Glance

Stage of Labor	Prelabor	First Stage Early (Latent) Phase	First Stage Late (Active) Phase
What you may experience	Nesting instinct. Braxton-Hicks contractions. Baby drops into pelvis. Backache; heaviness in pelvis. Frequent urination. Loose bowel movements. Menstrual-like cramps. Restlessness, light sleep. Weight loss. Vaginal discharge. Bloody show.	Contractions slow, steady, may not be a big deal. Mixed feelings — excited, but apprehensive: "This is it!" "How will it feel?" "How will I cope?" Desire to labor at home. Bloody show. Leaking or rupture of membranes (usually during next phase). Complacent, in-control feelings; chatty, enjoy company; contractions 5–30 minutes apart, last 30–45 seconds; increasingly stronger, but manageable. Go about your usual business.	Desire to go to birth place. Feelings: "Oh! This is serious business." Contractions accelerate: faster, harder, longer, demand your attention. Membranes may break — gush of fluid. More backache; whole body is involved in contractions; deep pelvic pressure. Take contractions more seriously; become private, retreat inward; touchy, irritable; quiet during contractions, less aware of surroundings. Contractions 3–5 minutes apart; last around 60 sec.; intense, not manageable by distraction only; need more pain-easing tools.
What you can do	Rest up — final event is near. Pack for birth. Tie up loose ends. Eat high-carbohydrate diet to store up energy. Mentally prepare for labor; rehearse relaxation techniques. Reread parts 2 and 3 of this book.	Putter around house; take a bath or shower. Rest; try to sleep; change positions, use pillows for comfort. Walk when rested. During contractions: embrace partner, lean against wall, kneel against chair or on hands and knees, side-lying. Between contractions: rest side-lying. Eat light meals, drink lots, snack frequently. Empty bladder. Birth partner: Be a "gofer" to prepare nest or to leave home; rub back, give massage, physical and emotional support. Call doctor or midwife.	During contractions: Begin experimenting with pain-easing positions: kneel, squat, dangle, hands and knees. Between contractions: rest side-lying or semisitting. Sit on toilet seat, use tub or shower for relaxation. Use pillows for comfort. Pull out more relaxation tools. Play music. Drink and snack. Empty bladder. Keep breathing relaxed. Request analgesia if needed. Birth partner: Massage, support, encourage; apply warm packs to back and/or lower abdomen.

Stage of Labor	Prelabor	First Stage Early (Latent) Phase	First Stage Late (Active) Phase
What's happening in your body	Cervix partially effaces and slightly dilates (1–2 cm.). Hormones prepare for birth: Progesterone decreases; estrogen, oxytocin, and prostaglandins increase. Pelvic ligaments relax. Vaginal wall tissues become more stretchable.	Cervix effaces nearly completely. Cervix dilates halfway or more. Baby's head descends lower into pelvis.	Cervix completely effaced. Baby's head descends lower, bulging and breaking membranes. Endorphins are released.
How long it may last	From a few hours to a few weeks.	From a few hours to a couple of days (average 8 hours for primips).	3–4 hours
How far along you may be	1–2 cm. dilated, partially effaced.	50–90 percent effaced 2–5 cm. dilated	100 percent effaced 5–8 cm. dilated
What's happening in birth canal	*Prelabor or early labor*	*"Bloody show"*	*Membranes bulging; effacing*	*Membranes ruptured; mostly effaced*

In the first illustration, labels read:
amniotic fluid
membrane
mucous plug
cervix
bladder
vagina
rectum

Labor at a Glance (cont.)

Stage of Labor	Transition	Second Stage	Third Stage
What you may experience	Shortest, but most intense phase. Feelings of doubt: "I can't go on"; confused and overwhelmed. Backache, bowel pressure, hot and cold flashes, shaking, nausea, vomiting, belching, aching thighs. May become unpleasable, hostile to birth partner and attendants; unaware of surroundings. Need to yell, groan. Contractions 1–3 minutes apart, last 60–90 seconds; intense, overwhelming, double peaks, relentless.	Irresistible urge to push. Brief lull in frequency and intensity of contractions. A "second wind" burst of energy. Rectal pressure and possible urge to defecate. Stretching, burning sensations as baby's head distends perineal tissues. Contractions often less intense and farther apart (3–5 minutes). Urge to reach down and touch baby's head while crowning.	So engrossed in baby you may be oblivious to placenta delivery. Cramping contractions. May notice a gush of blood as placenta separates. Overwhelming need to hold your baby. Relief that birth is over.
What you can do	During contractions: change positions for comfort, squat, kneel, sit leaning forward. Between contractions: Recharge; rest side-lying; suck ice chips, sip juice; meditate, be quiet and undisturbed. Use visual imagery: Focus on how short transition is; try a labor pool, tub or shower; imagine: "opening," "releasing," "surrendering." Play music. Relax pelvic muscles. Stay off your back. Increase epidural or I.V. medication in small doses if necessary. Birth partner: Model relaxation techniques; verbal encouragement; apply counterpressure on back; offer sips; remind mate that transition is hardest and shortest stage.	Short, frequent pushes (3–5 per contraction) are more efficient than prolonged pushing. Don't rush! Push when have urge, not when coached, unless you have an epidural. Avoid "purple pushing" — long, strained, breath-holding pushes. Rest between pushes. Relax pelvic muscles during pushing. Visualize: "opening," "releasing . . ." Improvise positions for comfort: squat, hands and knees, sitting on toilet. Allow anesthesia to wear off until you feel your urges to push. Resist pushing during crowning by panting or blowing.	Place baby skin-to-skin on abdomen; nestle cheek against your breast while attendant covers baby's exposed surface with warm blanket. Encourage baby to suck; nipple stimulation by baby or by hand releases oxytocin to contract uterus, help expel placenta, and stop bleeding. Massage your uterus to be sure it stays firm. Enjoy your baby while doctor or midwife attends to your perineum. Birth partner: take photos, videos of new family. Welcome and enjoy baby. Be calm, quiet; dim lights; stay warm.

Labor at a Glance (cont.)

Stage of Labor	Transition	Second Stage	Third Stage
What's happening in your body	Cervix dilates completely; baby's head squeezes through cervix into birth canal, begins to stretch vaginal canal and put pressure on rectal, pelvic, and back structures. Cervix is being pulled up over baby's head. Endorphins are released.	Birth partner: Remind mate to relax pelvic muscles; banish the "push harder" cheerleaders; remind mate to watch or touch baby's head emerging; wipe forehead, offer ice chips, moisten lips, rub back, support position changes. Perineal tissues stretch, preparing to accommodate baby, and triggering reflex urge to push. Oxytocin is released. Baby twists and turns through birth canal. Head eases out, attendant suctions mouth and nose, then maneuvers shoulders and body out.	Uterus is contracting or expelling the placenta and clamping uterine blood vessels to stop bleeding. Baby placed on mother's abdomen, wiped dry, cord cut; baby eased onto nipple. Mothering hormones are released to contract uterus, stimulate milk production, and enhance bonding.
How long it may last	15 minutes–1½ hours	½–3 hours	5–30 minutes
How far along you may be	8–10 cm. dilated	Fully effaced and dilated; baby navigates through birth canal.	Delivery of placenta
What's happening in birth canal	*Transition — dilation complete, pushing stage*	*Delivery of baby*	*Delivery of placenta*

with the first two stages. But your work isn't over yet. Delivery of the placenta can last from five to thirty minutes or so, depending on how quickly the birth attendant wants to wrap up the birth scene. Within a few minutes after delivery of your baby your uterus resumes contracting to expel the placenta. Some women feel these contractions as severe cramping. Others are oblivious to what's going on.

Your first skin-to-skin and eye contact with your baby releases oxytocin, the hormone that naturally helps your uterus contract and finish the job. Oxytocin is also released when the baby sucks at your breast. (For this reason you may feel uterine cramps each time you breastfeed in the first few days after birth.)

Even for this relatively simple third stage there are two opposing management schemes. In physiologic management, the birth attendant lets nature take its course. Baby is kept at the level of the placenta on mother's abdomen. The cord is clamped and cut when it quits pulsating and the mother's natural hormones contract the uterus expelling the placenta. If the delivery of the placenta is taking too long, you can help by squatting to give a few strong pushes.

In active management, the doctor may feel that nature is competent but slow. The cord is clamped right after delivery and the mother receives an injection of pitocin and ergot to contract her uterus. Some mothers may prefer active management because it gets the third stage over with quickly. In active management it seems as though some doctors believe that every woman will bleed to death if they don't intervene and give pitocin. But for the majority of women with uncomplicated deliveries, routine use of this medication is unnecessary. The body can do its job safely and you can assist by encouraging the baby to latch on and allowing him to suck as long as he wants. The top of your uterus, the fundus (found postpartum right about at your navel), will be firmly massaged to be sure it is contracting enough to expel the placenta. You will be instructed on how to massage your fundus yourself regularly until the danger of hemorrhage has passed.

If you don't ask to participate in the decision about the management of your third stage of labor, and you are delivering in the hospital, you are likely to get the active management treatment automatically. As with interventions during the first two stages of labor there is a trade-off. The incidence of retained placental fragments needing later removal with consequent infection is higher with active management. Active management does not imply hurried management — no one should ever pull on the cord to hasten the placenta, since this can result in hemorrhage or retained fragments.

The physical process of birth is now over, but the memory, and the reward, will last a lifetime.

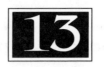

Composing Your Birth Plan

NO ONE BUT YOU knows the type of birth you want. No matter how well you plan and prepare, birth is full of surprises. But, in general, the better you plan, the more likely you are to get the birth you want.

WHY MAKE A PLAN?

Your birth plan helps you and your birth attendants. Just going through the exercise of organizing your thoughts on paper helps you work out the details of the birth you really want. Telling your birth attendants the kind of attention you want makes you more likely to get it. Obstetrical nurses, for example, attend mothers with a variety of birth wishes. Some want a medicated birth, others want the full experience.

Preparing Your Plan

Personalize your plan. Don't copy it from a book or class. Consider how individually written letters carry more weight than form letters. To be sure that you and your doctor are in agreement about your desires for your birth, make a first draft and work out the final plan in cooperation with your doctor

during a prenatal office visit. Consider including the following topics in your wish list:

Opening paragraph. Begin with a paragraph about you and your partner, your birth philosophy, and your degree of preparation for this birth. Convey any special needs or fears you have and any specific help you require. To win friends, put in a plug for why you chose this birth attendant and this birth facility.

List who will be at your birth. Include birth partner (usually husband), labor-support person (giving name and credentials if a professional labor assistant), photographer, relative, etc., as relevant.

List your preferences for the time of check-in. State whether you wish to enter the hospital walking or in a wheelchair, and ask for the option to return home if less than 5 centimeters dilated.

Specify preferences for people present. State that your labor-support person and partner are to be allowed to be present at all times.

Packing for Birth

In Back Seat of Car

- several pillows (cover pillows with small plastic garbage bags, then put on cases)
- towels
- blankets
- hot-water bottle
- pan or bowl (in case of nausea)
- baby's car seat, installed correctly ahead of time so you don't have any surprises

Labor-Saving Devices

- your favorite pillows
- watch for timing contractions
- cassette player with favorite music
- massage lotion or oil (unscented)
- paint roller and tennis balls for back rubs
- snacks, your favorite (e.g., lollipops, honey, dried and fresh fruit, juices, granola), plus sandwiches for father
- hot-water bottle

Toiletries (individual preferences)

- soap, deodorant, shampoo, conditioner (avoid perfumes; may upset baby)
- hairbrush, dryer, setting equipment
- toothbrush, toothpaste, lip balm

- sanitary napkins (also supplied by hospital)
- cosmetics
- glasses or contact lenses — or both (may not feel like dealing with contacts in labor)

Homecoming Clothes for Baby

- one undershirt
- socks or booties
- receiving blanket
- sleeper with legs (to fit into car seat)
- cap
- bunting with legs and heavy blanket if cold weather
- diapers

Other Items

- cameras (video and still)
- insurance forms
- hospital preadmittance forms
- fistful of change for telephone calls
- address book (for telephone numbers)
- favorite book and magazines
- "birthday" gift(s) for baby's sibling(s)
- one or more copies of your birth plan

Specify your room preference (e.g., LDR room).

List the comfort props that you desire or will bring along: pillows, shower, labor tub (page 152), bean bags (page 150), foam wedges (page 150), etc.

Describe the birth environment you desire. Mention lighting (dim, if desired); music (your own); quiet, no background chatter; equipment unobtrusively placed; no extraneous staff; privacy when desired, and attendance when needed; freedom to vocalize feelings in whatever way helps.

No time limits, please. State your preference that you not be hurried or given anxiety-producing time constraints as long as baby is tolerating labor well.

State your nutritional needs. Ask for clear juices and ice chips as desired, nutritional snacking if labor is prolonged. (See "Eating and Drinking During Labor, page 213.)

Present your medication mind-set. State type desired and not desired; epidural — say "yes," "no," or "maybe." Request freedom to use self-help alternatives to medication.

List your concerns about interventions. Mention electronic fetal monitoring (initial 20-minute test recording, none, by telemetry, or continuous); request freedom to use natural alternatives to pitocin if augmentation of labor is necessary; mention rupturing of membranes (natural or artificial); vaginal exams (frequent, or only as necessary); intravenous (request heparin or saline lock if an I.V. is necessary). Stress your desire for freedom of movement during labor and request that your freedom to improvise movements be uninhibited.

List your delivery preferences. Include positioning (vertical, squatting, side-lying, or semisitting); mirror positioned for mother's viewing of baby during delivery. Request freedom to touch baby during delivery and mother-directed instinctive pushing rather than coach-directed. Ask to take crowning stage slowly and controlled to avoid tearing. Request perineal support and massage to avoid episiotomy and that episiotomy be avoided unless absolutely necessary; ask to participate in the decision if it is. Consider alternatives to forceps, such as vacuum extraction, if necessary. Partner to announce sex of baby and cut cord if desired; put hand on baby's head during delivery if desired. Specify whether delivery of placenta should be natural or medically induced. (See placenta delivery, page 225.)

State preferences for first contact with baby. Ask that after suctioning baby be placed immediately on mother's abdomen and breasts if medically stable. Dim lights to protect newborn's eyes. Request freedom to initiate breastfeeding immediately and to assist in natural delivery of placenta; during private time for family bonding state that birth attendants and staff are to exit.

Say how you want to care for your newborn. State your preference — full rooming-in, modified rooming-in, or nursery care. Request that newborn routine procedures and exams (e.g., eye ointment) be delayed until after bonding time; baby be examined in presence of mother; bath be performed by mother or nurses. State feeding preferences — breast only, formula only, supplemental feedings of formula or water desired or undesired; preference for pacifier use, yes or no; circumcision or no circumcision, with or without local anesthesia; visits by baby's siblings (state age).

Presenting Your Plan

Don't present it like a terrorist with a list of nonnegotiable demands. You want everyone on your side. Boost your caregivers' egos by including your reasons for selecting them over others. Planting this positive message may get you a bit of extra attention. Consider these dos and don'ts.

Do be positive. Convey two messages. First, this is a well-researched baby, and you are a prepared and informed parent. You are doing everything you can do to take care of your health and the health of your baby. Second, you are asking your caregivers to do likewise. You view birth as a partnership — you just want to be sure everyone knows and fulfills his or her part. Also, convey that you are flexible about deviating from your plan if it is medically necessary, but you wish to be informed of the risks, benefits, and necessity of intervention and to participate in these decisions. Remember, a birth plan assumes that your birth will go normally — according to plan. But if it does not, have a contingency plan for decision making in case of problems. And, don't let yourself get angry if your birth doesn't go as planned. Anger triggers the tension-pain cycle (for explanation see page 143) and will cause your birth to deviate even further from your plan.

Don't be negative. Coming on defensively with a list of "I don't want"s is likely to earn you a "hands-off" reputation with birth attendants and a negative birth experience. If you were an obstetrical nurse, which message would you prefer to hear: "I would prefer to wear my own nightgown and be free to move about" or "I will not wear a hospital gown or be confined to bed"?

To avoid surprises be sure that your birth plan is signed by your obstetrician, presented to and agreed upon by his or her covering colleagues, and made a part of your office records and preregistration file at the hospital or birth center of your choice. A well–thought out birth plan benefits all birth helpers. Bear in mind that if you don't present your own birth plan, you run the risk of having the hospital give you theirs.

A SAMPLE BIRTH PLAN*

December 2, 1992

To: Our Kaiser Permanente Care Givers
      Obstetrical nursing staff of Shady
      Grove Adventist Hospital

From: Robert and Cheryl Sears, Maternity admit date approx. 2/4/93

We have chosen to give birth to our child at Shady Grove Adventist Hospital because of the progressive facilities and outstanding recommendations given to us by friends. We are also glad to have doctors of the Kaiser Permanente medical team assisting us through this joyous occasion. We realize that every birth experience is different. In our desire to have the most memorable and happiest birth possible, we have listed our preferences below. These decisions have been made after much research, consultation, and thought. Therefore, your help in attaining these goals is very much appreciated. You can be assured that in the unlikely event of complications, our full cooperation will be rendered after an informed discussion with the doctor has taken place, and adequate time for private consideration has been given us.

---

* *This plan is based on the plan to stay at home as long as possible before going to the hospital, so some items such as eating and drinking in labor, are not addressed. The plan could have a contingency added in case the couple decides to go to the hospital earlier in the labor.*

First-Stage Labor

- FHR monitored by fetoscope rather than ultrasound devices; no internal fetal monitoring please
- vaginal exams only upon consent, as few and as gently as possible to avoid premature rupture of membranes
- no augmentation of labor such as pitocin, amniotomy, or stripping of membranes
- husband and labor assistant to be present at all times
- no analgesia/anesthesia unless we ask for it
- freedom to move/walk around during labor
- use of tub and shower as desired prior to membrane rupture
- quiet room, dim lights, soft music (brought by us); no excess hospital staff please
- if I.V. prep deemed necessary, please use heparin lock

Second-Stage Labor

- choice of positions for pushing — no stirrups, please
- perineal massage with oil performed by labor assistant; hot compresses rather than episiotomy
- if assistance in delivery is necessary, please use suction rather than forceps
- husband to help "catch" baby
- husband to announce sex of baby
- please immediately place baby on mother's abdomen
- cord to be cut by husband, and not until pulsing has stopped
- baby to breastfeed immediately to assist in natural delivery of placenta. No pitocin, uterine massage, or pulling on the cord please

- no bright lights during bonding, please
- if stitching of perineum necessary, please use local anesthetic

After Birth

- newborn to stay with parents at all times; no nursery visits please
- please delay all routine exams to allow for bonding
- please perform all physical exams and procedures in room with mother
- if warming required, baby to be placed on mother's chest with blankets
- bath performed by mother if desired
- breastfeeding only; absolutely no bottles, pacifiers, artificial nipples, formula, or water
- father to remain with mother and baby through remainder of hospital stay
- if baby is a boy, no circumcision

We thank you in advance for your support and kind attention to our choices. We look forward to a wonderful birth.

(The story of this couple's birth is on page 237).

Sincerely,

_____   _____
Physician's signature   Robert W. Sears

_____   _____
Co-physician's   Cheryl Sears
signature

_____
Co-physician's
signature

SAMPLE BIRTH PLAN IN CASE A CESAREAN BECOMES NECESSARY

Prenatally

- Mother encouraged whenever possible to go into labor on her own before a scheduled cesarean is performed.
- For a scheduled cesarean, preoperative blood work and tests to be done on an out-patient basis.

Delivery

- Husband allowed in the OR at all times, if desired.
- Only the incision site and a small area on the back (for insertion of the regional anesthesia catheter) to be shaved.
- At least one of mother's hands to remain free (unstrapped).
- Low transverse uterine and abdominal incisions to be performed.
- Choices of anesthesia to be discussed. Long-acting morphine injection to be given in epidural for postoperative pain relief.
- Parents allowed the option of viewing birth (by mirror or by lowering the screen).
- If a general anesthesia becomes absolutely necessary, father to remain during the birth in order to greet baby.

After Birth

- Baby's health to be judged on its own merit. No special nursery care unless necessary.

- Immediately after the birth: as soon as baby's systems are stable, healthy baby to be held by father and placed against mother's cheek. Her free arm can be used to embrace baby.
- Unless baby requires special nursery care, baby can stay in recovery (preferably the LDRP room) with mother; father and nurse to supervise baby and help position baby to mother's breasts.
- If the baby is in need of special care, father may accompany baby to the nursery; baby and mother are to be reunited as soon as baby is stable and mother is able.
- Mother has option to refuse routine immediate postoperative medications.
- I.V. and catheter are to be removed from mother as soon as possible after birth.
- Nutritious food and drink to be made available to mother within a few hours after surgery.
- Parents and healthy baby to remain together in recovery and postpartum where breastfeeding can become established. 24-hour visitation for husband or other helper.
- Baby's siblings allowed to greet baby in mother's room as soon as possible.
- If mother develops noncontagious fever, baby allowed to remain with mother and continue breastfeeding.
- Mother to receive breastfeeding instruction and assistance from a lactation consultant. Supplemental formula, if needed, to be given by a supplemental nursing system (S.N.S.) rather than by bottle.

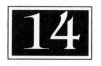

Birth Stories

THE FOURTEEN STORIES that follow are as individual as the mothers involved. Although no two are alike, these stories all illustrate how important it is for a couple to take responsibility for their birth.

I SHOULD HAVE SLEPT!

I'm not sure when my labor began. I was awakened on both Saturday and Sunday mornings around 3:00 A.M. with contractions that lasted thirty to forty-five seconds and were seven to ten minutes apart. These episodes lasted two to three hours, then faded away. At 8:00 A.M. Sunday morning I saw my first real sign — bloody show. I had mild, irregular contractions throughout the day on Sunday. I went to bed early to rest up for the big event. I was so excited that I had trouble resting.

Monday morning I was awakened about 3:00 A.M. After an hour of watching the clock, I forced myself to go back to sleep. At 6:00 A.M. I awoke and could no longer rest. My contractions were now six to seven minutes apart. They were slightly painful at their peak. At 9:00 A.M. they stopped being regular. I spent Monday cleaning and cooking, too excited to rest, knowing that it was only a matter of hours or days until our child's birth.

Monday night was very long and sleepless. At 4:00 A.M. Tuesday I noticed an increase in the frequency and intensity of my contractions. My husband and I were using relaxation to get through them and, although this method was working well, sleep or even lying down was out of the question. I thought this was *it.* We called our midwife/labor assistant, and she explained that the contractions would get even closer together and much more intense, and advised me to call back when they were too strong to talk through. At 10:00 A.M. the contractions started growing farther apart, so I decided to go for a walk to help speed things up. (I should have slept!) I walked for two hours with no improvement, so I decided to do some cleaning. (I should have slept!)

Bob's mother, Martha, arrived around 1:00 P.M. By 5:00 P.M. my contractions were four to seven minutes apart, lasting about one minute. At 10:00 P.M. Martha suggested taking a warm bath to help me relax and maybe even sleep because I was getting exhausted. Throughout the evening I had been moving around and trying various positions to find some comfort. I was very frustrated that the relaxing, lying on my side, listening to soft music, rubbing, and massaging that we had practiced were not helping. I didn't know what else to try. The bath slowed my labor and I slept for forty-five minutes in the tub. When I got out of the tub my contractions became consistently three to four minutes apart and lasted sixty to eighty seconds. After this point, I no longer remembered to eat or drink due to the intensity of the contractions.

At 1:00 A.M. Wednesday, I tried another bath to get some relief and rest. It worked, but only for half an hour. After that, the contractions were too difficult to handle in the small tub. At 3:00 A.M. I decided to call my midwife since the contractions seemed overwhelming. When she arrived at 5:00 A.M., I was 90 percent effaced, but only 2 centimeters dilated. This was the most discouraging thing I had ever heard! Our midwife was called away to an emergency, and I labored in severe pain for the next two hours — crying uncontrollably. The pain, disappointment, and exhaustion added up to misery. I was frustrated at how long I had been in labor with what I felt was very little progress. I was angry that no one had told me how painful it could be. The contractions overpowered me and fear set in. How could I make it through? I thought I would be almost done by now but I was just starting. About 7:00 A.M., I regained composure and control, with a new determination to make it through. From 7:00 to 11:00 A.M., I labored while leaning over the kitchen table, resting my forearms and head on a pillow during contractions. In between contractions, I sat straddled on a chair, resting my

head and arms on its back. The backup midwife arrived at 11:00 A.M. and checked my progress. I was 100 percent effaced, but still only 2 centimeters dilated. At 11:30 A.M., my water broke with a pop and a gush, bringing on contractions which were more severe and closer together. They were practically unbearable, and I felt that I was losing control again! A shower did no good. Exhausted and upset, I was crying again. It was time to go to the hospital. I wanted the pain to go away, and the doctors could make it go away.

We arrived at the hospital at 1:00 P.M. When the nurse checked me, I was at 6 centimeters — not enough to make me feel better. I wanted pain medication. I couldn't do it any longer. I was ready for an epidural. Bob tried to encourage me to use my "bag of tricks" for pain relief since these interventions certainly hadn't been in our birth plan. I refused. I wanted relief — he couldn't understand. He wasn't the one in excruciating pain, with no sleep for three days. The nurse, knowing from our birth plan the kind of birth we had hoped for, suggested a shot of Nubain, which would "take the edge off." It would mean an I.V., confinement to bed, and intermittent EFM, but it would last for only half an hour, and be long gone before it was time to push.

The Nubain helped very little, but it was enough to help me get back in control and stay on top of the contractions. I didn't want to stand or walk, so I wasn't bothered by confinement to bed. I continued laboring, sitting on the bed in a straddle position. In no time I felt that wonderful uncontrollable urge — the urge to push! I was at only 9½ centimeters, but there was no harm in pushing early, so I went for it. What relief! The pain was still there, but I was on top of it and my pushing was helping. I was on my hands and knees on the bed for the first half of second-stage labor. During the second half, I sat upright in the birthing bed. Bob and Martha were on either side, holding my legs up and helping me to pull them back during contractions, and in between contractions, I slept. After approximately one hour of pushing and no episiotomy, at 4:07 P.M. our beautiful baby boy, Andrew Robert Lee Sears, entered the world. Was it worth it? Every single second!

Our Comments: When labor starts you don't know how long it will last. This first-time mother (our daughter-in-law Cheryl) spent her energy in her early labor and was exhausted by the time she reached the point that required the most effort. She should have slept or at least rested. Unfortunately, her labor-support midwives did not pick up on her need for sleep, or they would have suggested using wine or calling for a sedative. If this had been included in the couple's birth plan, it could have been discussed prenatally with the doctor. Her exhaustion and discouragement could have set her up for a surgical birth, but she clicked into her birth plan, opened her pre-formulated bag of resources, and got a second wind. She used medical pain relief wisely — to enable herself to go on, to have the birth she wanted.

A "PURE" BIRTH

My husband and I were pleasantly shocked over how quickly I became pregnant. An incredible perfectionist, I found it a bit overwhelming to know I had only nine months to prepare myself for the major event of childbirth. Early in my pregnancy, I tried to exercise frequently and found that swimming gave me the best workout and a natural sense of well-being. During a good swim I was able to focus on the upcoming birth. Kegel exercises, squatting, pelvic tilts, and other postural toning techniques from my chiropractic training all became part of my day. I prefer a vegetarian diet, but I reluctantly increased my protein consumption to the recommended levels. After some research I also increased my intake of certain vitamins and minerals. I felt good throughout the pregnancy, although a touch of late-afternoon-to-early-evening sickness did shadow me for the first few months.

With some persuasion, my husband agreed to accompany me to not one but two full series of child-birthing classes. The one offered through the hospital clued us in on in-house procedures and reviewed the statistics on various interventions. The other was a private course with much more emphasis on what a true natural-birth experience could be. It included very specific methods to ensure as little medical intervention as possible.

One morning three weeks before my due date I woke to find myself going into labor. When I had gotten up to go to the bathroom I had noticed a small leak of clear fluid. I just figured that our fetus had matured more quickly than average and was ready to go. But I was not! My bag was not packed and I had not even decided what items to take.

For the first few hours, my contractions were mild and intermittent, and the water leaked out at a slow but steady pace. My OB confirmed that labor had begun and said that all looked fine. The only "not so uplifting" news was that if I didn't deliver by 7:00 A.M. the next morning I would need to be induced. But I felt that things were progressing at a good pace, so I didn't worry about that.

On our way home we stopped at a farm stand and I picked out light snacks to sustain me through labor. Whenever a contraction began, I would lean over a counter and pretend to be reading the display. About 3:00 P.M. my contractions were more regular and beginning to become uncomfortable. By 5:00 P.M. I had to lie on my bed, relax all my muscles, and really concentrate on my deep breathing. I felt comfortable and confident doing this at home since at my Bradley classes I had learned how to work with my body. I knew that the uterus was contracting as it should in a normal, healthy delivery and that my role at this point was to relax, stay out of its way, and let it do its thing.

We arrived at the hospital at 9:00 P.M. By this time I didn't feel like talking during the rather strong contractions. Unfortunately, our nurse behaved as though she had been trained by Attila the Hun. Everybody else was great, but her bedside manner left much to be desired. It took her half an hour to decide that I really was in labor, and about the time I was finally able to get comfortable, she informed me that she was now admitting me and that I needed to get up so that she could get my bed ready. I continued to concentrate very hard on relaxing and resting all my muscles and then breathing deeply through the contractions. At some point this became more difficult as I felt as if my uterus was on automatic pilot, and at a speed much quicker than I was in the mood for. I started shaking. I knew these were classic signs of the transition phase but couldn't believe I was already there. I had been in the hospital only two hours.

I would not call the next sensation a "sudden urge to push." It felt as if my insides were ready to explode out the bottom at any second. My husband was able to persuade a very kind nurse to come in and check me, and she very promptly informed us that our baby was coming any minute. I began pushing with the contractions, but I remember thinking "Why am I pushing? This baby could easily arrive on its own." The doctor arrived, and our little girl was born at 12:08 A.M., one half hour after I began pushing. She emerged calm and alert. I still remember the expression on her face.

I was glad I was lucid and drug-free for the whole thing. The first stage was a challenge I really enjoyed. Transition and second stage for me were somewhat frightening and painful, but, as I had learned, they lasted only a short period of time and were well worth what followed. I am so grateful for the fact that I was awake to see her born and that my husband and I were immediately able to welcome her into her new world. My last concerns melted away as she nuzzled up against my breast and began to feed. It was a very big day for all of us and it was wonderful to curl up for the first time as a family for a cozy, well-deserved, and truly relaxing night of sleep.

Our Comments: These super-prepared parents took two childbirth classes — one to familiarize themselves with hospital routines and another to increase their chances of achieving their goal of a drug-free birth. The mother's exercising, diet, focusing on the birth, and the fact that she really absorbed the material from the Bradley class helped her recognize the uncontrollable feelings that mark transition. All the effort paid off in a calm preg-

*nancy and a confident labor — not even
"Attila" threw them off course. In birth as
in life the more you invest the greater are
the returns.*

A MEDICALLY MANAGED BIRTH

At 6:00 P.M. on New Year's Day as I was
walking up to my front door my water
broke. There was only a small amount of
fluid, but it continued to leak, and I was having irregular contractions. I called my doctor, who told me to go to the hospital.

I was feeling anxious, but I was very surprised to find that I wasn't scared. My husband, Tom, and I got to the hospital at about
10:00 P.M. We were taken to the labor and
delivery room and we settled in. Hooked up
to a fetal monitor and an I.V., I was a little
disappointed that I was unable to move
around.

The nurse told me the doctor had prescribed a narcotic and an epidural. I
declined to have the narcotic. The nurse
told me I should try to get some sleep, but
I was much too excited. At 4:00 A.M., the
nurse came in and added pitocin to the I.V.,
since my contractions were still irregular
and not getting stronger.

It didn't take long before the contractions
were more severe and regular. Tom was
very supportive, helping me with my breathing and rubbing my back and forehead. I felt
very close to him. We had been to the Lamaze classes provided by the hospital and
thought we would use all the techniques we
had learned. When it came down to it, the
breathing was all we used — I never used
my focal point or the relaxation tape we had
bought.

The contractions were getting much
stronger and Tom was helping me breathe
through them. After a while, I was not feeling very sociable, and I was not able to handle the contractions as easily. Tom said,
"Come on, breathe," and I said, "I don't want
to breathe!" At this point I wasn't really
thinking about the baby — just about the
next contraction. I was starting to feel as if I
might not be able to do this.

The nurse came in and relieved Tom so
he could go get some coffee. The anesthesiologist came in and started the epidural —
I told him he was my best friend! It took
about fifteen minutes for the pain to subside
and during this time the contractions were
very strong and the nurse was extremely
helpful. When Tom returned, I was in a
much better mood and was feeling confident again.

When the nurse checked me again, I was
at 10 centimeters, and she said we were
ready to go. The doctor came in, and since I
was unable to move my legs, Tom pulled up
one leg and the nurse pulled up the other. I
did not feel the urge to push, but I could
feel a contraction coming on. Even though I
did not feel the pain, I found myself concentrating very hard and thinking only about
the baby I would finally be able to see. The
nurse had attached a fetal monitor to the
baby's head. Each time I pushed the baby's
heart rate slowed. The doctor said her cord
was wrapped around her neck, and that she
would use vacuum extraction to get her out
more quickly. I had been very confident up
to this point, but I started to worry that
everything wasn't going to be all right.

When I saw the baby's head, I felt a rush
of energy and a warm feeling of joy. After a
few more pushes, I had delivered and was
able to see my perfect baby girl. Because of

the cord around her neck, I wasn't able to hold her right away. I could see her from across the room. When I finally got to hold her and nurse her, I felt complete. I am still amazed how this perfect person came into my life.

Our Comments: Tracy was delighted with her American way of birth. We interviewed her about whether or not this style of birth left her "less fulfilled" as a woman. On the contrary, she felt that because she experienced little pain, she was left with mostly pleasant birth memories. There was no doubt in her mind she gave birth, and the fact she didn't experience the intense sensations of a drug-free birth did not lessen her fulfillment. For Tracy this was a "positive birth experience." The American way, unfortunately, did not give Tracy's body a chance to bring on natural gradual contractions. The rush to chemical induction set the stage for further interventions. We wonder whether her Lamaze instructor mentioned the importance of taking the contractions one at a time and of resting and releasing in between, thinking of the baby, not the next contraction.

I WITNESSED MYSELF BECOME A WOMAN — VBAC WATER BIRTH

When I was ten years old and I started menstruating, I was told that all the women in my family have a pelvic bone that doesn't move and hence, have to have cesareans.

When my first child was born, I lived up to the family history. I had a torturous thirty-six-hour labor. I had every intervention available. I was checked vaginally at least forty times (which gave me an infection that kept me in the hospital for seven days). By the end of this ordeal, I felt betrayed by everyone. I was told the reason for the cesarean was that my pelvis was too small and that I would never deliver a baby over five pounds! As they prepped me for surgery, the doctor said, "Your baby is in distress. We really needed to do all this." I told him while he was at it to cut my head off, too! I felt that all the interventions had caused the problems. Doctors just can't let nature do the work, and the woman is not even involved. We let them take over and ruin the experience that is our right as women.

After two miscarriages, I became pregnant again. By this time, I was highly educated about birth. I realized that my body could deliver a baby larger than five pounds. I learned to trust in nature and myself. I found a wonderful midwife who taught me that my body was perfect; she would attend our home birth.

At forty-one weeks my water broke. It was 4:00 A.M. I was so excited, since my previous labor had been induced. My contractions started right away. They were three minutes apart and a minute and a half long. My dream was about to come true.

The midwife arrived at about 7:30 A.M. I was dilated only to 2 centimeters. I was furious. The contractions were hard, and I was in an upright position the whole time. Eventually, I had the urge to push with the contractions. The midwife checked me: I was only 4 centimeters, but I had an urge to push! I stayed like that for hours.

On my way to the birthing tub, my midwife had me squat on the floor. In four contractions, I went from 4 to 8 centimeters. I got into the birthing tub at 9 centimeters, with a little piece of the cervix holding the baby back. As I pushed, my midwife pushed it over the baby's head. Bang! She was in the birth canal, and I could feel her moving down! I loved pushing! Earlier I had been afraid of it, but now it was great. Finally her head was fully crowned, and then was out. My parents, two friends, and Adam watched in amazement. My midwife and her assistant just let me run the whole show.

With the next contraction the body was out, and our baby came from the water into my arms. My husband, who was behind me in the tub, was crying. I looked at this little person who came from my body — all *nine pounds* of her. I did it! I did it for all the women before me, and for this precious new life. She will never be told that she will have to have a cesarean. We all witnessed a miracle, and I witnessed myself become a woman. I let my body birth the way it was intended.

My two births left me with completely different feelings. With my first I felt defeated. I thought everyone and everything had betrayed me. We have pictures of me right after the surgery. I look like I am dead. Someone even folded my hands over my stomach! I listened to my baby scream for two hours as they tortured him with all their "procedures."

With my VBAC home birth I felt elated. All I could say was "I did it! I did it!" I just proved three generations of women wrong! I shared the experience with everyone I loved. My baby cried for a second as she took her first breath, but after that she was quietly taking in the world. Now when I look back, I remember that wonderful feeling of being the first one to touch her. The first one to hold her. The first one to say "hello." The only positive factor of my C-section is that it taught me to become responsible for my birth and baby. I can finally say I'm a grown-up. I have felt terrific ever since!

Our Comments: *Cindi was one angry mom who spent three years educating herself to have the birth she wanted — and she got it. Instead of wallowing in a victim mentality she rose above her anger and did something about it. We would see this mother at ICAN meetings soaking up the information and support that empowered her to give birth the way she needed to. This story illustrates how birth is closely tied to a woman's sense of self-worth. The way she was treated in the first birth left her feeling humiliated and anxious. The second birth boosted her self-esteem and left her with good feelings that will last a lifetime.*

HIGH-RISK PREGNANCY — HIGH-RESPONSIBILITY BIRTH

It took us two years to conceive our baby. By that time I was thirty-nine years old, and we had undergone the trauma of infertility testing. I had been on Clomid (an ovulation-inducing drug) for nine months with no results. We had filed for adoption. At Christmas I decided to take a month off Clomid and see a new infertility guru in January. We conceived in December. So by the time I saw the infertility specialist in January he could only smile and shrug — I was already pregnant!

The months that followed were divine. I basked in the happiness of pregnancy. Morning sickness never showed its face to me. My friend took nude photos of me with my big belly. And I did my holistic things — healthy diet, regular massage and chiropractic adjustments, raspberry tea, perineal massages with olive oil (to prevent episiotomy), vitamin supplements, lots of Kegel exercises, and the appropriate yoga stretches. I had fantasized the birth of my child for years — natural, no drugs, a participatory experience with dim lights and soft music and no episiotomy. I imagined a midwife and birth at home, squatting on the wooden floor in our bedroom. I wanted my baby on my belly, skin to skin, breastfeeding. Eventually my fantasy of giving birth at home was modified at my husband's insistence — I contented myself by seeing a midwife at an alternative birthing center.

Six months into my pregnancy my midwife informed me that due to my consistently high blood pressure (since the third month) she would be unable to deliver my baby at the birthing center. I was "out of the scope of her practice" and considered high-risk. I was devastated, heartbroken to have to renounce the idea of using a midwife and seek out a doctor. But when I visited Dr. P. in my seventh month, I liked him immediately. When I shared my ideas about the birth I hoped for, he encouraged me to hire a labor coach, an R.N. with a private practice, to support us during the birth. She would be a familiar feminine presence for me, one who knew me and could be my advocate, freeing my husband to hold my hand and breathe with me.

Weeks later, our labor assistant visited our home and sat down with my husband and me. Did my husband want to cut the cord? Would I be breastfeeding? Did I want an epidural? She helped us know what to expect and assisted us in detailing our choices. Together we wrote a birth plan, which my husband and I discussed with Dr. P., and

which he forwarded to the hospital with my preadmittance file.

In the weeks that followed, Dr. P. told me some of what might happen during the birth as a result of my high blood pressure, but neither of us could have foreseen what happened. In the seventh month, due to my high blood pressure, I was restricted to bed six hours per day. By the ninth month I was on complete bed rest. I was seeing my doctor twice a week to monitor my blood pressure, continuing to take homeopathic supplements, and seeing a massage therapist who did a special treatment to the lymph system to help lower my blood pressure. All the while I maintained my hope for a completely natural, drug-free birth.

At thirty-nine weeks Dr. P. informed me that we needed to induce labor. "Your blood pressure has become too high," he said. "With contractions, it is bound to go even higher. It is becoming dangerous for you and for the baby. I want you to meet me at the hospital tonight." I was stunned. No bag of waters breaking in the middle of the night for me. No waking my husband: "Surprise, honey! It's time!" I called my labor assistant. She encouraged me to ask Dr. P. to administer prostaglandin gel to my cervix. This, she said, would help my cervix ripen and increase my chances of having a vaginal delivery. Otherwise, inducing labor often initiates contractions but the cervix doesn't soften, often leading to a C-section. Reality was beginning to hit me.

Friday evening Dr. P. administered prostaglandin gel to my cervix and began an I.V. of magnesium to lower my blood pressure and another I.V. of a low dose of pitocin to get my contractions started. My bag of waters broke around 5:00 A.M. Saturday, and with that, my own contractions began. As the contractions increased, I felt a greater need to walk around, squat, and test the labor positions I had learned in my childbirth class. But much to my dismay, even sitting up made my blood pressure shoot up to dangerously high levels. Magnesium has the side effect of rubbery legs, so even if my blood pressure had allowed it, I would not have been able to stand and walk during labor. My blood-pressure readings increased dramatically in any position but lying down, so down I stayed with my husband and assistant breathing me through those painful contractions as best they could.

During the day my blood pressure began to rise again as a result of the pain I was experiencing with the contractions. My doctor told me the magnesium was not having the desired effect, that my blood pressure was getting dangerously high again ($^{207}/_{119}$), and that he recommended an epidural because one of its side effects is to lower the blood pressure dramatically. In my foggy magnesium-induced state, it took me a while to comprehend that I must have an epidural to maintain my chances of a vaginal delivery. If things went on the way they were, my blood pressure would necessitate a C-section.

An epidural — just what I had hoped to avoid! I cried through the injection and the insertion of the epidural needle, not because it hurt, but because I was feeling so lost and so tired. What happened to the birth I had imagined? It became even more remote with the insertion of a urinary catheter, necessary because the epidural removes the sensation to urinate. To make matters worse, the "variables" on the baby's heartbeat, monitored by an external belt, were no longer clearly discernible. There had been a fall in the heartbeat caused by a decrease in fluid as the umbilical cord was now compressed with each contraction. To protect and pad the

baby during the remainder of the labor and to allow a clear reading of the baby's vitals, my doctor recommended an amnioinfusion. This involved a vaginal catheter to reinfuse water into the amniotic sac. In addition, a scalp electrode became necessary to ensure an accurate reading of the baby's state.

So there I was at the height of my labor, flat on my back with two I.V.s in my arm, an I.V. in my spine, two vaginal catheters, a urinary catheter, and an oxygen mask (to be sure enough oxygen got to the baby). This was surely not the birth I imagined, and I cried off and on without shame. My husband and coach sympathetically helped me to take each step. My doctor remained steady and firm about what we must do and never told me that if I didn't go along with his advice, a C-section would be inevitable.

Late Saturday night, when the contractions were at their height, I developed a "hot spot" — a place where the epidural did not take effect. The pain in this area around my right ovary was excruciating, and once again my blood pressure began to rise. My husband and coach were fast asleep, exhausted from the intensity of supporting me for such a long time. I spent a couple of hours breathing through the contractions until the hot spot became too much. When the anesthesiologist suggested a second epidural, I consented.

It took a total of thirty-five hours for me to dilate fully. At about 4:30 A.M. on Sunday Dr. P. told me it was time to push. Push? You've got to be kidding. Between my lack of sleep, the magnesium's fuzzy effect, and the numbing of my lower body by the epidural, I couldn't believe I would be able to push this baby out. The doctor checked the baby's position. "High. Very high. This little guy has got a long way to go." He looked skeptical. For the first time I felt fear. How long, I wondered, would he let me push? How long before a C-section was suggested? "Now you've got to get really mad and push that baby out," he told me.

My assistant and a nurse propped me up in a semisitting position in an adjustable labor bed. Foot pedals were set up. It seemed like just a few pushes later (it was a little over an hour) that I got a glimpse of my baby's head crowning. I couldn't believe what I saw in the mirror when a little face emerged. The lights were dimmed and music softened the sound of voices. Moments later, our son "shot into the world," as my husband said.

There was no episiotomy, just a stitch for a tiny tear. The baby was put immediately to my breast. The nurses waited as long as possible to perform the routine checks and bath. I could not believe what was handed to me — a perfect little boy with skin and hair the color of a peach. My husband and I laughed for joy.

The next day Dr. P. came to check on me. With incredible kindness he asked if I was disappointed that the birth had not turned out the way I had expected. My eyes filled with tears. What I felt was not disappointment. In that moment I could not have been happier. I had experienced the incredible *power* of pushing my baby out into the world.

In the days and weeks that followed, I came to appreciate the many lessons for me in this birth. I had educated myself and made a plan based on informed choices, but then I had to abandon my plan and trust in my doctor to help me when I could no longer help myself. I did not have the birth I imagined, but I am grateful to my doctor for his judicious use of the technology that helped me to bring our son into the world.

In my heart I know I had the best birth I could have had — my birth.

Our Comments: *Leah had enough medical problems to set her up for a surgical birth. Instead of becoming a passive patient in the high-risk category, she took high responsibility in educating herself to get the birth she wanted. She trusted her doctors to do their part and she trusted her body to do its part. Despite her medical condition, this mother got to experience the power of pushing her baby out and the joy of holding him in her arms right from the start.*

A PAINLESS BIRTH

They say Sunday is the day of rest. Well it can be, even when you're in labor. I know because it happened to me.

On Sunday, December 30, we got up and went to church, just like every Sunday. After church we went to the mall to do a little bit of walking. I had lost part of my mucous plug a few days before, so we thought a walk would speed things up a bit. During our walk I had a few mild contractions here and there, but I barely noticed them. We then went home and relaxed for the rest of the afternoon. Later on that evening I had a little bit of spotting so I called my doctor. She said it might just be more of the mucous plug and told me not to worry. I was still having a few mild contractions here and there, but they were painless and undisturbing. At about 8:00 P.M. the spotting got heavier and the contractions a little bit stronger, but they were still very manageable and irregular. Our doctor told us to go to the hospital to get checked out. When we got there the nurses checked me around 10:00 P.M. and found I was dilated to 4 centimeters. We were shocked! I had no idea I was actually in labor. I thought I was supposed to feel pain, but all I was feeling was a little bit of pelvic pressure.

My doctor thought I still had a little while to go, so the nurses said I could go home or check in to my room. We decided to check in, and at 10:15 P.M. I was admitted to my room to await my doctor's arrival. The nurse, a friend of mine, stayed in the room with me while my husband went to the car to get the bags. The pelvic pressure I was feeling was getting a little bit stronger now, so I lay on the bed and chatted with my friend.

At about 10:30 P.M. mid-sentence, I felt a gush of water and something between my legs. I had my leg in the air and I yelled, "Help! What's going on?" My friend laughed and said it was just the baby. I yelled, "Oh no! Go get my husband!" I was trying to hold the baby in. A few nurses ran in, and my husband got there just in time to see our baby boy, Caleb Jonathan, born at 10:35 P.M. One of the nurses caught the baby, and my husband and I were totally shocked. It was over before we thought it had begun. What a great joy and relief to have a painless delivery! Our doctor got there shortly after the birth. I hadn't had time for a monitor, an I.V., or anything. Later on that night, the nurse was still working on my admitting papers, and we all laughed when a man came into the room a few hours later and asked, "Did someone in here need an epidural?"

Our Comments: Is birth supposed to be this easy or was this woman just lucky? One thing that contributed to Kathy's pain- *less delivery was the fact that she didn't fear her labor. Women we know who have had painless births approach birth with confidence in their body's ability to perform the way it was designed to.*

HIGH-TECH CONCEPTION — HIGH-TOUCH BIRTH

After a long period of infertility treatment, my husband and I decided to try ZIFT (Zygote Intra-Fallopian Transfer), which would give us a three-in-one chance of conceiving. We found a wonderful doctor who involved my husband, Ken, in every step. Ken gave me the injections daily at home, for four months, watched the eggs mature in my ovaries through ultrasound, saw the removal of the eggs, saw the four zygotes transferred back. Several weeks later he was with me when we saw the twins on the ultrasound.

Knowing I would be confined to bed for three months, I had gathered a stack of books to read. Dr. Michel Odent's book convinced me there were other ways to deliver than the traditional hospital route.

At nine weeks, I miscarried one twin. We had lost our natural fertility, and now we had lost one twin. We did not want to lose the birth we wanted.

Our friends who had used the Natural Childbirth Institute told us of their wonderful experience. We met with several midwives, and chose Nancy because of her professional practice and her experience. My prenatal care was excellent.

At twenty-six weeks I started preterm labor, which Nancy stopped with rehydration. At thirty-three weeks I started preterm labor again and went to the hospital to see my backup doctor. The hospital was filled with laboring women yelling and the doctors yelling back at them. The coaching sounded more like fans yelling at players. In one hour my husband and I were so tense that we knew this was no place to have a baby and longed to be back at the calm, comforting, birth center. The contractions stopped and we were able to return safely to the care of Nancy.

On the Saturday before Easter Sunday, my lower back began to ache. I went to sleep Saturday night at 10:00 P.M., but I awoke at 2:00 A.M. with a low backache. Then my water broke. We called Nancy and planned to meet her at 3:00 A.M. at the birth center to be checked. I was 4 centimeters and baby was face up. Nancy filled the laboring tub, turned the lights down, and put soft music on as Ken unpacked our car.

My contractions were five minutes apart, and I felt mild pressure as I sat in the tub brushing my teeth, drinking, eating, and enjoying the excitement with my husband. Nancy checked on us, but waited in the other room. We treasured the privacy.

At 4:00 A.M. another woman arrived and delivered at 5:00 A.M. I heard her "sounding" and I tried it. This helped me release the pressure I felt.

At 6:00 A.M. the contractions slowed to seven minutes apart. Nancy suggested I walk around for a change. One contraction out of the tub, and I realized how much pain the tub took away. It was 8:00 A.M. and I was 8 centimeters. The baby had turned face down, so I crawled back into the tub. The water gave me relief during the contractions, and in between Ken rubbed my back and put cool cloths on my head.

At 9:00 A.M. the pressure increased, so I "sounded" my way loudly through the contractions. This upset my husband as he felt helpless to ease my struggle. The midwife reassured us by saying it was normal, and our baby was soon to be here.

At 9:45 A.M. Nancy announced the baby was on the way. My husband put on his swim shorts, and we went into the delivery tub. The water was warm, the room was dim. Ken crawled in behind me, supporting me through the five pushes it took to deliver the baby's head.

The midwife freed his neck from the umbilical cord and out came his body at 10:02 A.M. Nancy held his face out of the water as I scooped up his body. His eyes opened as he looked at mom and dad, and he wiggled his arms and legs in the water. We sat in the tub for twenty minutes or so and adored our miracle. Dad cut the cord, the placenta came out, and we moved to the bed to repair a tear. We packed and left for home at 11:50 A.M., Easter Sunday. We were not nervous about leaving with our young son because throughout prenatal care the midwife made him our responsibility. He came from our bodies to our arms and stayed in our arms.

In the beginning we were called crazy so many times for wanting a natural birth that we started to believe it. But we followed our hearts. We appreciate the medical establishment for the highly skilled, warm doctor that helped us conceive our son. We also appreciate the medical establishment for giving us the highly skilled warm midwife who helped us have a wonderful birth.

Our Comments: *Couples who have special pregnancies (infertility, surrogates, senior parents, and so on) often become convinced that they need high-tech obstetrics all the way. They seek out the "best," often* *feeling more secure at a prominent university hospital under the care of a widely published doctor. The price of this birth security may often be a less than satisfying birth experience. While some special pregnancies need this kind of intensive care, others don't.*

BIRTH THE SCHEDULED WAY

Thoughts from Erin's baby book: "It's a week past your due date, and, like your brother, you don't want to leave your cocoon. The doctor says you are so "low" you may fall out! Tomorrow he is going to induce labor.

"Dad likes having a baby this way. He says it's more calm and controlled. You can get a good night's sleep, then just check in to the hospital and have a baby. No wild car rides rushing to the hospital. No water breaking at the most unwelcome time. I, on the other hand, was hoping to begin labor on my own. My first pregnancy was induced, and I wanted to experience the onset of labor naturally this time, without drugs or doctor interference. But I trust my doctor, and he says it's time.

"Well, today will be your birthday. We arrive at the hospital at 7:00 A.M. The doctor breaks my water, and I begin to have mild contractions. With the help of a 'pit' I.V. drip, my contractions get progressively stronger, and within hours I am ready to push you out. It's 5:30 P.M., and after a rather easy vaginal delivery, I am holding you in my arms. For a second time my labor was induced. I had hoped for a different beginning. But what is most important is how healthy and beautiful you are, my sweet baby girl."

Our Comments: Diane was happy about her healthy baby but sad about her birth experience. A few weeks after delivery we counseled her about these birth feelings. Knowing she was in the hands of a very competent obstetrician who exercised good judgment, respecting parents' birth wishes but not jeopardizing the health of babies, we helped her work through these feelings. Diane would have felt better about her birth if the reasons for the induction and the risks of waiting had been more thoroughly explained to her. She then could have participated more in the decision to induce. While this induced birth had a happy ending, some do not. The methods of judging when a pregnancy is at "term" and "ready" are not precise. Babies are sometimes delivered before they're ready and end up spending the next few days or weeks in a newborn intensive care unit when they should have been left to mature within the mother.

A NO-REGRETS CESAREAN

We had been married for seven years and knew we wanted children, but postponed it until the "ideal" time arrived. I deeply desired to do all I could to create a support system around us that would help us become ideal parents, and I did a lot of reading about parenting and the birthing process. I realized the importance of selecting a professional labor assistant. I also felt it was important to have an obstetrician with whom my husband and I could establish a trusting relationship rather than the adversarial relationship that many couples seemed to have with their doctor. Early in my pregnancy I selected both a labor-support professional and an obstetrician whom we felt we could trust completely.

We approached this pregnancy prayerfully and systematically. We prepared a birth plan, and submitted it to our obstetrician for his review and approval. Our desire was to give birth vaginally with as little medical intervention as possible. I wanted to participate in this birth to the fullest. And with the wonderful support, encouragement, love, and prayers of my support system, I achieved this goal.

As my labor progressed and approached the 24-hour safety margin for ruptured membranes, it was evident that we were on borrowed time, according to the medical profession. But because our baby was so strong on the fetal monitor, our doctor allowed us to continue to labor so that we might achieve our goal of a vaginal delivery. I dilated fully and pushed with little success for three hours. As we approached the twenty-ninth hour after my membranes ruptured, it was becoming clear that the baby was too high to consider using forceps or vacuum extraction. An epidural was given as a last-ditch effort to relax my pelvis enough for the baby to pass through. This attempt was unsuccessful. We were exhausted and found it hard to believe that this baby would ever be born, as preparations were made for a cesarean. My husband and our labor assistant could not hold back the tears of disappointment.

Was I another statistic of unnecessary cesarean birth? A resounding no! We learned that the C-section was necessary because the baby was wedged in my pelvis. Pictures of her reflect how I had pushed, creating a "shelf" on her forehead. In our case, medical intervention was necessary to achieve a healthy baby and delivery. This was not part of our plan, but I know I did everything I could before, during, and after birth to achieve a healthy birth and relationship with our daughter.

Our Comments: I (Bill) had the privilege of meeting this couple prenatally, attending their birth, and helping them work through their feelings after birth. This was one of the most responsible birth couples I have ever known. They did all their necessary homework, chose the right obstetrician and professional labor assistant for them, and worked out their birth philosophy and birth plan. Their key to a no-regrets surgical birth is that in their minds these parents believed they had done all they could do. There was no one to blame (except perhaps a quirk of nature), and these parents rested in the satisfaction that their thorough preparations for birth, while not giving them a vaginal birth, gave them a satisfying birth.

Ironically, two reporters from the Los Angeles Times *were present during this labor and birth in order to write a story about labor assistants. The theme of their article was how the use of these "new" labor-support persons could lower the chances of the mother needing a cesarean birth. Initially, they were disappointed because this birth turned out to be a cesarean despite the use of an excellent professional labor assistant. I reassured these reporters that the main purpose of a professional labor assistant was to help a couple achieve a satisfying birth experience. And certainly this couple achieved their desire. The story was printed.*

EPIDURAL GONE WRONG

For the birth of our first child my husband and I planned to have a natural, unmedicated birth within a hospital setting. We prepared ourselves by reading books on the subject of natural childbirth and by attending classes in the Bradley and Lamaze methods. We planned to arrive at the hospital toward the end of labor so that I would receive as little medical intervention as possible. However, my bag of waters broke at the beginning of my labor and the on-call doctor advised us to go to the hospital immediately.

When we arrived at the hospital, the nurse put me in bed and hooked me up to a fetal monitor. I was not happy about this, because being confined in bed inhibited my labor. After twenty minutes of monitoring at the top of each hour, I was allowed to get out of bed and move about freely. The pain was manageable as long as I was mobile and could change positions.

After ten hours of natural labor, my doctor did not feel I was progressing, so she ordered a pitocin I.V. Once the pitocin flowed into my bloodstream, the pain became unbearable. I felt as if I were out of my head. I endured it as long as I could, but there was no letup and I was seriously afraid of losing consciousness. Since my ultimate fear was going under the knife, I consented to an epidural hoping to avoid a C-section.

Once the epidural took effect, I felt great relief. A few hours later, I felt the urge to push. The pushing stage was the most enjoyable. Even though I had the epidural, I still felt each contraction and was able to push our baby out into the world naturally. It was the most significant moment in my entire life.

Later that day I began to feel excruciating pain in the back of my head, which radiated down my neck and spine. The doctors determined that I was suffering from a dural puncture. Two forms of treatment were proposed. The first was a caffeine drip, which relieved the pain only temporarily. The second treatment was an epidural patch in which my own blood was injected into the spinal space. This intervention was also unsuccessful, and, in fact, actually caused a second dural puncture. I opted to allow this to heal naturally even though it took several weeks. During this time I was flat on my back and unable to care for my baby except to breastfeed and hold her.

All of the side effects I encountered during my labor, delivery, and recovery period were due to medical interventions. Hence, having my first baby was a great learning experience.

Our Comments: *Stephanie learned what not to do for her next birth. Her doctor had told her to go to the hospital too soon. Checking into the hospital before labor was well established and progressing opened the door to the domino effect of medical interventions. Being confined in bed to be monitored slowed her labor, which necessitated pitocin to get the labor going, which led to an epidural because the pain was unbearable. The epidural caused the prolonged spinal headache and a painful postpartum entry into motherhood. Despite all the intervention, Stephanie felt she gave birth "naturally" because she avoided a surgical birth and was able to participate during the pushing stage.*

MAKING A BIRTH OUT OF A CESAREAN

My first child was born by cesarean section because baby was in a frank breech position. I was uninformed and assumed that when I asked my physicians for a "natural birth" they would do everything for me to ensure that end. The emotional scars are still with me. But I started reading. Most of my information on "true natural childbirth" came from attending La Leche League meetings and borrowing books from their lending library. I learned that most OBs know a lot about intervention and very little about natural childbirth. I also learned that the medical interventions often created the problems.

For two years I read and networked with people who had similar beliefs. Finally, I became pregnant again. I was determined not to have another C-section. During my pregnancy I changed providers four times, as my situation changed. It was a roller coaster, but I wanted to ensure my VBAC.

Initially, I chose a lay midwife. I knew it was a controversial choice, but I felt safe — until I began bleeding early on in the pregnancy. Then I wanted all the medical technology available. The problem was diagnosed as a low progesterone level and a partial separation of the placenta. The doctor prescribed progesterone and a little bed rest. By my seventh month, however, I was terrified that I would not be able to achieve a nonmedicated birth with this provider; the hospital I would be delivering in had a 32 percent C-section rate. The labor assistant I had hired acted as a sounding board for all my confusion at this point. It was a hard decision to make so far along, but I decided to switch to a birth center. It felt right. I knew that there I could attain the deep relaxation necessary to endure the rigors of labor. I never labored with my first child, so I was scared about the unknown pains of labor.

At thirty-five weeks, on a Saturday night while I slept, the baby turned from head down to breech. One of my reasons for choosing the birth center was that the OB there was willing to deliver breech babies vaginally and also had a good success rate in doing external versions (turning the baby in the womb back into a head-down position). At thirty-six weeks we went to the hospital to try to turn the baby. I was so emotional at this point that all I could see was another C-section despite my having worked so hard to avoid one. The version would be attempted as long as the cord was not around the baby's neck. I believed deep down inside that everything had to work my way because I had worked so hard to make everything right.

The cord turned out to be around the baby's neck, and to make it worse, I had a double-footling breech. We couldn't turn the baby or deliver her vaginally because of the risk of a prolapsed cord. Without the head or buttocks down in the pelvis, there was too great a chance that the cord would come down first once my water broke. I cried and cried. My husband had never seen me hurt so much. For three days I stayed in bed depressed. I feared I'd be angry at this little baby for not letting me birth her. My labor assistant, who had been present at the attempted version, called and suggested we get a second opinion. Back I went to my original OB. The cord was definitely around the neck, but this doctor felt it was safe to attempt the version. Again, I was totally optimistic that I was going to have my VBAC. But the birth-center doctor called to convince me not to attempt such a risky procedure. By this point, I was scared about how far I'd go to have a VBAC. Was I endangering my baby's life so that I could have the birth I envisioned? I decided against the version, but every day I lay in the breech tilt position trying to turn her. At the same time I was scared that I'd make her turn and tighten the cord around her neck.

We scheduled the C-section for thirty-nine weeks' gestation, giving the baby two more weeks to turn on her own. Through talking with my Bradley instructor, I regained some sense of peace, and mostly a feeling of being in control of my birth. If I was going to have a C-section, I needed a new birth plan that would meet my needs. The hardest part of my first C-section was not having my baby with me until six hours after the birth. More than anything I wanted to have continuous physical contact with my baby. Arrangements were made with my pediatrician, and as it turned out, I held Alexandra on the operating table, nursed her in the recovery room, and slept with her from the first night. The nurses tried to take her to the nursery, but doctor's orders called for her to remain safely in my arms.

My eyes still fill with tears, and my inner soul yearns to have birthed my beautiful Alexandra. But I know that this C-section was necessary. Tomorrow she'll be six months old, and I know she is with us because of medical technology. I am not hurting this time because I was informed and took control of my birth.

Our Comments: *Despite her emotional roller coaster, this mother had a no-blame C-section because she took the time and energy to explore her options. She participated in the decision about what was best for her baby, and came to terms with the need for the cesarean and then worked to get what was important to her — having her baby with her.*

A FAMILY BIRTH

It was a hot August night and I was one week past my due date when I felt the twinge in my womb signaling me that labor would begin soon. My two sons were tucked into bed and my husband and mother were taking care of last-minute details. My certified nurse-midwife arrived at 10:00 P.M. to find me already dilated to 5 centimeters. The bedroom was ready with all of the necessary birthing supplies and the peaceful mood was enhanced with candles, flowers, and soft music. I took a shower and tried to relax and calm myself as much as possible. From past experience I knew I would need my energy later.

Before the contractions became extremely demanding, I called friends who would be praying for me. It was empowering to know that my friends were with me in spirit. I continued to walk around the room and massage my belly. When the waves of contractions came I would concentrate and visualize my cervix opening, and I thought about how soon I would be loving my baby. My attentive husband was completely available to me. He massaged my back and feet, held my hands, and breathed softly with me during the contractions. As my body worked harder and harder to open up I found that standing was the most comfortable position. My midwife had left us alone until I voiced a deep birthing sound, and soon she was upstairs to check me. How well she knew the calls of birthing women, for I was now fully dilated and ready to push. My husband sat in the chair telling me how great I was doing and how much he loved me while I stood leaning against him for support. My mother woke our two sons, and they came into the room just as the baby was crowning. My midwife worked with me and a few moments later at 1:00 A.M. I delivered a 10½-pound, perfectly healthy baby boy.

As soon as he slipped out she handed him to me and I sat down on the bed. My four-year-old and six-year-old sons came over to see him, touched his feet, and said how tender he was. Our baby latched on to my breast immediately and nursed while I delivered the placenta. We then all snuggled together on the bed just watching our new family member. The older boys became sleepy and returned to their room while the midwife finished checking over the baby and me. It was a very peaceful birth, relaxed, loving, and natural. We celebrated with juice and tea. Then the midwife returned home, and my mother went to bed. My husband and I and our new baby boy enjoyed the afterglow of birth and marveled at the miracle we had just experienced.

Our Comments: This family birth shows how calm birth can be. A high-touch, low-tech delivery while the mother stood supported by her husband is far different from the frantic birth scenes you see in the movies.

A FEARLESS BIRTH

My pregnancy was wonderful! I continued to play tennis three to four days a week and do step-aerobics two or three days a week. I felt that continuing to exercise would better prepare my body for labor.

Phil and I attended six Lamaze classes. We did some home practice, but not as much as I thought we should. Phil was supportive and interested in all aspects of the preg-

nancy. He even came to most of my prenatal visits.

On the Tuesday before the birth I slept all day long. On Wednesday and Thursday the "nesting" instinct set in and I finished the baby's room, cleaned house, and so on.

I woke up on Friday at 5:30 A.M. with back and abdominal pain. My contractions were seven minutes apart, then five minutes apart. I called the doctor, took a shower, dressed, and went to the hospital to be checked. I was dilated to 3 centimeters and was 90 percent effaced. I found myself breathing deeply and concentrating throughout each contraction. They felt like cramps, and I looked forward to the "breaks" in between.

We decided to go home to labor for a while since we lived only fifteen minutes from the hospital. I ate a waffle, yogurt, and juice, then went for a walk. My neighbors videotaped our early labor. At 1:00 P.M. we went back to the hospital.

The nurse asked me what my plans were regarding medication. When I said I wanted to do it naturally, she said "okay" in a tone indicating that I might change my mind.

During the early contractions, I wanted silence and no movement around me. My husband was quick to convey my wishes to those around. By 2:00 P.M. my sister had arrived. The doctor also came in to check me. I was almost at 4 centimeters and 100 percent effaced. He recommended breaking my water. I wasn't sure about this, but we finally decided that it would be best. My contractions intensified by 3:00 P.M. I realized that they were more painful in bed, so I got back up to lean against the window sill. I stared at one focal point near the window and did knee bends while deliberately breathing in through my nose and out through my mouth. Contractions came more frequently and with increased intensity. At 4:00 P.M. I had dilated to 6 centimeters. I tried a few other positions — kneeling on a pillow and leaning over the recliner were okay, but I didn't like sitting or lying down. I remember looking at the clock and being amazed at how much time had passed by. Phil suggested that I go into the shower since I liked standing and he thought the warm water would keep me relaxed.

In the shower, contractions increased to less than one minute apart. My breathing rhythm drastically increased. I felt like I had to have a bowel movement. The doctor came and checked me at 5:15 P.M. I was at 10 centimeters and ready to push! I had just gone through transition and didn't realize it. I had been thinking I would have to endure more intense pain. I pushed on the birthing bed, then stood up to lean against it. This proved to be the better position as the baby's head moved down. I think the force of gravity and moving with the contractions helped me. Teresa (the nurse) helped me to focus on where I needed to push. Phil, as always, encouraged me with very positive statements.

The baby's head became visible, so the doctor came in to help. We had discussed the fact that I didn't want an episiotomy unless necessary. He told me to push in a very controlled manner as I watched in the mirror. After the head was born, I really needed to concentrate on the shoulders. One, then the other — WOW! I heard Phil yell, "It's a boy, it's a boy!" and they placed him on my stomach. It is an indescribable feeling to know we delivered this little guy without medication.

One thing that helped me go through labor so well was the way I confronted it. I wasn't going to be a martyr, but at the same time I took the word "try" out of "I'm going to do it naturally." Having the positive mental outlook was the key. There were times when I said, "This is hard; this is hard." But I never said I wouldn't do it. There really wasn't time to think about it because I had to concentrate with each contraction.

Phil was such a support. He seemed to enjoy the Lamaze classes, and learned to support me unconditionally throughout the pregnancy and especially during labor. I couldn't have done it without him.

Our Comments: *This woman had a satisfying birth mainly because she trusted her body and* didn't fear birth. *Relaxed birthing muscles and a confident mind work better at birth than tension and fear. What strikes us in this story is her confidence that helped her stay focused, even though she realized labor is hard. She tried different things, felt confident to stick with what worked for her, and used the help available to her. She just kept going from one contraction to the next.*

COACH OF THE YEAR*

When our pregnancy was about five months along we heard about The Bradley Method®. This natural method, which encourages non-drug use, extreme relaxation during labor, and healthy eating habits, appealed to us, and we decided to give it a try.

When I found out that it was a twelve-week class I was less than pleased. I didn't feel like I had that kind of time. But the amount of knowledge I received in just one

---

* *This birth story was written by the baby's father.*

class was great. I learned that even in the birth of our child we are consumers with choices, and that if we don't take the time to learn about childbirth and our options, someone else will make those decisions for us. As part of our class we designed a birth plan detailing our desires for our birthing experience, which we had gone over with our doctor. Toward our due date he approved it and then faxed it over to the hospital to be put in our file.

When we were one week from our due date, our doctor said everything was fine and that we should plan on the baby's being about a week late. The next day at 1:30 P.M., my wife, Vicky, called me at work to say that she had lost her mucous plug and to ask if I would come home because she didn't want to be alone. (She had no idea she was in labor.) I got home about an hour later to find my wife leaking water, and the color of the water indicated the presence of meconium, so there was some concern. We called our doctor and he told us to come down to his office. While Vicky was sliding into his chair to be examined about 3:00 P.M., her water broke completely — all over his foot. "I guess I won't need to do this exam," he said, and sent us over to the hospital.

Once we were settled, our nurse came in and put Vicky on the fetal monitor even though both she and baby were doing fine. She told Vicky that she would put in an I.V. to get glucose to the baby so he would be active, and that she would give her some pitocin to "move your labor along." Both these things were against our birth plan. From our class we knew these types of things were done and we were prepared for this situation. I let the nurse know these things had been previously discussed with our doctor and that we would not consent

to these procedures without first talking to him personally. At this point we were left alone to labor privately in a quiet, peaceful atmosphere. We were hardly disturbed for the next two hours, in which time the contractions rapidly went to two minutes apart and 1½ minutes long, becoming much more intense.

At about this time Vicky's labor started to peak in intensity and she was in intense pain at the peak of contractions, although our relaxation techniques helped reduce the pain. We know this because at one point Vicky lost the method for about three contractions. By this I mean that she stopped trying intense relaxation and was fighting her pain by tensing up almost into a ball, which tightens all the muscles and slows labor. I talked to her calmly and reminded her of all our practicing, telling her that we had to get back to relaxing. After that the difference in the contractions amazed me. With our relaxation techniques, the rest of the contractions were manageable. I kept listening to Vicky's directions, to what she desired. She wanted me to keep touching her, and I did.

The nurse came in and began preparing a needle with pitocin to help the uterus contract again after the birth. I explained to her that we had discussed this with our doctor and that Vicky would be breastfeeding immediately after birth, which contracts the uterus naturally, and we would prefer that no pitocin was given. We agreed to discuss it with our doctor to see if he felt it was necessary.

By 8:30 P.M. Vicky was feeling the urge to push, and she did. She pushed for half an hour, in which time our doctor prepared for the birth. What an intense joy to see our baby's head coming as mom worked so very hard to give him life. At 9:05 P.M. our Jonathan Daniel was born — totally healthy, totally alert, and totally drug-free!

I cannot say enough about The Bradley Method® and its ability to make parents knowledgeable consumers, involved in the birth of their baby instead of watching from the sidelines.

It makes birth such a team effort for the husband and wife. Thank you, Victoria, for being so brave, tough, and wonderful. I am very proud of you! Vicky says that she couldn't have done it without me. That makes me very proud!

Our Comments: *Statements like "our pregnancy" and "we had a vaginal exam" leave no doubt that Walt was really into this birth. His involvement not only helped Vicky have a more comfortable labor, but it also made Walt and Vicky more sensitive to each other. This mutual sensitivity is a great prelude to parenting.*

Queen for a Month

AS YOU HOLD this precious person in your arms whom you labored to bring into the world, your mind will be filled with both wonderful and scary thoughts. Even as you bask in the miracle before you and your accomplishment, it is normal also to have those "Will I be a good enough mother?" feelings. You will, as long as you set the conditions that allow your natural mothering abilities to unfold.

Just as hormones got you through birth, hormones will get you into mothering, and, as with birthing, there are things you can do to get these biological helpers working for you. Rooming-in with your baby, breastfeeding and holding her, and responding to her cues will all put your hormones to work for you in your transition into mothering. Just as you created the environment and selected the help that gave you the best odds for a satisfying birth experience, you can also orchestrate your postpartum environment to have a satisfying mothering experience. The birth-day feelings of "Queen for a Day" should be extended to "Queen for a Month." Martha advises expectant mothers in her childbirth class, "Don't

take your nightgown off for at least two weeks. Sit in your rocking chair nursing your baby and let yourself be pampered." You deserve to luxuriate in a month-long baby shower, complete with a full-time "servant" at your beck and call and "meals-on-wheels" provided by your friends.

After birth, your body and soul undergo tremendous changes. The afterglow of birth wanes into the reality of around-the-clock new-baby care. Along with being a time to work through feelings of fatigue and self-doubt, postpartum period is also a time to work through your birth feelings. One reason we stress the value of having a satisfying birth experience is the realization that how a woman gives birth influences how she approaches mothering. If you had a less than satisfying birth experience, you are a setup for postpartum depression. Recognize this vulnerability and seek professional counseling quickly if your feelings begin to overwhelm you.

How to thrive and survive the postpartum period and get the best start with your baby is covered in our companion volume *The Baby Book.* There we take an approach similar to the one in this book — we give you the tools to develop a style of parenting that brings out the best in your baby and yourself. The life you labored so hard to birth is now the person you will work so hard to nurture. Throughout your life you will have various roles, but none will be so rich and so lasting as that of mother.

References and Additional Reading

General Reference

Chalmers, I., M. Enkin, and J. N. Keirse, eds. 1989. *Effective Care in Pregnancy and Childbirth.* Vol. 1–2. New York: Oxford University Press. (a 1,500-page review of the most important topics in obstetrics)

Chapter 1: Our Birth Experiences — What We Have Learned
Chapter 2: Birth — Then and Now

De Lee, J. B. 1920. "The Prophylactic Forceps Operation." *Am. J. Obstet. Gynecol.* 1:34–44.
Wertz, R. W., and D. C. Wertz. 1977. *Lying-In: A History of Childbirth in America.* New Haven: Yale University Press.
Wessel, H. 1981. *Under the Apple Tree.* Fresno, Calif.: Bookmates International.

Chapter 3: Choices in Childbirth

Bradley, Robert A. 1981. *Husband-Coached Childbirth.* New York: Harper & Row.
Dick-Read, Grantly. 1944. *Childbirth Without Fear.* 5th ed., edited by Helen Wessel and Harlan Ellis. New York: Harper & Row, 1984.
Flanagin, A. 1990. "Home Births and Medical Interventions." *JAMA* 264:2203–8.
Kennell, J., et al. 1991. "Continuous Emotional Support During Labor in a U.S. Hospital. A Randomized Controlled Trial." *JAMA* 265:2197–2201.
Klaus, M., et al. 1986. "Effects of Social Support During Parturition on Maternal and Infant Morbidity." *Brit. Med. J.* 293 (6547):585–87.
Rooks, J. P., et al. 1989. "Outcomes of Care in Birth Centers." The National Birth Center Study. *N. Engl. J. Med.* 321:1804–11.
Sousa, R., et al. 1980. "The Effect of a Supportive Companion on Perinatal Problems, Length of Labor and Mother-Infant Interaction." *N. Engl. J. Med.* 303:597–600.
Tyson, H. 1991. "Outcomes of 1,001 Midwife-Attended Home Births in Toronto 1983–1988." *Birth* 18:1 (March).

Chapter 4: Getting Your Body Ready for Birth

Brewer, G. S., and T. Brewer. 1983. *The Brewer Medical Diet for Normal and High-Risk Pregnancies.* New York: Simon & Schuster.
Diakow, Peter R. P., et al. 1991. "Back Pain During Pregnancy and Labor." *J. Manipulative and Physiological Therapeutics* 14 (2):116.
Paolone, A., and S. Worthington. 1985. "Cautions and Advice on Exercise During Pregnancy." *Contemp. OB/GYN* 25:150–62.

Chapter 5: Tests, Technology, and Other Interventions That Happen on the Way to Birth

Banta, H. D., and S. B. Thacker. 1982. "Benefits and Risks of Episiotomy." *Birth* 9 (1):25–30.

Bidgood, K. A., and P. J. Steen. 1987. "A Randomized Control Study of Oxytocin Augmentation of Labor 1. Obstetric Outcome." *Br. J. Obstet. Gynaecol.* 94:518–22.

Boylan, P. C. 1989. "Active Management of Labor: Results in Dublin, Houston, London, New Brunswick, Singapore, and Valparaiso." *Birth* 16:3 (September).

Freeman, R. 1990. "Intrapartum fetal monitoring — A Disappointing Story." *N. Engl. J. Med.* 322:624–26.

Hemrinki, E., et al. 1985. "Ambulation Versus Oxytocin in Protracted Labor: A Pilot Study." *Eur. J. Obstet. Gynecol. Reprod. Biol.* 20:199–208.

Intrapartum Fetal Monitoring. 1989. ACOG Technical Bulletin no. 132.

Klein, M., et al. 1992. "Does Episiotomy Prevent Trauma and Pelvic Floor Relaxation?" *Online J. Curr. Clin. Trials* (July 1).

Levenu, K. J., et al. 1986. "A Prospective Comparison of Selective and Universal Electronic Fetal Monitoring in 34,995 Pregnancies." *N. Engl. J. Med.* 315:615–19.

MacDonald, D. W. 1985. "Continuous EFM: Are the Benefits Proven?" *Contemp. OB/GYN* 26:37–52.

Owen, J., and J. C. Hauth. 1992. "Oxytocin for the Induction or Augmentation of Labor." *Clin. Obstet. and Gynecol.* 35:464–75.

Petitti, D. 1984. "Ultrasound Exposure in Humans, Effects in Utero." *Birth* 11:3 (fall).

Platt, L. D. 1989. "Assessing the Fetus with Doppler Ultrasound." *Contemp. OB/GYN* 168–99 (January).

Read, J. A., et al. 1981. "A Randomized Trial of Ambulation Versus Oxytocin for Labor Enhancement." *Am. J. Obstet. Gynecol.* 139:669–72.

Santini, D. L., et al. 1990. "The Impact of Universal Screening for Gestational Glucose Intolerance on Outcome of Pregnancy." *Surg. Gynec. Obs.* 170:427–36.

Schifrin, B., and D. Clement. 1990. "Why Fetal Monitoring Remains a Good Idea." *Contemp. OB/GYN* 70–86 (February).

Shalev, E., et al. 1985. "Psychogenic Stress in Women During Fetal Monitoring." *Acta Obstet. Gynecol. Scand.* 64:417–20.

Shearer, M. A. 1984. "A Summary and Analysis of the NIH Consensus Development Conference on Ultrasound Imaging in Pregnancy." *Birth* 11:1 (spring).

Sleep, J., and A. Grant. 1987. "West Berkshire Perineal Management Trial." *Br. Med. J.* 32:181–83.

Whitfield, C. R. 1985. "Ultrasonography: Routine for All Pregnancies." *Contemp. OB/GYN* 91–94 (June).

Chapter 6: Cesarean Births
Chapter 7: VBAC — Yes, You Can! (Vaginal Birth After Cesarean)

Clark, S. L. 1988. "Rupture of a Scarred Uterus." *Ob. Gyn. Clin. N. Amer.* 15 (4):737–44.

Demott, R. K., and H. F. Sandmire. 1990. "The Green Bay Cesarean Section Study. The Physician Factor as a Determinant of Cesarean Birth Rates." *Am. J. Obstet. Gynecol.* 162:1593–1602.

Flamm, B. L. 1990. *Birth After Cesarean: The Medical Facts.* New York: Prentice Hall.

———, et al. 1988. "VBAC: Results of a Multicenter Study." *Am. J. Obstet. Gynecol.* 158:1079–84.

Queenan, J. T., et al. 1988. "Today's High C/S Rate: Can We Reduce It?" *Contemp. OB/GYN* 154–66 (July).

Sadousky, E., et al. 1987. "Managing Breech Delivery." *Contemp. OB/GYN* 47–58 (July).

Weiner, C. P. 1992. "Vaginal Breech Delivery in the 1990s." *Clin. Obstet. and Gynecol.* 35:559–69.

Chapter 8: Why Birth Hurts — Why It Doesn't Have To

Kelly, J. 1962. "The Effect of Fear and Uterine Motility." *Am. J. Obstet. Gynecol.* 83:576–81.

Simpkin, P. T. 1986. "Stress, Pain, and Catecholamines in Labor." *Birth* 13 (4):227–39.

———. 1992. "Overcoming the Legacy of Childhood Sexual Abuse: The Role of Caregivers and Childbirth Educators." *Birth* 19 (4):224–25.

Wardlaw, S. L., et al. 1979. "Plasma B-Endorphins and B-Lipotropin in the Human Fetus at Delivery: Correlation with Arterial $_pH$ and $_pO_2$." *J. Clin. Endocrinol. Metab.* 49:888–91.

Chapter 9: Relaxing for Birth

Church, L. K. 1989. "Water Birth: One Birth Center's Observations." *J. Nurs. Midwifery* 34:165–70.

Hanser, S. B., et al. 1983. "The Effect of Music on Relaxation of Expectant Mothers During Labor." *J. Music Therapy* 20 (2):50–58.

Lenstrup, C., et al. 1987. "Warm Tub Bath During Delivery." *Acta Obstet. Gynecol. Scand.* 66:709–12.

Rosenthal, M. J. 1991. "Warm-Water Immersion in Labor and Birth." *Female Patient* 16:35–47.

Smitt, R. 1983. "Music to Labor To." *Brit. Med. J.* 287:1984–85.

Chapter 10: Easing Birth Pains — How the Doctor Can Help

Abboud, T. K., et al. 1983. "Effects of Epidural Anesthesia on Maternal Plasma Beta-Endorphin Levels." *J. Anesthesiology* 59:1–5.

American College of Obstetrics and Gynecologists. 1988. Committee Opinion on Obstetrical Forceps. no. 59.

Berg, T. G., and W. F. Rayburn. 1992. "Effects of Analgesia on Labor." *Clin. Obstet. and Gynecol.* 35:457–63.

Chestnut, D. H., et al. 1987. "The Influence of Continuous Epidural Bupivicaine Analgesia on the Second Stage of Labor and Method of Delivery in Nulliparous Women." *Anesthesiology* 66:774–80.

Curran, M. 1990. "Epidural Analgesia for Labor and Delivery." *Anest. Clin. NA* 8:55–75.

Goodfellow, C. F., et al. 1983. "Oxytocin Deficiency at Delivery with Epidural Analgesia." *Br. J. Obstet. Gynaecol.* 90:214–19.

MacArthur, C., et al. 1990. "Epidural Anesthesia and Long-term Backache After Childbirth." *Br. Med. J.* 301: 9–12.

Macaulay, J. H., et al. 1992. "Epidural Analgesia in Labor and Fetal Hyperthermia." *Obstet. Gynecol.* 80:665–69.

Writer, D. 1992. "Epidural Analgesia for Labor." *Anest. Clin. NA* 10:59–85.

Chapter 11: Best Birthing Positions

Caldeyro-Barcia, R., et al. 1960. "Effect of Position Changes on the Intensity and Frequency of Uterine Contractions During Labor." *Am. J. Obstet. Gynecol.* 80:284.

Gordosi, J., et al. 1989. "Randomized Controlled Trial of Squatting in the Second Stage of Labor." *Lancet* 74–77 (July 8).

McKay, S. 1984. "Squatting: An Alternative Position for the Second Stage of Labor." *Maternal Child Nursing* 9:181–83.

————, and C. S. Mahan. 1984. "Laboring Patients Need More Freedom to Move." *Contemp. OB/GYN* 24:90–119.

Roberts, J., et al. 1983. "The Effects of Maternal Position on Uterine Contractility and Efficiency." *Birth* 10 (4):243–49.

Russell, J. G. B. 1969. "Moulding of the Pelvic Outlet." *J. Obstet. Gynaec. Brit. Cwlth.* 76:817–20.

Chapter 12: Labor and Delivery

Flynn, A. M., et al. "Ambulation in Labor." *Brit. Med. J.* 2:591–93.

Hannah, M. E., et al. 1992. "Induction of Labor as Compared with Serial Antenatal Monitoring in Post-term Pregnancy." *N. Engl. J. Med.* 326:1587–92.

Hazle, N. R. 1986. "Hydration in Labor: Is Routine Intravenous Necessary?" *J. Nurs. Midwifery* 31 (4):171–76.

McKay, S., and C. S. Mahan. 1984. "Are We Overmanaging the Second Stage of Labor?" *Contemp. OB/GYN* 24:37–63.

Odent, Michel. 1984. *Birth Reborn.* New York: Pantheon.

Smith, M. A., et al. 1993. "The Rational Management of Labor." *Amer. Fam. Phys.* 47:1471–81.

Index

References to main discussion are printed in boldface type.